Hartman's Nursing Assistant Care

The Basics

Hartman Publishing, Inc.
with Jetta Fuzy, RN, MS

FIFTH EDITION

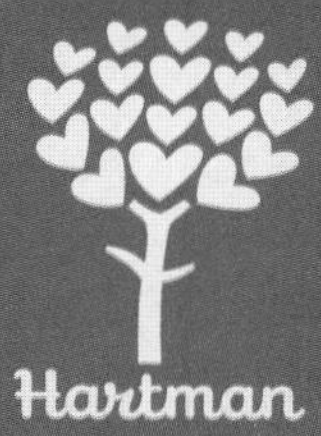

Credits

Managing Editor
Susan Alvare Hedman

Designer
Kirsten Browne

Cover Illustrator
Iveta Vaicule

Photography
Matt Pence, Pat Berrett, Art Clifton, and Dick Ruddy

Proofreaders
Sara Alexander, Sapna Desai, and Joanna Owusu

Editorial Assistant
Angela Storey

Sales/Marketing
Deborah Rinker, Kendra Robertson, Erika Walker, Belinda Midyette, and Carol Castillo

Customer Service
Fran Desmond, Thomas Noble, Col Foley, Brian Fejer, and Henry Bullis

Information Technology
Eliza Martin

Warehouse Coordinator
Chris Midyette

Copyright Information

1313 Iron Ave SW
Albuquerque, NM 87102
(505) 291-1274
web: hartmanonline.com
email: orders@hartmanonline.com
Twitter: @HartmanPub

ISBN 978-1-60425-100-5

PRINTED IN CANADA

Third Printing, 2021

Notice to Readers

Though the guidelines and procedures contained in this text are based on consultations with healthcare professionals, they should not be considered absolute recommendations. The instructor and readers should follow employer, local, state, and federal guidelines concerning healthcare practices. These guidelines change, and it is the reader's responsibility to be aware of these changes and of the policies and procedures of his or her healthcare facility.

The publisher, authors, editors, and reviewers cannot accept any responsibility for errors or omissions or for any consequences from application of the information in this book and make no warranty, express or implied, with respect to the contents of the book. The publisher does not warrant or guarantee any of the products described herein or perform any analysis in connection with any of the product information contained herein.

Special Thanks

A heartfelt thank you goes to our insightful and wonderful reviewers, listed in alphabetical order:

Theresa DeBon, BS, RN
Tulsa, OK

Tamie Hodges, BSN, RN
Benton, KY

Charles Illian, BSN, RN
Orlando, FL

Wendy Marlene Pickard, RN, BS, ONC
Round Rock, TX

Alice Sorrell-Thompson, MBA, BSN, RN, PHN
Los Angeles, CA

Lori A Spiezio, RN, WCC
Telford, PA

We are very appreciative of the many sources who shared their informative photos with us:

- Briggs Corporation
- Detecto
- Dreamstime
- Exergen Corporation
- Harrisburg Area Community College
- Hollister Incorporated
- Invacare Corporation
- Medline Industries
- National Pressure Ulcer Advisory Panel
- North Coast Medical, Inc.
- Nova Medical Products
- RG Medical Diagnostics of Wixom, MI
- Sage Products LLC
- TIDI Products LLC
- Vancare, Inc.
- Welch Allyn

Gender Usage

This textbook uses gender pronouns interchangeably to denote care team members and residents.

Please email corrections and suggestions to editor@hartmanonline.com.

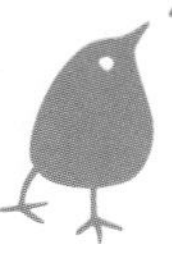

Contents

Page | Learning Objective | Page

1 The Nursing Assistant in Long-Term Care

1. Compare long-term care to other healthcare settings 1
2. Describe a typical long-term care facility 2
3. Explain Medicare and Medicaid 3
4. Describe the nursing assistant's role 4
5. Describe the care team and the chain of command 5
6. Define policies, procedures, and professionalism 8
7. List examples of legal and ethical behavior and explain Residents' Rights 10
8. Explain legal aspects of the resident's medical record 18
9. Explain the Minimum Data Set (MDS) 20
10. Discuss incident reports 20

2 Foundations of Resident Care

1. Understand the importance of verbal and written communications 21
2. Describe barriers to communication 24
3. List guidelines for communicating with residents with special needs 26
4. Identify ways to promote safety and handle non-medical emergencies 31
5. Demonstrate how to recognize and respond to medical emergencies 37
6. Describe and demonstrate infection prevention and control practices 45

3 Understanding Residents

1. Identify basic human needs 60
2. Define *holistic care* 62
3. Explain why promoting independence and self-care is important 62
4. Identify ways to accommodate cultural differences 63
5. Describe the need for activity 64
6. Discuss family roles and their significance in health care 65
7. Describe the stages of human growth and development 66
8. Discuss developmental disabilities 69
9. Describe some types of mental health disorders 70
10. Explain how to care for residents who are dying 72
11. Define the goals of a hospice program 76

4 Body Systems and Related Conditions

1. Describe the integumentary system 79
2. Describe the musculoskeletal system and related conditions 80
3. Describe the nervous system and related conditions 84
4. Describe the circulatory system and related conditions 90
5. Describe the respiratory system and related conditions 94
6. Describe the urinary system and related conditions 96
7. Describe the gastrointestinal system and related conditions 98
8. Describe the endocrine system and related conditions 102
9. Describe the reproductive system and related conditions 104
10. Describe the immune and lymphatic systems and related conditions 106

5 Confusion, Dementia, and Alzheimer's Disease

1. Discuss confusion and delirium 111
2. Describe dementia and discuss Alzheimer's disease 112
3. List strategies for better communication with residents with Alzheimer's disease 114
4. List and describe interventions for problems with common activities of daily living (ADLs) 116
5. List and describe interventions for common difficult behaviors related to Alzheimer's disease 118
6. Describe creative therapies for residents with Alzheimer's disease 122

Learning Objective — *Page*

6 Personal Care Skills

1. Explain personal care of residents 124
2. Identify guidelines for providing skin care and preventing pressure injuries 125
3. Describe guidelines for assisting with bathing 129
4. Describe guidelines for assisting with grooming 138
5. List guidelines for assisting with dressing 143
6. Identify guidelines for proper oral hygiene 147
7. Explain guidelines for assisting with toileting 152
8. Explain guidelines for safely positioning and moving residents 157

7 Basic Nursing Skills

1. Explain admission, transfer, and discharge of a resident 169
2. Explain the importance of monitoring vital signs 173
3. Explain how to measure weight and height 186
4. Explain restraints and how to promote a restraint-free environment 188
5. Define *fluid balance* and explain intake and output (I&O) 190
6. Explain care guidelines for urinary catheters, oxygen therapy, and IV therapy 196
7. Discuss a resident's unit and related care 200
8. Explain the importance of sleep and perform proper bedmaking 202
9. Discuss dressings and bandages 207

8 Nutrition and Hydration

1. Identify the six basic nutrients and explain MyPlate 209
2. Describe factors that influence food preferences 213
3. Explain special diets 213
4. Describe how to assist residents in maintaining fluid balance 216
5. List ways to identify and prevent unintended weight loss 218
6. Identify ways to promote appetites at mealtime 219
7. Demonstrate how to assist with eating 219
8. Identify signs and symptoms of swallowing problems 222
9. Describe how to assist residents with special needs 225

9 Rehabilitation and Restorative Care

1. Discuss rehabilitation and restorative care 227
2. Describe the importance of promoting independence and list ways exercise improves health 228
3. Discuss ambulation and describe assistive devices and equipment 229
4. Explain guidelines for maintaining proper body alignment 232
5. Describe care guidelines for prosthetic devices 233
6. Describe how to assist with range of motion exercises 234
7. List guidelines for assisting with bladder and bowel retraining 239

10 Caring for Yourself

1. Describe how to find a job 241
2. Describe a standard job description and explain how to manage time and assignments 243
3. Discuss how to manage and resolve conflict 244
4. Describe employee evaluations and discuss appropriate responses to feedback 245
5. Discuss certification and explain the state's registry 246
6. Describe continuing education 246
7. Explain ways to manage stress 247

Abbreviations **250**

Glossary **251**

Index **262**

Procedure *Page*

Procedures

Performing abdominal thrusts for the conscious person 38
Responding to shock 39
Responding to a myocardial infarction 40
Controlling bleeding 40
Treating burns 41
Responding to fainting 42
Responding to seizures 43
Responding to vomiting 45
Washing hands (hand hygiene) 49
Putting on (donning) and removing (doffing) gown 51
Putting on (donning) mask and goggles 52
Putting on (donning) gloves 53
Removing (doffing) gloves 53
Caring for an ostomy 101
Giving a complete bed bath 129
Giving a back rub 133
Shampooing hair in bed 134
Giving a shower or a tub bath 136
Providing fingernail care 138
Providing foot care 139
Combing or brushing hair 141
Shaving a resident 142
Dressing a resident 144
Applying knee-high elastic stockings 146
Providing oral care 147
Providing oral care for the unconscious resident 149
Flossing teeth 150
Cleaning and storing dentures 151
Assisting a resident with the use of a bedpan 153
Assisting a male resident with a urinal 154
Assisting a resident to use a portable commode or toilet 156
Moving a resident up in bed 158
Moving a resident to the side of the bed 158

Procedure *Page*

Positioning a resident on his side 159
Logrolling a resident 161
Assisting resident to sit up on side of bed: dangling 162
Transferring a resident from bed to wheelchair 165
Transferring a resident using a mechanical lift 167
Admitting a resident 170
Transferring a resident 171
Discharging a resident 172
Measuring and recording an oral temperature 175
Measuring and recording a rectal temperature 177
Measuring and recording a tympanic temperature 178
Measuring and recording an axillary temperature 179
Counting and recording radial pulse and counting and recording respirations 181
Measuring and recording blood pressure (one-step method) 183
Measuring and recording weight of an ambulatory resident 186
Measuring and recording height of an ambulatory resident 187
Measuring and recording urinary output 191
Collecting a routine urine specimen 192
Collecting a clean-catch (mid-stream) urine specimen 194
Collecting a stool specimen 195
Providing catheter care 196
Emptying the catheter drainage bag 198
Making an occupied bed 203
Making an unoccupied bed 206
Changing a dry dressing using non-sterile technique 207
Serving fresh water 217
Feeding a resident 221
Assisting a resident to ambulate 229
Assisting with ambulation for a resident using a cane, walker, or crutches 231
Assisting with passive range of motion exercises 235

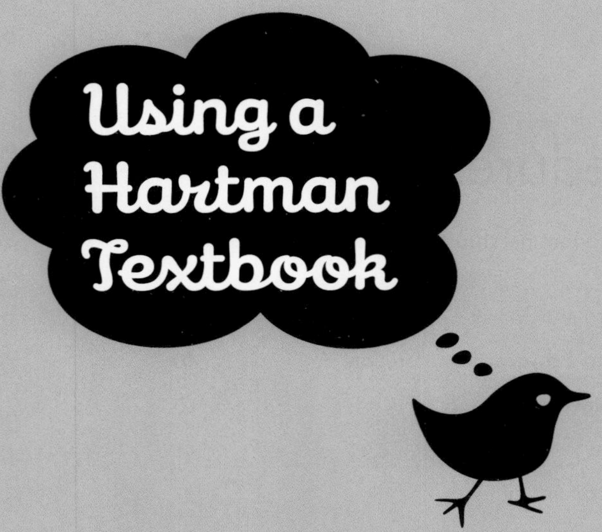

Understanding how this book is organized and what its special features are will help you make the most of this resource!

We have assigned each chapter its own colored tab. Each colored tab contains the chapter number and title, and it is on the side of every page.

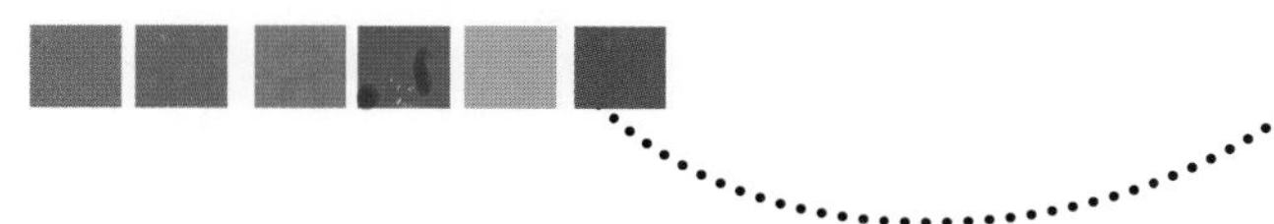

1. List examples of legal and ethical behavior	Everything in this book, the student workbook, and the instructor's teaching material is organized around learning objectives. A learning objective is a very specific piece of knowledge or a very specific skill. After reading the text, if you can do what the learning objective says, you know you have mastered the material.
bloodborne pathogens	Bold key terms are located throughout the text, followed by their definitions. They are also listed in the glossary at the back of this book.
Making an occupied bed	All care procedures are highlighted by the same black bar for easy recognition.
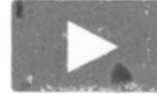	This icon indicates that Hartman Publishing offers a corresponding video for this skill.
Guidelines: Preventing Falls	Guidelines and Observing and Reporting lists are colored green for easy reference.
Residents' Rights Abuse and Alzheimer's Disease	These boxes teach important information about how to support and promote Residents' Rights and person-centered care.

Beginning and ending steps in care procedures

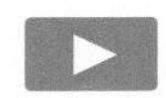

For most care procedures, these steps should be performed. Understanding why they are important will help you remember to perform each step every time care is provided.

Beginning Steps	
Identify yourself by name. Identify the resident by name.	A resident's room is his home. Residents have a legal right to privacy. Before any procedure, knock and wait for permission to enter the resident's room. Upon entering his room, identify yourself and state your title. Residents have the right to know who is providing their care. Identify and greet the resident. This shows courtesy and respect. It also establishes correct identification. This prevents care from being performed on the wrong person.
Wash your hands.	Handwashing provides for infection prevention. Nothing fights infection in facilities like performing consistent, proper hand hygiene. Handwashing may need to be done more than once during a procedure. Practice Standard Precautions with every resident.
Explain procedure to resident. Speak clearly, slowly, and directly. Maintain face-to-face contact whenever possible.	Residents have a legal right to know exactly what care you will provide. It promotes understanding, cooperation, and independence. Residents are able to do more for themselves if they know what needs to happen.
Provide for the resident's privacy with a curtain, screen, or door.	Doing this maintains the resident's right to privacy and dignity. Providing for privacy in a facility is not simply a courtesy; it is a legal right.
Adjust the bed to a safe level, usually waist high. Lock the bed wheels.	Locking the bed wheels is an important safety measure. It ensures that the bed will not move as you are performing care. Raising the bed helps you to remember to use proper body mechanics. This prevents injury to you and to residents.

Ending Steps

Return bed to lowest position. Remove privacy measures.	Lowering the bed provides for the resident's safety. Remove extra privacy measures added during the procedure. This includes anything you may have draped over and around the resident, as well as privacy screens.
Place call light within resident's reach.	A call light allows the resident to communicate with staff as necessary. It must always be left within the resident's reach. You must respond to call lights promptly.
Wash your hands.	Handwashing is the most important thing you can do to prevent the spread of infection.
Report any changes in resident to the nurse. Document procedure using facility guidelines.	You will often be the person who spends the most time with a resident, so you are in the best position to note any changes in a resident's condition. Every time you provide care, observe the resident's physical and mental capabilities, as well as the condition of his or her body. For example, a change in a resident's ability to dress himself may signal a greater problem. After you have finished giving care, document the care using facility guidelines. Do not record care before it is given. If you do not document the care you gave, legally it did not happen.

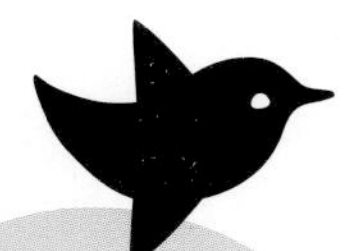

In addition to the beginning and ending steps listed above, remember to follow infection prevention guidelines. Even if a procedure in this book does not tell you to wear gloves or other PPE, there may be times when it is appropriate.

A few procedures in this book mention positioning side rails on beds, but most references to side rails have been omitted. This is due to the decline in their use because of risk of injury. Follow your facility's policies regarding side rails.

1 The Nursing Assistant in Long-Term Care

1. Compare long-term care to other healthcare settings

Welcome to the world of health care! Health care happens in many places. Nursing assistants work in many of these settings. In each setting similar tasks will be performed. However, each setting is also unique.

This textbook will focus on long-term care. **Long-term care** (**LTC**) is given in long-term care facilities for people who need 24-hour skilled care. **Skilled care** is medically necessary care given by a skilled nurse or therapist; it is available 24 hours a day. It is ordered by a doctor and involves a treatment plan. This type of care is given to people who need a high level of care for ongoing conditions. The term *nursing homes* was once widely used to refer to these facilities. Now they are often known as *long-term care facilities, skilled nursing facilities, rehabilitation centers*, or *extended care facilities.*

People who live in long-term care facilities may be disabled. They are often elderly, but younger adults sometimes require long-term care, too. They may arrive from hospitals or other healthcare settings. Their **length of stay** (the number of days a person stays in a care facility) may be short, such as a few days or months, or longer than six months. Some of these people will have a **terminal illness**. This means that the illness will eventually cause death. Other people may recover and return to their homes or to other care facilities or situations.

Most people who live in long-term care facilities have **chronic** conditions. This means the condition lasts a long period of time, even a lifetime. Chronic conditions include physical disabilities, heart disease, and dementia. (Chapters 4 and 5 have more information about these disorders and diseases.) People who live in these facilities are usually referred to as *residents* because the facility is where they reside or live. These places are their homes for the duration of their stay (Fig. 1-1).

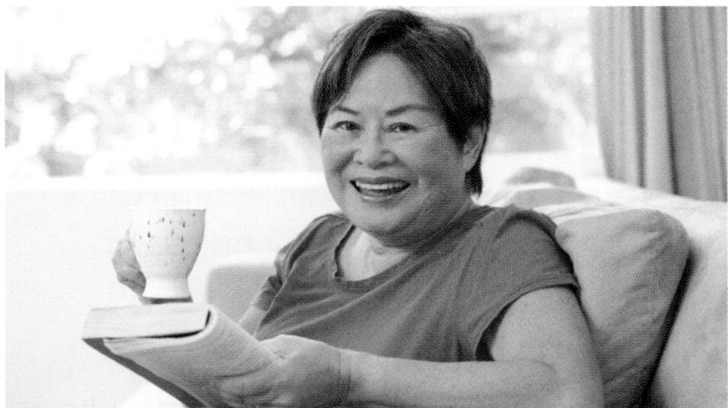

Fig. 1-1. *People who live in long-term care facilities are called residents because the facility is where they reside for the duration of their stay.*

People who need long-term care will have different **diagnoses**, or medical conditions determined by a doctor. The stages of illness or disease affect how sick people are and how much care they will need. The tasks nursing assistants perform will also vary. This is due to the fact that each resident has different symptoms, abilities, and needs.

Other healthcare settings include the following:

Home health care, or home care, is provided in a person's home (Fig. 1-2). This type of care is generally given to people who are older and are chronically ill but who are able to and wish to remain at home. Home care may also be needed when a person is weak after a recent hospital stay. Home care includes many of the services offered in other settings.

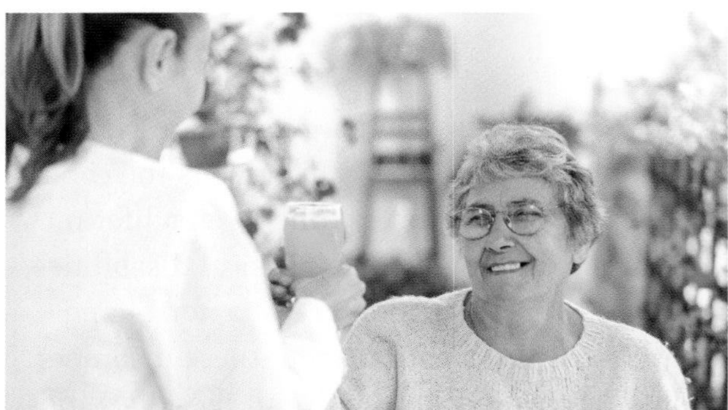

Fig. 1-2. *Home care is performed in a person's home.*

Assisted living facilities are residences for people who need some help with daily tasks, such as showering, eating, and dressing. Help with medications may also be given. People who live in these facilities do not need 24-hour skilled care. Assisted living facilities allow more independent living in a homelike environment. An assisted living facility may be attached to a long-term care facility, or it may stand alone.

Adult day services are for people who need some help and supervision during certain hours, but who do not live in the facility where care is provided. Generally, adult day services are for people who need some help but are not seriously ill or disabled. Adult day services can also provide a break for spouses, family members, and friends.

Acute care is 24-hour skilled care given in hospitals and ambulatory surgical centers. It is for people who require short-term, immediate care for illnesses or injuries (Fig. 1-3). People are also admitted for short stays for surgery.

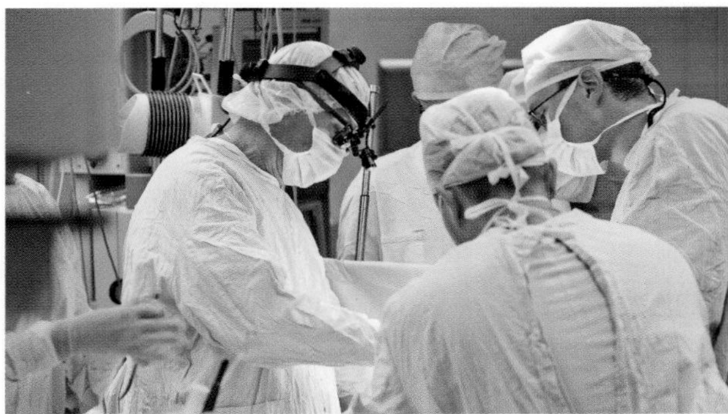

Fig. 1-3. *Acute care is performed in hospitals for illnesses or injuries that require immediate care.*

Subacute care is care given in hospitals or long-term care facilities. It is used for people who need less care than for an acute (sudden onset, short-term) illness, but more care than for a chronic (long-term) illness. Treatment usually ends when the condition has stabilized or after the set time for treatment has been completed. The cost is usually less than for acute care but more than for long-term care.

Outpatient care is usually given to people who have had treatments, procedures, or surgeries and need short-term skilled care. They do not require an overnight stay in a hospital or other care facility.

Rehabilitation is care given by specialists. Physical, occupational, and speech therapists help restore or improve function after an illness or injury. Information about rehabilitation is located in Chapter 9.

Hospice care is given in facilities or homes for people who have about six months or less to live. Hospice workers give physical and emotional care and comfort until a person dies. They also support families during this process. More information may be found in Chapter 3.

2. Describe a typical long-term care facility

Long-term care facilities are businesses that provide skilled nursing care 24 hours a day. These facilities may offer assisted living housing, dementia care, or subacute care. Some facilities offer specialized care. Others care for all types of residents. The typical long-term care facility offers personal care for all residents and focused care for residents with special needs. Personal care includes bathing; skin, nail, and hair care; mouth care; and assistance with walking, eating and drinking, dressing, transferring, and elimination. All of these daily personal care tasks are called **activities of daily living**, or **ADLs**. Other common services offered at these facilities include the following:

- Physical, occupational, and speech therapy
- Wound care
- Care of different types of tubes, such as catheters (thin tubes inserted into the body to drain fluids or inject fluids)
- Nutrition therapy
- Management of chronic diseases, such as Alzheimer's disease, acquired immunodeficiency syndrome (AIDS), diabetes, chronic obstructive pulmonary disease (COPD), cancer, and congestive heart failure (CHF)

When specialized care is offered at long-term care facilities, the employees must have special training. Residents with similar needs may be placed in units together. Nonprofit companies or for-profit companies can own long-term care facilities.

Residents' Rights

Culture Change and Person-Centered Care

Many long-term care facilities promote meaningful environments with individualized approaches to care. **Culture change** is a term given to the process of transforming services for elders so that they are based on the values and practices of the person receiving care. Culture change involves respecting both elders and those working with them. Core values are promoting choice, dignity, respect, self-determination, and purposeful living. To honor culture change, care settings may need to change their organization, practices, physical environments, and relationships. **Person-centered care** emphasizes the individuality of the person who needs care, and recognizes and develops his or her capabilities. Person-centered care revolves around the resident and promotes his or her individual preferences, choices, dignity, and interests. Each person's background, culture, language, beliefs, and traditions are respected. Improving each resident's quality of life is an important goal. Giving person-centered care will be an ongoing focus throughout this textbook.

3. Explain Medicare and Medicaid

The Centers for Medicare & Medicaid Services (CMS, cms.gov) is a federal agency within the US Department of Health and Human Services. CMS runs two national healthcare programs—Medicare and Medicaid. They both help pay for health care and health insurance for millions of Americans. CMS has many other responsibilities as well.

Medicare (medicare.gov) is a federal health insurance program that was established in 1965 for people aged 65 or older. It also covers people of any age with permanent kidney failure or certain disabilities. Medicare has four parts. Part A helps pay for care in a hospital or skilled nursing facility or for care from a home health agency or hospice. Part B helps pay for doctor services and other medical services and equipment. Part C allows private health insurance companies to provide Medicare benefits. Part D helps pay for medications prescribed for treatment. Medicare will only pay for care it determines to be medically necessary.

Medicaid (medicaid.gov) is a medical assistance program for people who have a low income, as well as for people with disabilities. It is funded by both the federal government and each state. Eligibility is determined by income and special circumstances. People must qualify for this program.

Medicare and Medicaid pay long-term care facilities a fixed amount for services. This amount is based on the resident's needs upon admission and throughout his stay at the facility.

4. Describe the nursing assistant's role

A nursing assistant can have many different titles. *Nurse aide, certified nurse aide, patient care technician,* and *certified nursing assistant* are some examples. The title given varies by state requirements. This textbook uses the term *nursing assistant.*

A nursing assistant (NA) performs assigned nursing tasks, such as taking a resident's temperature. A nursing assistant also provides personal care, such as bathing residents and helping with hair care. Promoting independence and self-care are other very important tasks that a nursing assistant does. Common nursing assistant duties include the following:

- Bathing residents
- Helping residents with elimination needs
- Assisting with range of motion exercises and ambulation (walking)
- Transferring residents from a bed to a chair or wheelchair
- Measuring vital signs (temperature, pulse rate, respiratory rate, and blood pressure)
- Assisting with meals (Fig. 1-4)

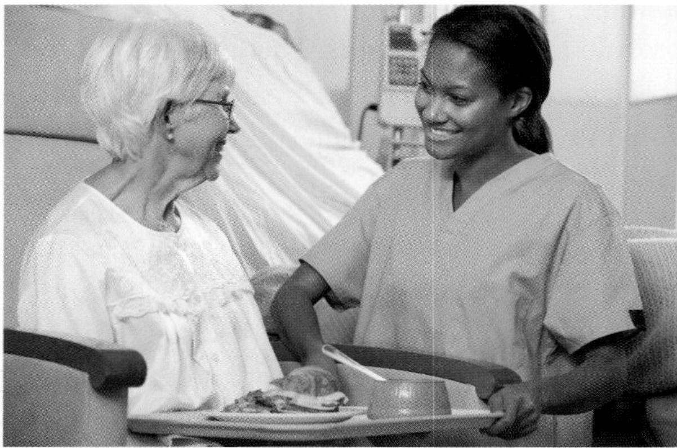

Fig. 1-4. *Helping residents eat and drink is an important part of an NA's job.*

- Helping residents dress and undress
- Giving back rubs
- Helping with mouth care
- Making and changing beds
- Keeping residents' living areas neat and clean
- Caring for supplies and equipment

Nursing assistants are not allowed to insert or remove tubes, give tube feedings, or change sterile dressings. Some states allow nursing assistants to give medications if they have completed an additional, specialized course for medications and meet the requirements of the individual facility.

Nursing assistants spend more time with residents than other care team members. They act as the "eyes and ears" of the team. Observing changes in a resident's condition and reporting them is a very important duty of the NA. Residents' care can be revised or updated as conditions change. Another duty of the NA is noting important information about the resident (Fig. 1-5). This is called **charting**, or documenting.

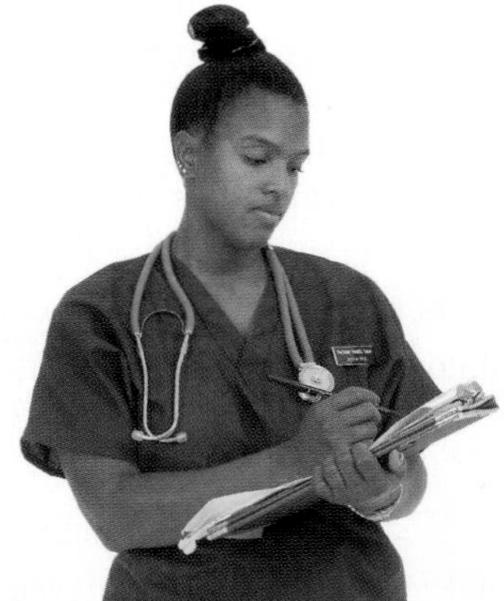

Fig. 1-5. *Observing carefully and reporting accurately are some of the NA's most important duties.*

Nursing assistants are part of a team of health professionals. The team includes doctors, nurses, social workers, therapists, dietitians, and specialists. The resident and resident's family are part of the team too. Everyone, including the resident, works closely together to meet goals. Goals include helping residents to recover from illnesses and to do as much as possible for themselves.

Residents' Rights

Responsibility for Residents

All residents are the responsibility of each nursing assistant. An NA will receive assignments to perform tasks, care, and other duties for specific residents. If he sees a resident who needs help, even if the resident is not on his assignment sheet, the NA should provide the needed care.

5. Describe the care team and the chain of command

Residents will have different needs and problems. Healthcare professionals with a wide range of education and experience will help care for them. This group is known as the *care team*. Members of the care team include the following:

Nursing Assistant (NA) or Certified Nursing Assistant (CNA): The nursing assistant performs assigned tasks, such as taking vital signs. The NA also provides or assists with personal care, such as bathing residents and helping with elimination needs. Nursing assistants must have at least 75 hours of training, and in many states, training exceeds 100 hours.

Registered Nurse (RN): In a long-term care facility, a registered nurse coordinates, manages, and provides skilled nursing care. This includes giving special treatments and medications as prescribed by a doctor. A registered nurse also assigns tasks and supervises daily care of residents by nursing assistants. A registered nurse is a licensed professional who has graduated from a two- to four-year (associate's or bachelor's) nursing program. RNs have diplomas or college degrees. They have passed a national licensure examination. Registered nurses may have additional academic degrees or education in specialty areas.

Licensed Practical Nurse (LPN) or Licensed Vocational Nurse (LVN): A licensed practical nurse or licensed vocational nurse gives medications and treatments. An LPN or LVN is a licensed professional who has completed one to two years of education and has passed a national licensure examination.

Physician or Doctor (MD [medical doctor] or DO [doctor of osteopathy]): A doctor diagnoses disease or disability and prescribes treatment (Fig. 1-6). Doctors have graduated from four-year medical schools, which they attend after receiving bachelor's degrees. Many doctors also attend specialized training programs after medical school.

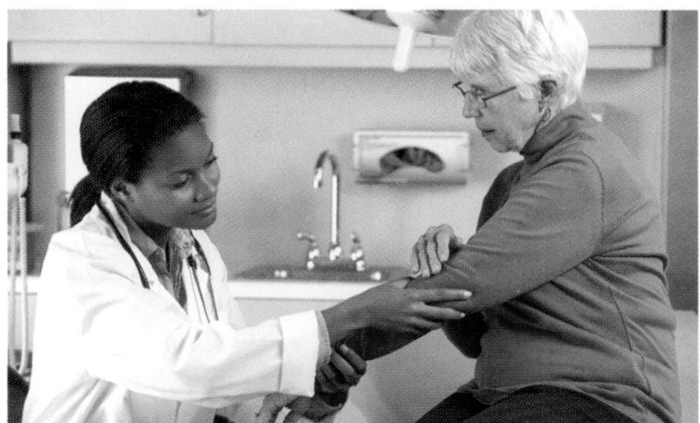

Fig. 1-6. *A doctor makes a diagnosis and prescribes treatment.*

Physical Therapist (PT or DPT): A physical therapist evaluates a person and develops a treatment plan. Goals are to increase movement, improve circulation, promote healing, reduce pain, prevent disability, and regain or maintain mobility (Fig. 1-7). A PT gives therapy in the form of heat, cold, massage, ultrasound, electrical stimulation, and exercise to muscles, bones, and joints. A physical therapist has graduated from a three-year doctoral degree program (doctor of physical therapy, or DPT) after receiving an undergraduate degree. PTs have to pass a national licensure examination before they can practice.

Occupational Therapist (OT): An occupational therapist helps residents learn to adapt to disabilities. An OT may help train residents to perform activities of daily living, such as bathing, dressing, and eating. This often involves the use of equipment called **assistive** or **adaptive devices**. The OT evaluates the resident's needs and plans a treatment program. Occupational therapists have earned a master's degree. OTs must pass a national licensure examination before they can practice.

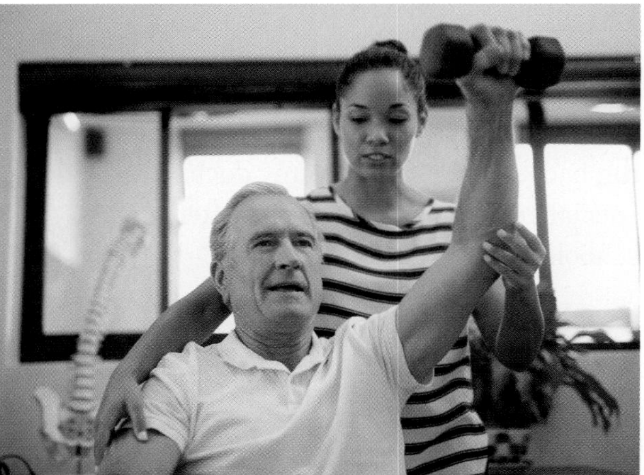

Fig. 1-7. A physical therapist helps exercise muscles, bones, and joints to improve strength or restore abilities.

Speech-Language Pathologist (SLP): A speech-language pathologist, or speech therapist, identifies communication disorders, addresses factors involved in recovery, and develops a plan of care to meet goals. An SLP teaches exercises to help the resident improve or overcome speech problems. An SLP also evaluates a person's ability to swallow food and drink. Speech-language pathologists have earned a master's degree in speech-language pathology and are licensed or certified to work.

Registered Dietitian (RD or RDN): A registered dietitian (RD) or registered dietitian nutritionist (RDN) assesses a resident's nutritional status and develops a treatment plan to improve health and manage illness. An RD creates diets to meet residents' special needs and may also supervise the preparation of food and educate people about nutrition. Registered dietitians have completed a bachelor's degree or master's degree and must pass a national licensure examination.

Medical Social Worker (MSW): A medical social worker determines residents' needs and helps get them support services, such as counseling and financial assistance. He may help residents obtain clothing and personal items if the family is not involved or does not visit often. A medical social worker may book appointments and transportation. MSWs have usually earned a master's degree in social work.

Activities Director: The activities director plans activities for residents to help them socialize and stay active. These activities are meant to improve and maintain residents' well-being and to prevent further complications from illness or disability. Games, performances, and arts and crafts are some types of activities that the activities director may plan or lead. An activities director has usually earned a bachelor's degree; however, she may have an associate's degree or qualifying work experience. An activities director may be called a *recreational therapist* or *recreation worker*, depending upon education and experience.

Resident and Resident's Family: The resident is an important member of the care team. Providing person-centered care means placing the resident's well-being first, and giving her the right to make decisions and choices about her own care. The resident helps plan care, and the resident's family may also be involved in these decisions. The family is a great source of information. They know the resident's personal preferences, history, diet, habits, and routines.

Residents' Rights

Resident as Member of Care Team

All members of the care team should focus on the resident. The team revolves around the resident and his or her condition, treatment, and progress. Without the resident, there is no care team.

A nursing assistant carries out instructions given to her by a nurse. The nurse is acting on the instructions of a doctor or other member of the care team. This is called the **chain of command**. It describes the line of authority and helps to make sure that residents get proper health care. The chain of command also protects employees and employers from liability. **Liability** is a legal term. It means that someone can be held responsible for harming someone else. For example, imagine that a task an NA does for a resident harms that resident. However, the task was in the care plan and was done according to policy and procedure. In this case, the NA may not be liable, or responsible, for hurting the resident. However, if the NA does something not in the care plan that harms a resident, she could be held responsible. That is why it is important for the team to follow instructions and for the facility to have a chain of command (Fig. 1-8).

Administrator: manages non-medical aspects of the facility, administers finances, and coordinates policy in consultation with medical professionals

Medical Director (MD): reviews and consults on medical aspects of care, coordinating with attending physicians and nursing staff and encouraging quality care

Director of Nursing (DON): manages the nursing staff at a facility

Assistant Director of Nursing (ADON): assists the DON with the management of nursing staff

Staff Development Coordinator: directs the training of employees at a facility

Minimum Data Set (MDS) Coordinator/Resident Assessment Coordinator: manages the assessment of resident needs and delivery of required care in a long-term care facility (usually a specially trained nurse)

Nursing Supervisor: supervises and supports nursing staff of the entire facility or multiple nursing units, assisting with resident care as needed

Charge Nurse: supervises and supports nursing staff of a particular unit and treats a limited number of residents

Staff Nurses (RNs, LPNs/LVNs): provide nursing care as prescribed by a physician

Nursing Assistants (NAs, CNAs): perform assigned nursing tasks, assist with routine personal care, and observe and report any changes in residents' conditions and abilities

Other Services

Physical Therapist (PT): administers therapy to increase movement, promote healing, reduce pain, and prevent disability

Occupational Therapist (OT): helps residents learn to adapt to disabilities and trains them to perform ADLs

Speech-Language Pathologist (SLP): identifies communication disorders and swallowing problems and develops a plan of care

Fig. 1-8. *The chain of command describes the line of authority and helps ensure that the resident receives proper care.*

Nursing assistants must understand what they can and cannot do. This is so that they do not harm residents or involve themselves or their employers in lawsuits. Some states certify that nursing assistants are qualified to work. However, nursing assistants are not licensed healthcare providers. Everything they do in their job is assigned to them by a licensed healthcare professional. That is why these professionals will show great interest in what NAs do and how they do it.

Every state grants the right to practice various jobs in health care through licensure. Examples include a license to practice nursing, medicine, or physical therapy. Each member of the care team works within his or her scope of practice. A **scope of practice** defines the tasks that healthcare providers are legally allowed to do as permitted by state or federal law. Laws and regulations about what NAs can and cannot do vary from state to state. It is important that NAs know which tasks are outside their scope of practice and not perform them.

The **care plan** is individualized for each resident. It is developed to help achieve the goals of care. The care plan lists the tasks that team members, including NAs, must perform. It states how often these tasks should be performed and how they should be carried out.

Care planning should involve input from the resident and/or the family, as well as from health professionals. Person-centered care places special emphasis on the importance of the resident's input.

The care plan is a guide to help the resident be as healthy as possible. It must be followed carefully. It is critical that NAs make observations and report them to the nurse. Even simple observations can be very important. The information that NAs collect and the changes they observe help determine how care plans may need to change. NAs spend so much time with residents; they are likely to have valuable information that will help in care planning.

6. Define policies, procedures, and professionalism

All facilities have manuals outlining their policies and procedures. A **policy** is a course of action that should be taken every time a certain situation occurs. For example, a very basic policy is that healthcare information must remain confidential. A **procedure** is a method, or way, of doing something. For example, a facility will have a procedure for reporting information about residents. The procedure explains what form to complete, when and how often to complete it, and to whom it is given. New employees will be told where to find a list of policies and procedures that all staff are expected to follow. Common policies at long-term care facilities include the following:

- All resident information must remain confidential. This is not only a facility rule; it is also the law. More information about confidentiality, including the Health Insurance Portability and Accountability Act (HIPAA), can be found later in the chapter.
- The care plan must always be followed. **Tasks not listed in the care plan or approved by the nurse should not be performed.**
- Nursing assistants should not do tasks that are not included in their job description.
- Nursing assistants must report important events or changes in residents to a nurse.
- Nursing assistants should not discuss their personal problems with residents or residents' families.
- Nursing assistants should not take money or gifts from residents or their families.
- Nursing assistants must be on time for work and must be dependable.

Employers will have policies and procedures for every resident care situation. These have been developed to give quality care and protect resident safety. Procedures may seem long and complicated, but each step is important. NAs must become familiar with and always follow policies and procedures.

Professional means having to do with work or a job. **Personal** refers to life outside a job, such as family, friends, and home life. **Professionalism** is behaving properly when on the job. It includes dressing appropriately and speaking well. It also includes being on time, completing tasks, and reporting to the nurse. For an NA, professionalism means following the care plan, making careful observations, and reporting accurately. Following policies and procedures is an important part of professionalism. Residents, coworkers, and supervisors respect employees who behave professionally. Professionalism helps people keep their jobs. It may also help them earn promotions and raises.

A professional relationship with residents includes the following:

- Providing person-centered care
- Keeping a positive attitude
- Doing only the assigned tasks that are in the care plan and that the NA is trained to do
- Keeping all residents' information confidential
- Always being polite and cheerful (Fig. 1-9)
- Not discussing personal problems

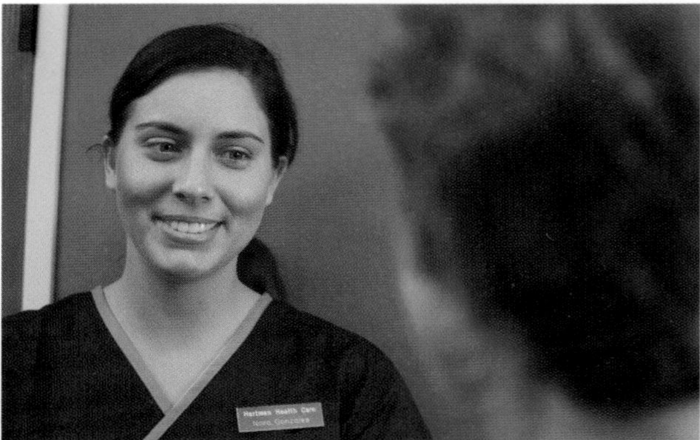

Fig. 1-9. *Nursing assistants are expected to always be polite and cheerful.*

- Not using personal phones in residents' rooms or in any resident care area
- Not using profanity, even if a resident does
- Listening to the resident
- Calling a resident *Mr., Mrs., Ms.,* or *Miss,* and his or her last name, or by the name he or she prefers; terms such as *sweetie, honey, dearie,* etc., are disrespectful and should not be used
- Never giving or accepting gifts
- Always explaining care before providing it
- Following practices, such as handwashing, to protect oneself and residents

A professional relationship with employers includes the following:

- Completing tasks efficiently
- Always following all policies and procedures
- Documenting and reporting carefully and correctly
- Reporting problems with residents or tasks
- Reporting anything that keeps an NA from completing duties
- Asking questions when the NA does not know or understand something
- Taking directions or feedback without becoming upset
- Being clean and neatly dressed and groomed
- Always being on time
- Telling the employer if the NA cannot report for work
- Following the chain of command
- Participating in education programs
- Being a positive role model for the facility

Nursing assistants must be:

- **Compassionate:** Being **compassionate** is being caring, concerned, empathetic, and understanding. Demonstrating **empathy** means identifying with the feelings of others. People who are compassionate understand others' problems. They care about them. Compassionate people are also sympathetic. Showing **sympathy** means sharing in the feelings and difficulties of others.
- **Honest**: An honest person tells the truth and can be trusted. Residents need to feel that they can trust those who care for them. The care team depends on honesty in planning care. Employers count on truthful records of care given and observations made.
- **Tactful**: Being **tactful** means showing sensitivity and having a sense of what is appropriate when dealing with others.
- **Conscientious**: People who are **conscientious** try to do their best. They are guided by a sense of right and wrong. They are alert, observant, accurate, and responsible. Giving conscientious care means making accurate observations and reports, following the care plan, and taking responsibility for one's actions (Fig. 1-10).

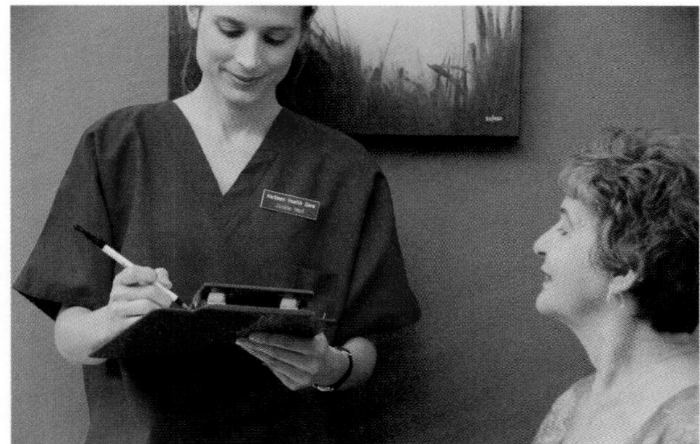

Fig. 1-10. *Nursing assistants must be conscientious about documenting observations and procedures.*

- **Dependable:** NAs must be able to make and keep commitments. They must be at work on time. They must skillfully do tasks, avoid absences, and help their peers when needed.
- **Patient**: People who are patient do not lose their temper easily. They do not act irritated or complain when things are hard. Residents are often elderly and may be sick or in pain.

They may take a long time to do things. They may become upset. NAs must not rush residents or act annoyed.

- **Respectful:** Being respectful means valuing other people's individuality. This includes their age, religion, culture, feelings, practices, and beliefs. People who are respectful treat others politely and kindly.
- **Unprejudiced:** NAs work with people from many different backgrounds. They must give each resident the same quality care regardless of age, gender, sexual orientation, religion, race, ethnicity, or condition.
- **Tolerant**: Being tolerant means respecting others' beliefs and practices and not judging them. NAs may not like or agree with things that residents or their families do or have done. However, their job is to care for each resident as assigned, not to judge him or her. NAs should put aside their opinions. They should see each resident as an individual who needs their care.

7. List examples of legal and ethical behavior and explain Residents' Rights

Ethics and laws guide behavior. **Ethics** are the knowledge of right and wrong. An ethical person has a sense of duty toward others. He tries to do what is right. **Laws** are rules set by the government to help people live peacefully together and to ensure order and safety. Ethics and laws are very important in health care. They protect people receiving care and guide those giving care. NAs and all care team members should be guided by a code of ethics. They must know the laws that apply to their jobs.

Guidelines: Legal and Ethical Behavior

- G Be honest at all times.
- G Protect residents' privacy and confidentiality. Do not discuss their cases except with other members of the care team.
- G Keep staff information confidential.
- G Report abuse or suspected abuse of residents. Help residents report abuse if they wish to make a complaint of abuse.
- G Follow the care plan and assignments. If you make a mistake, report it promptly.
- G Do not perform any tasks outside your scope of practice.
- G Report all resident observations and incidents to the nurse.
- G Document accurately and promptly.
- G Follow rules about safety and infection prevention (see Chapter 2).
- G Do not accept gifts or tips (Fig. 1-11).
- G Do not get personally or sexually involved with residents or their family members or friends.

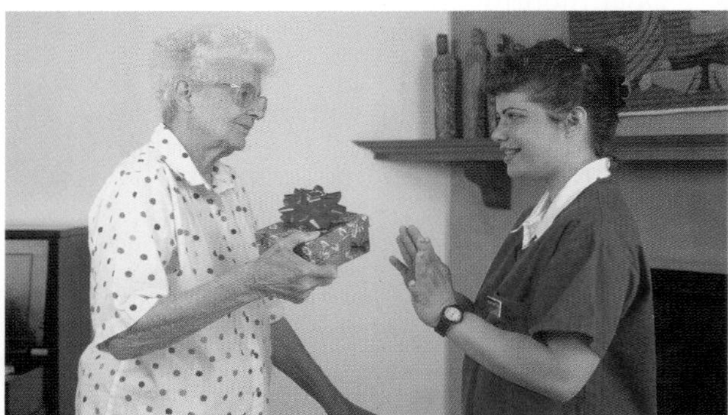

Fig. 1-11. *Nursing assistants should not accept money or gifts because it is unprofessional and may lead to conflict.*

The **Omnibus Budget Reconciliation Act (OBRA)** was passed in 1987. It has been updated several times since. OBRA was passed in response to reports of poor care and abuse in long-term care facilities. Congress decided to set minimum standards of care, which included standardized training of nursing assistants.

OBRA requires that the Nurse Aide Training and Competency Evaluation Program (NATCEP) set minimum standards for nursing assistant training. NAs must complete at least 75 hours of training that covers topics like communication, preventing infections, safety and emergency procedures, and promoting residents' independence and legal rights. Training must also include basic nursing skills, such as how to measure vital signs. NAs must also know how to respond to mental health and social services needs, rehabilitative needs, and how to care for residents who are cognitively impaired.

OBRA requires that NAs pass a competency evaluation (testing program) before they can be employed. NAs must also attend regular in-service education (a minimum of 12 hours per year) to keep their skills updated.

OBRA also requires that states keep a current list of nursing assistants in a state registry. In addition, OBRA identifies standards that instructors must meet in order to train nursing assistants. OBRA sets guidelines for minimum staff requirements and specific services that long-term care facilities must provide.

The resident assessment requirements are another important part of OBRA. OBRA requires that complete assessments be done on every resident. The assessment forms are the same for every facility.

OBRA made major changes in the survey process. Surveys are inspections to help make sure that long-term care facilities follow state and federal regulations. Surveys are done periodically by the state agency that licenses facilities. They may be done more often if a facility has been cited for problems. To **cite** means to find a problem through a survey. Inspections may be done less often if the facility has a good record. Inspection teams include a variety of trained healthcare professionals. The results from surveys are available to the public and posted in the facility.

OBRA also identifies important rights for residents in long-term care facilities. **Residents' Rights** specify how residents must be treated while living in a facility. They are an ethical code of conduct for healthcare workers. Facility staff give residents a list of these rights and review each right with them. In 2016, the Centers for Medicare and Medicaid Services (CMS) finalized a rule to improve the care and safety of residents in long-term care facilities. It was the first comprehensive update since 1991. It includes strengthening the rights of residents who live in long-term care facilities. NAs must be familiar with these legal rights. Residents' Rights include the following:

Quality of life: Residents have the right to the best care available. Dignity, choice, and independence are important parts of quality of life. The facility must give equal access to quality care regardless of a resident's condition, diagnosis, or payment source.

Services and activities to maintain a high level of wellness: Residents must receive the correct care. Healthcare professionals at facilities must develop a care plan for residents, and their care should keep them as healthy as possible. A baseline care plan for residents, which includes instructions for providing person-centered care, must be developed within 48 hours of admission. Residents' health should not decline as a direct result of the care given at the facility.

The right to be fully informed about rights and services: Residents must be told what services are available. They must be told the fee for each service. They must be informed of charges both orally and in writing. Residents must be given a written copy of their legal rights, along with the facility's rules. Legal rights must be explained in a language they can understand. Residents must be given contact information for state agencies relating to quality of care, such as the ombudsman program (more information may be found later in the chapter). When requested, survey results must be shared with residents. Residents have the right to be notified about any change of room or roommate. They have the right to communicate with someone who speaks their language. They have the right to assistance for any sensory impairment, such as vision loss.

The right to participate in their own care: Residents have the right to participate in planning their treatment, care, and discharge. Residents have the right to see and sign their care plans after all significant changes. Residents have the right to be informed of risks and benefits of care and treatment, including treatment options and alternatives, and to choose the options they prefer. They have the right to request, refuse, and/or discontinue treatment and care. They can refuse restraints and refuse to participate in experimental research.

Residents have the right to be told of changes in their condition. They have the right to review their medical record. They have the right to choose and change their care providers at any time.

Informed consent is a concept that is part of participating in one's own care. A person has the legal and ethical right to direct what happens to his or her body. Doctors also have an ethical duty to involve the person in his or her health care. **Informed consent** is the process by which a person, with the help of a doctor, makes informed decisions about his or her health care.

The right to make independent choices: Residents can make choices about their doctors, care, and treatments. They can make personal decisions, such as what to wear and how to spend their time. They can join in community activities, both inside and outside the care facility. They have the right to a reasonable accommodation of their needs and preferences. They have a right to participate in resident or family groups, such as a Resident Council. A Resident Council is a group of residents who meet regularly to discuss issues related to the long-term care facility. This council gives residents a voice in facility operations and an opportunity to provide suggestions on improving the quality of care.

The right to privacy and confidentiality: Residents have the right to speak privately with anyone, the right to privacy during care, and the right to confidentiality regarding every aspect of their lives (Fig. 1-12). Their medical, personal, and financial information cannot be shared with anyone but the care team.

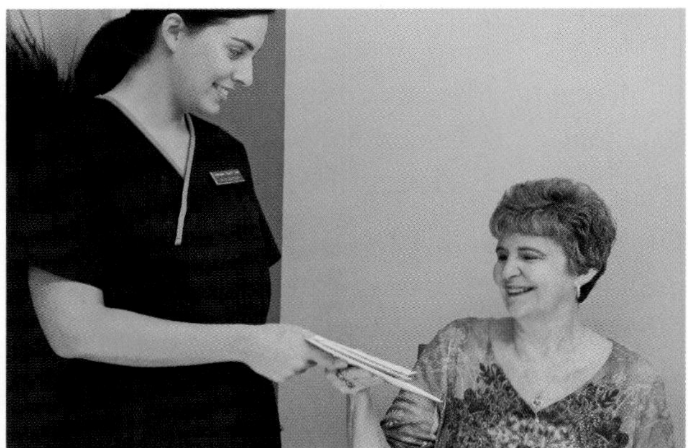

***Fig. 1-12.** Residents have the right to privacy, which includes private communication with anyone. They have the right to send and receive mail that is unopened.*

The right to dignity, respect, and freedom: Residents must be respected and treated with dignity by caregivers. Residents must not be abused, mistreated, or neglected in any way.

The right to security of possessions: Residents' personal possessions must be safe at all times. Facilities must make an effort to protect residents' property from loss or theft. Possessions cannot be taken or used by anyone without a resident's permission. Residents have the right to manage their own finances or choose someone else to do it for them. Residents can request that the facility handle their money. If the care facility handles residents' financial affairs, residents must have access to their accounts and financial records, and they must receive quarterly statements, among other things. Residents have the right to not be charged for any care that is covered by Medicaid or Medicare.

Rights during transfers and discharges: Residents have the right to be informed of and to consent to any location changes. Residents have the right to stay in a facility unless a transfer or discharge is needed. Residents can be moved from the facility due to safety reasons (their safety or others' safety), if their health has improved or worsened, or if payment for care has not been received for a determined period of time.

The facility must develop an effective discharge plan for residents that involves each resident's goals and preferences. This plan must be regularly reviewed and updated as appropriate. If the resident is planning to stay at the facility long term, discharge planning still needs to occur, keeping the resident's preferences in mind.

The right to complain: Residents have the right to make complaints and voice grievances without fear for their safety or care. Facilities must work quickly to address their concerns.

The right to visits: Residents have the right to visits from doctors, family members (including spouses and domestic partners), friends, ombudsmen, clergy members, legal representatives, or any other person. Visits cannot be restricted, limited, or denied on the basis of race, color, national origin, religion, sex, gender identity, sexual orientation, or disability.

Rights with regard to social services: The facility must provide residents with access to social services. This includes counseling, assistance in solving problems with others, and help contacting legal and financial professionals.

Guidelines: Protecting Residents' Rights

- **G** Never abuse a resident physically, emotionally, verbally, or sexually. Watch for and immediately report any signs of abuse or neglect.
- **G** Call the resident by the name he or she prefers.
- **G** Involve residents in planning. Allow residents to make as many choices as possible about when, where, and how care is performed.
- **G** Always explain a procedure to a resident before performing it.
- **G** Do not unnecessarily expose a resident while giving care.
- **G** Respect a resident's refusal of care. Residents have a legal right to refuse treatment and care. However, report the refusal to the nurse immediately.
- **G** Tell the nurse if a resident has questions, concerns, or complaints about treatment or the goals of care.
- **G** Be truthful when documenting care.
- **G** Do not talk or gossip about residents. Keep all resident information confidential.
- **G** Knock and ask for permission before entering a resident's room (Fig. 1-13).

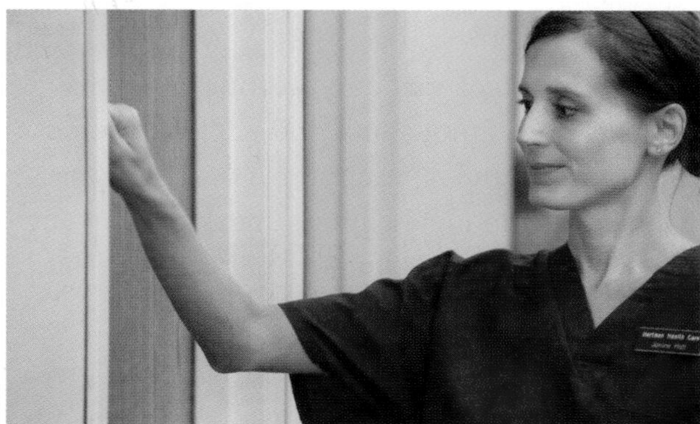

Fig. 1-13. *Always respect residents' privacy. Knock before entering their rooms, even if the door is open.*

- **G** Do not accept gifts or money from residents.
- **G** Do not open a resident's mail or look through his belongings.
- **G** Respect residents' personal possessions. Handle them gently and carefully. Keep personal items labeled and stored according to facility policy.
- **G** Report observations about a resident's condition or care.
- **G** Help resolve disputes by reporting them to the nurse.

Residents' Rights

Maintaining Boundaries

In professional relationships, boundaries must be set. Boundaries are the limits to or within relationships. Nursing assistants are guided by ethics and laws that set limits for their relationships with residents. These boundaries help support a healthy resident-staff relationship. Working closely with residents on a regular basis may make it more difficult to honor the boundaries of professional relationships. Residents may feel that NAs are their friends. If a staff member and resident become personally involved with each other, it becomes more difficult to enforce rules. The resident may expect the NA to break the rules because she thinks they are friends. Emotional attachments to residents are unprofessional and may weaken an NA's judgment. NAs should be friendly, warm, and caring with residents. But they should behave professionally and stay within the limits of set boundaries. Facility rules and the care plan's instructions should be followed. They are in place for everyone's protection.

A very important part of protecting residents' rights is preventing abuse and neglect. **Abuse** is purposeful mistreatment that causes physical, mental, or emotional pain or injury to someone. There are many forms of abuse, including the following:

- **Physical abuse** is any treatment, intentional or not, that causes harm to a person's body. This includes slapping, bruising, cutting, burning, physically restraining, pushing, shoving, or even rough handling.
- **Psychological abuse** is emotional harm caused by threatening, scaring, humiliating, intimidating, isolating, or insulting a person, or by treating him or her as a child.
- **Verbal abuse** is the use of spoken or written words, pictures, or gestures that threaten, embarrass, or insult a person.
- **Sexual abuse** is the forcing of a person to perform or participate in sexual acts against his or her will. This includes unwanted touching or exposing oneself to a person. It also includes sharing pornographic material.
- **Financial abuse** is the improper or illegal use of a person's money, possessions, property, or other assets.
- **Assault** is a threat to harm a person, resulting in the person feeling fearful that he or she will be harmed. Telling a resident that she will be slapped if she does not stop yelling is an example of assault.
- **Battery** is the intentional touching of a person without his or her consent. An example is an NA hitting or pushing a resident. This is also considered physical abuse. Forcing a resident to eat a meal is another example of battery.
- **Domestic violence** is abuse by spouses, intimate partners, or family members. It can be physical, sexual, or emotional. The victim can be a man or woman of any age or a child.
- **False imprisonment** is unlawful restraint that affects a person's freedom of movement. Both the threat of being physically restrained and actually being physically restrained are types of false imprisonment. Not allowing a resident to leave the facility is also considered false imprisonment.
- **Involuntary seclusion** is the separation of a person from others against the person's will. An example is an NA confining a resident to his room.
- **Workplace violence** is abuse of staff by other staff members, residents, or visitors. It can be verbal, physical, or sexual. This includes improper touching and discussion about sexual subjects.
- **Sexual harassment** is any unwelcome sexual advance or behavior that creates an intimidating, hostile, or offensive working environment. Requests for sexual favors, unwanted touching, and other acts of a sexual nature are examples of sexual harassment.
- **Substance abuse** is the repeated use of legal or illegal drugs, cigarettes, or alcohol in a way that harms oneself or others. For the NA, substance abuse can lead to unsafe

practices that result in negligence, malpractice, neglect, and abuse. It can also lead to the loss of the NA's certification.

Neglect is the failure to provide needed care that results in physical, mental, or emotional harm to a person. Neglect can be put into two categories: active neglect and passive neglect. **Active neglect** is the purposeful failure to provide needed care, resulting in harm to a person. **Passive neglect** is the unintentional failure to provide needed care, resulting in physical, mental, or emotional harm to a person. The caregiver may not know how to properly care for the resident, or may not understand the resident's needs.

Negligence means actions, or the failure to act or provide the proper care for a resident, resulting in unintended injury. An example of negligence is an NA forgetting to lock a resident's wheelchair before transferring her. The resident falls and is injured. **Malpractice** occurs when a person is injured due to professional misconduct through negligence, carelessness, or lack of skill.

Nursing assistants must never abuse residents in any way. They must also try to protect residents from others who abuse them. If an NA ever sees or suspects that another caregiver, family member, or resident is abusing a resident, she must report this immediately to the nurse in charge. **Reporting abuse or suspected abuse is not an option—it is the law.**

Observing and Reporting: Abuse and Neglect

The following injuries are considered suspicious and should be reported:

- O/R Poisoning or traumatic injury
- O/R Teeth marks
- O/R Belt buckle or strap marks
- O/R Bruises, contusions, or welts
- O/R Scars
- O/R Fractures or dislocations
- O/R Burns of unusual shape and in unusual locations, or cigarette burns
- O/R Scalding burns
- O/R Scratches or puncture wounds
- O/R Scalp tenderness or patches of missing hair
- O/R Swelling in the face, broken teeth, or nasal discharge
- O/R Bruises, bleeding, or discharge from the vaginal area

These signs could indicate abuse:

- O/R Yelling obscenities
- O/R Fear, apprehension, or fear of being alone
- O/R Poor self-control
- O/R Constant pain
- O/R Threatening to hurt others
- O/R Withdrawal or apathy (Fig. 1-14)

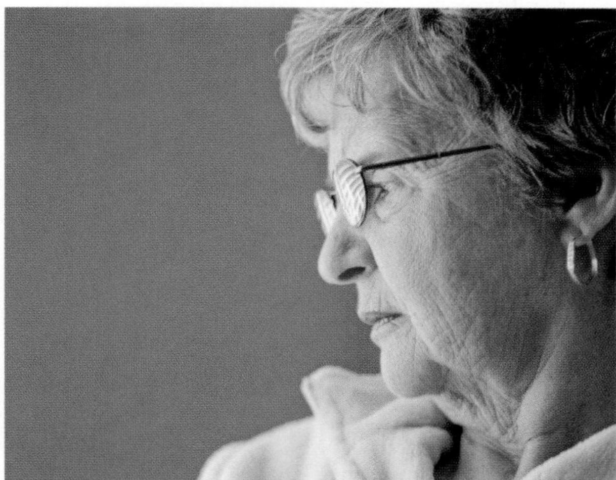

Fig. 1-14. *Withdrawing from others is an important change to report.*

- O/R Alcohol or drug abuse
- O/R Agitation, anxiety, or signs of stress
- O/R Low self-esteem
- O/R Mood changes, confusion, or disorientation

- O/R Private conversations are not allowed, or the family member/caregiver is present during all conversations
- O/R Reports of questionable care by the resident or her family

These signs could indicate neglect:

- O/R Pressure injuries
- O/R Unclean body
- O/R Body lice
- O/R Unanswered call lights
- O/R Soiled bedding or incontinence briefs not being changed
- O/R Poorly-fitting clothing
- O/R Unmet needs relating to hearing aids, eyeglasses, etc.
- O/R Weight loss or poor appetite
- O/R Uneaten food
- O/R Dehydration
- O/R Fresh water or beverages not being offered regularly
- O/R Reports of not receiving prescribed medication by the resident or her family

Nursing assistants are in an excellent position to observe and report abuse or neglect. NAs have an ethical and legal responsibility to observe for signs of abuse and to report suspected cases to the proper person. NAs must follow the chain of command when reporting abuse. If action is not taken, the NA should keep reporting up the chain of command until action is taken. If no action is taken at the facility level, she can call the state abuse hotline or contact the proper state agency. Abuse can be reported anonymously. If a life-or-death situation is witnessed, the NA should remove the resident to a safe place if possible. The NA should get help immediately or have someone go for help. The resident should not be left alone.

If abuse is suspected or observed, the NA should give the nurse as much information as possible. If a resident wants to make a complaint of abuse, the NA must help her in every way. This includes telling the resident about the process and her rights. NAs must never retaliate against (punish) residents complaining of abuse. If an NA sees someone being cruel or abusive to a resident who made a complaint, she must report it. All care team members are responsible for residents' safety and should take this responsibility seriously.

In long-term care facilities in the United States, an **ombudsman** is assigned by law as the legal advocate for residents (ltcombudsman.org). The Older Americans Act (OAA) is a federal law that requires all states to have an ombudsman program. An ombudsman visits facilities and listens to residents. He or she decides what action to take if there are problems. Ombudsmen can help resolve conflicts and settle disputes concerning residents' health, safety, welfare, and rights. The ombudsman will gather information and try to resolve the problem on the resident's behalf and may suggest ways to solve the problem. Ombudsmen provide an ongoing presence in long-term care facilities. They monitor care and conditions (Fig. 1-15).

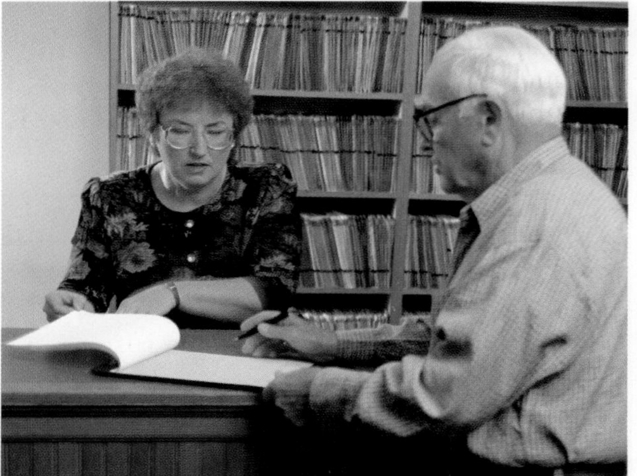

Fig. 1-15. *An ombudsman is a legal advocate for residents. He or she visits the facility and listens to residents, and may work with other agencies to resolve complaints.*

To respect **confidentiality** means to keep private things private. Nursing assistants will learn confidential (private) information about residents. They may learn about a resident's health, finances, and relationships. Ethically and legally, they must protect this information. NAs should not share information about residents with anyone other than the care team.

Congress passed the **Health Insurance Portability and Accountability Act (HIPAA)** (hhs.gov/hipaa) in 1996. It has been further defined and revised since then. One reason this law was passed is to help keep health information private and secure. All healthcare organizations must take special steps to protect health information. Their employees can be fined and/or imprisoned if they do not follow rules to protect patient privacy.

Under this law, a person's health information must be kept private. **Protected health information (PHI)** is information that can be used to identify a person and relates to the patient's condition, any health care that the person has had, and payment for that health care. Examples of PHI include a person's name, address, telephone number, social security number, email address, and medical record number. Only people who must have information to provide care or to process records should know a person's private health information. They must protect the information. It must not become known or used by anyone else. It must be kept confidential.

HIPAA applies to all healthcare providers, including doctors, nurses, nursing assistants, and any other care team members. NAs cannot give out any information about a resident to anyone who is not directly involved in the resident's care unless the resident gives official consent or unless the law requires it. For example, if a neighbor asks an NA how a resident is doing, she should reply, "I'm sorry, but I cannot share that information. It's confidential." That is the correct response to anyone who does not have a legal reason to know about the resident.

Guidelines: Protecting Privacy

- **G** Make sure you are in a private area when you listen to or read your messages.
- **G** Know with whom you are speaking on the phone. If you are not sure, get a name and number. Call back after you find out it is all right to share information with this person.
- **G** Do not talk about residents in public (Fig. 1-16). Public areas include elevators, grocery stores, lounges, waiting rooms, parking garages, schools, restaurants, etc.

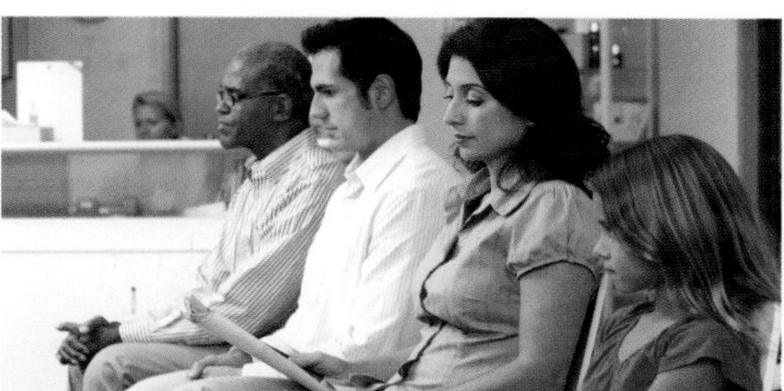

Fig. 1-16. NAs should not discuss any information about residents in public places.

- **G** Use confidential rooms for reports to other care team members.
- **G** If you see a resident's family member or a former resident in public, be careful with your greeting. He or she may not want others to know about the family member or that he or she has been a resident.
- **G** Do not bring family or friends to the facility to meet residents.
- **G** Make sure nobody can see protected health or personal information on your computer screen while you are working. Log out and/or exit the browser when finished with any computer work.
- **G** Do not give confidential information in emails. You do not know who has access to your messages.
- **G** Do not share resident information, photos, or videos on any social networking site, such as Facebook, Twitter, Instagram, or Pinterest.

G Make sure fax numbers are correct before faxing information. Use a cover sheet with a confidentiality statement.

G Do not leave documents where others may see them.

G Store, file, or shred documents according to facility policy. If you find documents with a resident's information, give them to the nurse.

All healthcare workers must follow HIPAA regulations no matter where they are or what they are doing. There are serious penalties for violating these rules, including the following:

- Fines ranging from $100 to $1.5 million
- Prison sentences of up to ten years

Maintaining confidentiality is a legal and ethical obligation. It is part of respecting residents and their rights. Discussing a resident's care or personal affairs with anyone other than members of the care team violates the law.

8. Explain legal aspects of the resident's medical record

The resident's medical record or chart is a legal document. What is documented in the chart is considered in court to be what actually happened. In general, if something does not appear in a resident's chart, it did not legally happen. Failing to document care could cause very serious legal problems for NAs and their employers. It could also harm residents. NAs must remember that if it was not documented, it was not done. Careful charting is important for these reasons:

- It is the only way to guarantee clear and complete communication among all the members of the care team.
- Documentation is a legal record of every part of a resident's treatment. Medical charts can be used in court as legal evidence.
- Documentation helps protect nursing assistants and their employers from liability by proving what they did when caring for residents.
- Documentation gives an up-to-date record of the status and care of each resident.

Guidelines: Careful Documentation

G Document care immediately after it is given. This makes details easier to remember. **Do not record any care before it has been done.**

G Think about what you want to say before documenting. Be as brief and as clear as possible.

G Use facts, not opinions.

G Use black ink when documenting by hand. Write as neatly as you can.

G If you make a mistake, draw one line through it. Write the correct information. Put your initials and the date (Fig. 1-17). Do not erase what you have written. Do not use correction fluid. Documentation done on a computer is time-stamped; it can only be changed by entering another notation.

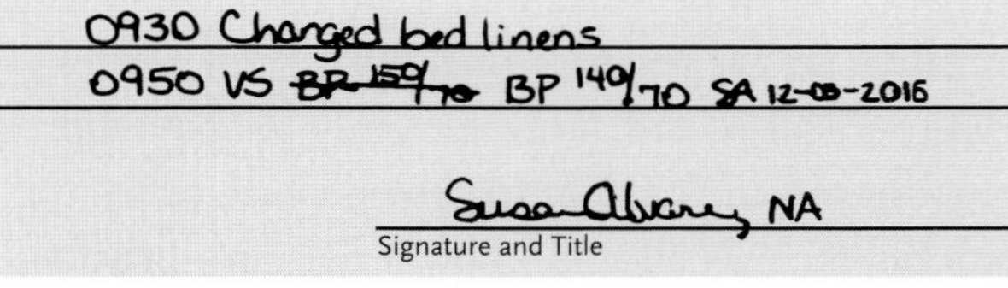

Fig. 1-17. One example of how to correct a mistake.

G Sign your full name and title (for example, Sara Martinez, NA). Write the correct date.

G Document as specified in the care plan. Documentation may be done by code. For example, when documenting activities of daily living (ADLs) on a flow sheet, you may need to choose a code to explain what the resident was able to do. Zero may be classified as independent, 1 as needs supervision, 2 as needs limited assistance, 3 as needs extensive assistance, and 4 as total dependence. You will be trained to document properly at your facility.

G Documentation may need to be done using the 24-hour clock, or military time (Fig. 1-18). Regular time uses the numbers 1 to 12 to show each of the 24 hours in a day. In military time, the hours are numbered from 00 to 23. Midnight is expressed as 0000 (or 2400), 1:00 a.m. is 0100, 1:00 p.m. is 1300, and so on.

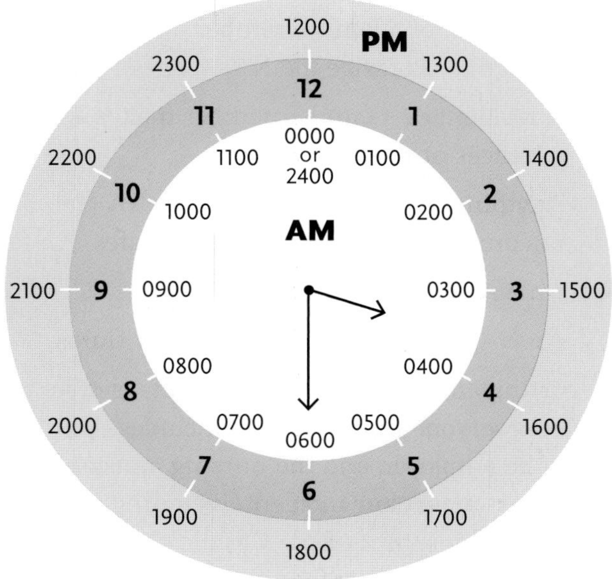

Fig. 1-18. Divisions in the 24-hour clock.

Both regular and military time list minutes and seconds the same way. The minutes and seconds do not change when converting from regular to military time. The abbreviations a.m. and p.m. are used in regular time to show what time of day it is. However, these are not used in military time, since specific numbers show each hour of the day. For example, to change 4:22 p.m. to military time, add 4 + 12. The minutes do not change. The time is expressed as 1622 (sixteen twenty-two) hours.

To change the hours between 1:00 p.m. to 11:59 p.m. to military time, add 12 to the regular time. For example, to change 3:00 p.m. to military time, add 3 + 12. The time is expressed as 1500 (fifteen hundred) hours.

Midnight is the only time that differs. It can be written as 0000, or it can be written as 2400. This follows the rule of adding 12 to the regular time. Follow facility policy on how to express midnight.

To change from military time to regular time, subtract 12. The minutes do not change. For example, to change 2200 hours to standard time, subtract 12 from 22. The answer is 10:00 p.m.

G At some facilities, computers or tablets are used for documentation. Computers record and store information that can be retrieved when needed. This is faster and more accurate than writing information by hand. A computer may remain in a resident's room for care team members to input information each time they visit the room. A computer may be in the hallway or other common area. A computer or tablet may also be carried from room to room. Some general guidelines for computer documentation are listed below:

- If your facility uses computers for documentation, you will be trained to use them. Always ask questions if you do not know or understand something. Some facilities use both handwritten and electronic records. Even when facilities require electronic/computer documentation, training often includes how to document by hand in case there is a system failure.
- Legal documentation rules apply to both electronic and paper medical charts.
- HIPAA privacy guidelines apply to electronic documentation. Make sure nobody can see protected health information on your computer screen. Do not share your log-in information with anyone.
- Do not have someone else enter information for you, even if it is more convenient.
- Make sure you are logged in to the correct resident's chart before beginning to document. Log out and/or exit a resident's chart when finished with documentation.
- Some computer software automatically fills in certain fields with information that has

been entered before (autofill). Be sure that you are documenting correctly and that any autofill entries are accurate. Check your entries before exiting a resident's chart.

- Treat computers carefully.
- Do not use the facility's computers or tablets to browse the internet or access any personal accounts.

9. Explain the Minimum Data Set (MDS)

The federal government developed a resident assessment system in 1990 and has revised it periodically. It is called the **Minimum Data Set (MDS)**. The MDS is a detailed form with guidelines for assessing residents. It also lists what to do if resident problems are identified. Nurses must complete the MDS for each resident within 14 days of admission and again each year. In addition, the MDS for each resident must be reviewed every three months. A new MDS must be done when there is any major change in the resident's condition. NAs contribute to the MDS by reporting changes in residents promptly and documenting accurately. Doing this means a new MDS can be completed when needed.

10. Discuss incident reports

An **incident** is an accident, problem, or unexpected event during the course of care. It is something that is not part of the normal routine. A mistake in care, such as feeding a resident from the wrong meal tray, is an incident. A resident fall or injury is another type of incident. Accusations made by residents against staff, as well as employee injuries, are other types of incidents. State and federal guidelines require that incidents be recorded in an incident report. An incident report (also called an *occurrence, accident, accident/incident,* or *event report*) is a report that documents the incident and the response to it. The information in an incident report is confidential. It is intended for internal use to help prevent future incidents. Incident reports should be filed when any of the following occur:

- A resident falls (all falls must be reported, even if the resident says he or she is fine)
- An NA or a resident breaks or damages something
- An NA makes a mistake in care
- A resident or a family member makes a request that is outside the NA's scope of practice
- A resident or a family member makes sexual advances or remarks
- Anything happens that makes an NA feel uncomfortable, threatened, or unsafe
- An NA gets injured on the job
- An NA is exposed to blood or body fluids

Reporting and documenting incidents is done to protect everyone involved. This includes the resident, the employer, and the nursing assistant. NAs must report any incident, including job-related injuries, immediately to the charge nurse. When documenting incidents, NAs should complete the report as soon as possible and give it to the charge nurse. This is important so that details are not forgotten.

If a resident falls and the NA did not see it, he should not document "Mr. G fell." Instead he should document "Found Mr. G on the floor" or "Mr. G states that he fell." NAs should write brief and accurate descriptions of the events as they happened. They should not place blame or liability within the report.

Guidelines: Incident Reporting

- G Tell what happened. State the time and the mental and physical condition of the person.
- G Describe the person's reaction to the incident.
- G State the facts; do not give opinions.
- G Do not document that an incident report was completed on the medical record.
- G Describe the action taken to give care.

2 Foundations of Resident Care

1. Understand the importance of verbal and written communications

Effective communication is a critical part of a nursing assistant's job. Nursing assistants must communicate with supervisors, the care team, residents, and family members. A resident's health depends on how well an NA communicates observations and concerns to the nurse.

Communication is the process of exchanging information with others. It is a process of sending and receiving messages. People communicate with signs and symbols, such as words, drawings, and pictures. They also communicate through their behavior.

Verbal communication uses spoken or written words. Oral reports are an example of verbal communication. **Nonverbal communication** is communicating without using words. An example is a person shrugging his shoulders. Nonverbal communication also includes how a person says something. Body language is another form of nonverbal communication. Movements, facial expressions, and posture can express different attitudes or emotions (Fig. 2-1).

> **Residents' Rights**
>
> **Different Languages**
>
> When caring for residents, NAs should speak in a language that residents can understand or find an interpreter (someone who speaks the resident's language). Picture cards or gestures can help with communication. NAs should not use a different language when speaking with staff in front of residents.

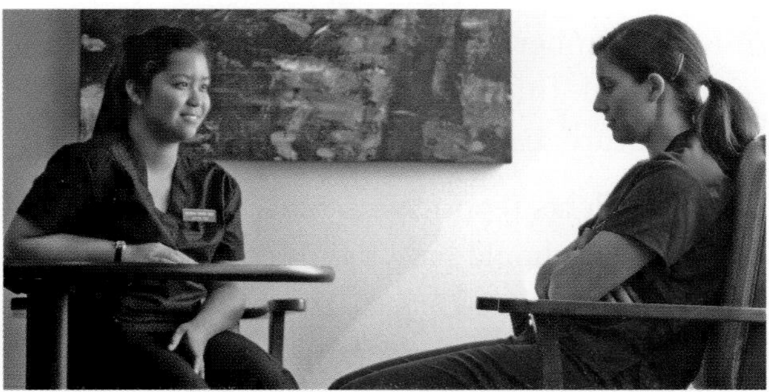

Fig. 2-1. *Body language sends messages just as words do. Which of these people seems more interested in their conversation—the person on the right who is looking down with her arms crossed or the person on the left who is sitting up straight and smiling?*

Nursing assistants must make brief, accurate oral and written reports to residents and staff. Careful observations are used to make these reports and are important to the health and well-being of all residents. Signs and symptoms that should be reported will be discussed throughout this textbook. Some observations will need to be reported immediately to the nurse. Deciding what to report immediately involves critical thinking. Anything that endangers residents should be reported immediately, including the following:

- Falls
- Chest pain
- Severe headache
- Trouble breathing
- Abnormal pulse, respiration, or blood pressure
- Change in mental status

- Sudden weakness or loss of mobility
- Fever
- Loss of consciousness
- Change in level of consciousness
- Bleeding
- Swelling of a body part
- Change in resident's condition
- Bruises, abrasions, or other signs of possible abuse

When making reports about residents, NAs must remember that all resident information is confidential. Information should only be shared with the care team.

When residents report symptoms, events, or feelings, the NA should have them repeat what they have said. He should ask for more information. The NA should ask open-ended questions that need more than a "yes" or "no" answer. For example, an NA should not ask, "Did you sleep well last night?" Instead, he should ask, "Can you tell me about your night and how you slept?" This will encourage the resident to offer facts and details.

Proper Communication

When communicating with residents, the NA should remember to use these tips:

- Always greet the resident by his or her preferred name.
- Identify himself.
- Focus on the topic to be discussed.
- Face the resident while speaking and avoid talking into space.
- Talk with the resident, not other staff members, while giving care.
- Listen and respond when the resident speaks.
- Praise the resident and smile often.
- Encourage the resident to interact with him and others.
- Be courteous.
- Tell the resident when he is leaving the room.

Residents' Rights

Names

NAs should call residents by the names residents prefer. NAs should not refer to residents by their first names unless a resident has asked them to do so. Terms such as *sweetie*, *honey*, or *dearie* are disrespectful and should not be used.

When making any report, the right information must be collected before documenting it. Facts, not opinions, are most useful to the nurse and the care team. Two kinds of factual information are needed in reporting. **Objective information** is based on what a person sees, hears, touches, or smells. Objective information is collected by using the senses. It is also called *signs*. **Subjective information** is something a person cannot or did not observe. It is based on something that the resident reported that may or may not be true. It is also called *symptoms*. An example of objective information is "Mr. Hartman is holding his head and rubbing his temples." A subjective report of the same situation might be "Mr. Hartman says he has a headache." The nurse needs factual information in order to make decisions about care and treatment. Both objective and subjective reports are valuable.

In any report, what is observed (signs) and what the resident reports (symptoms) need to be clearly noted. "Ms. Scott reports pain in left shoulder" is an example of clear reporting. NAs are not expected to make diagnoses based on signs they observe. Their observations, however, can alert the care team to possible problems. In order to report accurately, NAs must observe residents accurately. To observe accurately, as many senses as possible should be used to gather information (Fig. 2-2).

Sight. The NA should look for changes in the resident's appearance. These include rashes, redness, paleness, swelling, discharge, weakness, sunken eyes, and posture or gait (walking) changes.

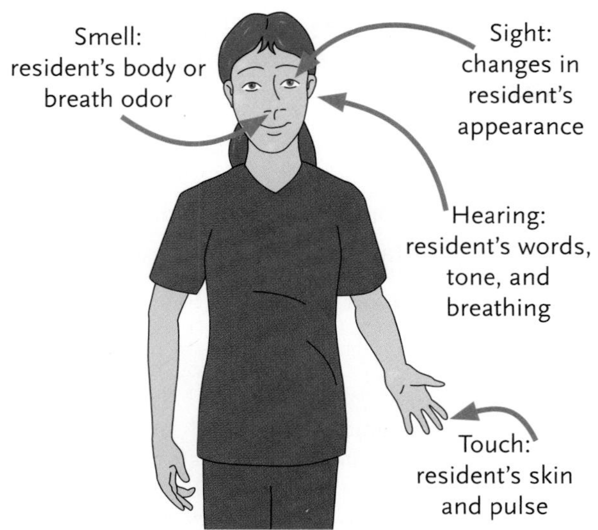

***Fig. 2-2.** Reporting observations accurately requires using more than one sense.*

Hearing. The NA should listen to what the resident says about his condition, family, or needs. Is the resident speaking clearly and making sense? Does he show emotions, such as anger, frustration, or sadness? Is his breathing normal? Does he wheeze, gasp, or cough? Is the area quiet enough for him to rest as needed?

Touch. Does the resident's skin feel hot or cool, moist or dry? Is the pulse rate normal?

Smell. Are there any odors coming from the resident's body? Odors could suggest poor bathing, infections, or incontinence. **Incontinence** is the inability to control the bladder or bowels. Breath odor could suggest use of alcohol or tobacco, indigestion, or poor mouth care.

For oral reports, the NA should write notes so that important details are not forgotten (Fig. 2-3). When needing to give an oral report, unless the situation is urgent, the NA should approach the nurse and wait for the nurse to complete the task she is currently doing. Once the nurse has acknowledged the NA, she can briefly state the message and deliver the written summary as well if there is one. Waiting until the nurse is done helps reduce the risk of error. Following an oral report, the NA must document when, why, about what, and to whom an oral report was given. Documentation should always occur after the report is given, not before.

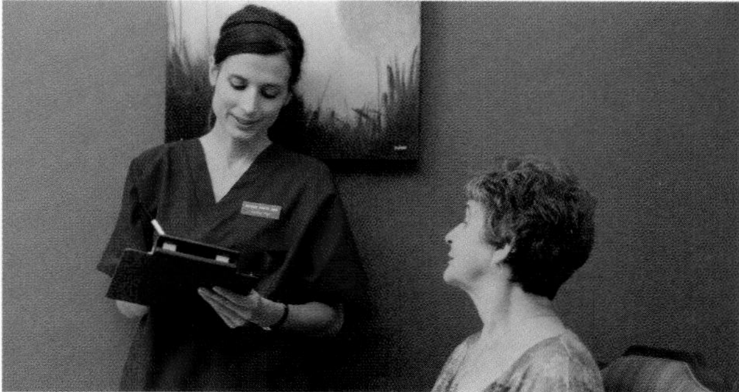

***Fig. 2-3.** Taking notes helps nursing assistants remember facts and report accurately.*

Sometimes the nurse or another member of the care team will give an NA a brief oral report on one of her residents. The NA should listen carefully and take notes. She should ask about anything she does not understand. At the end of the report, the NA can restate what she has been told to make sure she understands.

Throughout an NA's training, she will learn medical terms for specific conditions. Medical terms are often made up of roots, prefixes, and suffixes. A root is a part of a word that contains its basic meaning. The prefix is the word part that comes before the root to help form a new word. The suffix is the word part added to the end of a root that helps form a new word. Prefixes and suffixes are called *affixes* because they are attached, or affixed, to a root. Here are some examples:

- The root *derm* or *derma* means skin. The suffix *itis* means inflammation. Dermatitis is an inflammation of the skin.
- The prefix *brady* means slow. The root *cardia* means heart. Bradycardia is slow heartbeat or pulse.
- The suffix *pathy* means disease. The root *neuro* means of the nerve or nervous system. Neuropathy is a nerve disease or disease of the nervous system.

When speaking with residents and their families, NAs should use simple, non-medical terms. Medical terms should not be used because they may not be understood. But when speaking with the care team, using medical terminology will help give more complete information.

Abbreviations are another way to help the care team communicate more efficiently with each other. For example, the abbreviation *prn* means *as necessary*. NAs should learn the standard medical abbreviations their facility uses. They can use them to report information briefly and accurately. NAs may need to know these abbreviations to read assignments or care plans. A brief list of abbreviations is located at the end of this textbook. There may be other terms in use at a facility, so NAs should follow facility policy.

Telephone Communication

Nursing assistants may be asked to make a call or answer the telephone at their facility.

Guidelines: Telephone Communication

- G Always identify your facility's name, your name, and your position. Be friendly and professional.
- G If you need to find the person the caller wishes to speak with, place the caller on hold after asking if it is okay to do so.
- G If the caller has to leave a message, write it down and repeat it to make sure you have the correct message. Ask for proper spellings of names. Do not ask for more information than the person needs to return the call: a name, short message, and phone number is enough. Do not give out any information about staff or residents. If someone is calling to give a doctor's order for a resident, find the nurse or take a message for the nurse.
- G Thank the person for calling. Say goodbye.

Call Lights

Long-term care facilities are required to have a call system, often called *call lights*, so that residents can call for help whenever they need it. They are in resident rooms and bathrooms. Some have strings for residents to pull, and others have buttons to push. The signal is usually both a light outside the room and a sound that can be heard in the nurses' station. This is the primary way a resident can call for help. NAs must always respond immediately when they see the light or hear the sound. They should do so even if the resident who needs help is not on their assignment sheet. All residents are the responsibility of each NA. NAs should respond to call lights in a courteous and respectful manner. They must check each time before leaving a room to make sure that the call light is within reach of the resident's stronger hand and that the resident knows how to use it.

2. Describe barriers to communication

Communication can be blocked or disrupted in many ways (Fig. 2-4). These are some barriers and ways for a nursing assistant to avoid them:

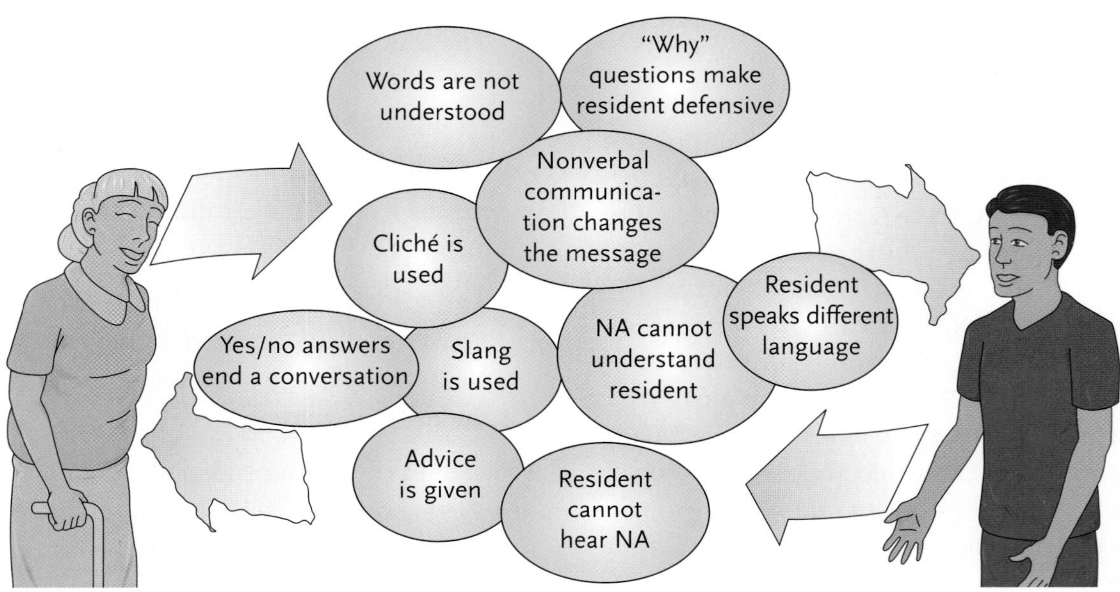

Fig. 2-4. *Barriers to communication.*

Resident does not hear NA, does not hear correctly, or does not understand. The NA should face the resident. He should speak slowly and clearly. He should not shout, whisper, or mumble. The NA should speak in a low voice, using a pleasant tone. If the resident wears a hearing aid, the NA should check that it is on and is working.

Resident is difficult to understand. The NA should be patient and take time to listen. He can ask the resident to repeat or explain the message. He should then state the message in his own words to make sure he has understood.

NA, resident, or others use words that are not understood. An NA should not use medical terms with residents or their families. He should speak in simple, everyday words and ask what a word means if he is not sure.

NA uses slang or profanity. The NA should avoid using slang words. They are unprofessional and may not be understood. He should not use profanity, even if the resident does.

NA uses clichés. Clichés are phrases that are used over and over again and do not really mean anything. For example, "Everything will be fine" is a cliché. Instead of using a cliché, the NA should listen to what a resident is really saying. He should respond with a meaningful message.

NA responds with "Why?" The NA should avoid asking "Why?" when a resident makes a statement. "Why" questions make people feel defensive.

NA gives advice. The NA should not offer his opinion or give advice. Giving medical advice is not within an NA's scope of practice. It could be dangerous.

NA asks questions that only require yes/no answers. The NA should ask open-ended questions that need more than a "yes" or "no" answer. Yes and no answers end conversation. For example, if an NA wants to know what a resident likes to eat, he should not ask, "Do you like vegetables?" Instead, he should ask, "Which vegetables do you like best?"

Resident speaks a different language. If a resident speaks a different language than the NA does, the NA should speak slowly and clearly. He should keep his messages short and simple. He should be alert for words the resident understands, as well as signs that the resident is only pretending to understand. He may need to use pictures or gestures to communicate. The NA can ask the resident's family or other staff members who speak the resident's language for help. He should be patient and calm.

NA or resident uses nonverbal communication. Nonverbal communication can change a message. The NA should be aware of his body language and gestures. He can look for nonverbal messages from residents and clarify them. For example, "Mr. Feldman, you say you're feeling fine but you seem to be in pain. Can I help?"

Defense mechanisms may be considered barriers to communication. **Defense mechanisms** are unconscious behaviors used to release tension or cope with stress. They help to block uncomfortable or threatening feelings. These are some common defense mechanisms:

- **Denial**: Completely rejecting the thought or feeling—"I'm not upset with you!"
- **Projection**: Seeing feelings in others that are really one's own—"My teacher hates me."
- **Displacement**: Transferring a strong negative feeling to a safer situation—for example, an unhappy employee cannot yell at his boss for fear of losing his job. He later yells at his wife.
- **Rationalization**: Making excuses to justify a situation—for example, after stealing something, saying "Everybody does it."
- **Repression**: Blocking painful thoughts or feelings from the mind—for example, not remembering a traumatic experience.
- **Regression**: Going back to an old, usually immature behavior—for example, throwing a temper tantrum as an adult.

Culture can affect communication. A **culture** is a system of learned beliefs and behaviors that is practiced by a group of people. Each culture may have different knowledge, behaviors, beliefs, values, attitudes, religions, and customs. When an NA communicates with residents from different cultures, she should ask herself these questions:

- What information do I need to communicate to this person?
- Does this person speak English as a first or second language?
- Do I speak this person's language, or do I need an interpreter?
- Does this person have any cultural practices about touch or gestures I should adapt to?

It is important for NAs to be sensitive to each resident's needs. This is key to providing professional, person-centered care. Learning each resident's behavior and preferences can be a challenge. However, it is an important part of communication. It is especially vital in a multicultural society (a society made up of many cultures), such as the United States. The NA should be aware of all the messages sent and received. Listening and observing carefully will help an NA better understand residents' needs and feelings.

3. List guidelines for communicating with residents with special needs

Due to illness or impairments, some residents need special techniques to aid communication. An **impairment** is a loss of function or ability; it can be a partial or complete loss. Special techniques for different conditions are listed below. Information about Alzheimer's disease and related communication tips is in Chapter 5.

Hearing Impairment

There are many different kinds of hearing loss. A person may be born with hearing impairment or it may happen gradually. People who have a hearing impairment may use a hearing aid, read lips, or use sign language. People with impaired hearing also closely observe the facial expressions and body language of others to add to their knowledge of what is being said.

Guidelines: Hearing Impairment

G If the person has a hearing aid, make sure he or she is wearing it and that it is turned on.

G There are many types of hearing aids (Fig. 2-5). Follow the manufacturer's directions for cleaning. In general, the hearing aid needs to be cleaned daily. Wipe it with special cleaning solution and a soft cloth. Do not put the hearing aid in water. Handle it carefully; do not drop it. Always store it inside its case when it is not being worn. Turn it off when it is not in use. Remove it before bathing, showering, or shampooing hair. Some hearing aids have rechargeable batteries. Some need to be recharged nightly. Follow instructions in the care plan.

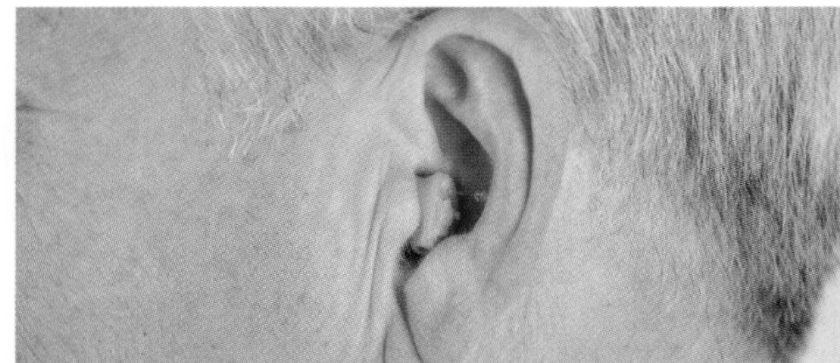

Fig. 2-5. *One type of hearing aid.*

G Reduce or remove noise, such as TVs, radios, and loud speech. Close doors if needed.

G Get the resident's attention before speaking. Do not startle residents by approaching from behind. Walk in front or touch them lightly on the arm to let them know you are near.

G Speak clearly, slowly, and in good lighting. Directly face the person (Fig. 2-6). The light should be on your face, not on the resident's. Ask if she can hear what you are saying.

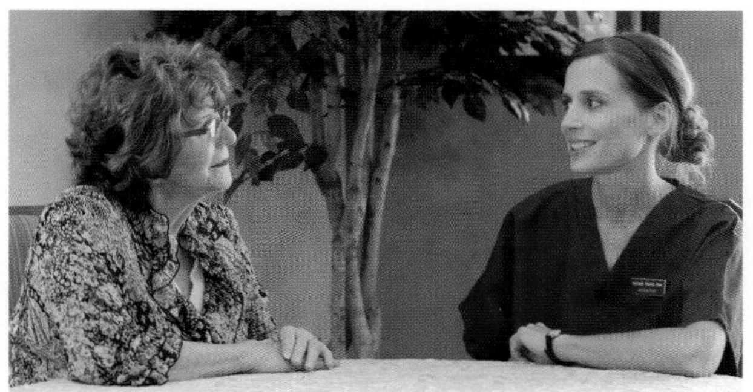

Fig. 2-6. Speak face-to-face in good light.

- Do not shout. Do not mouth the words in an exaggerated way.
- Keep the pitch of your voice low.
- Residents may read lips, so do not chew gum or eat while speaking. Keep your hands away from your face while talking.
- If the resident hears better out of one ear, try to speak and stand on that side.
- Use short sentences and simple words. Avoid sudden topic changes.
- Repeat what you have said, using different words when needed. Some people who are hearing impaired want you to repeat exactly what you said. This is because they miss only a few words.
- Use picture cards or a notepad as needed.
- Residents who have a hearing impairment may hear less when they are tired or ill. This is true of everyone. Be patient and empathetic. Avoid long, tiring conversations.
- Some residents who are hearing impaired have speech problems and may be difficult to understand. Do not pretend you understand if you do not. Ask the resident to repeat what was said. Observe the lips, facial expressions, and body language. Then tell the resident what you think you heard. You can also request that the resident write down words.
- Hearing decline can be a normal aspect of aging. Be understanding and supportive.

Vision Impairment

Vision impairment can affect people of all ages. It can exist at birth or develop gradually. It can occur in one eye or in both. It can also be the result of injury, illness, or aging. Some vision impairment causes people to wear corrective lenses, such as contact lenses or eyeglasses. Some people need to wear eyeglasses all the time. Others only need them to read or for activities that require seeing distant objects, such as driving.

Guidelines: Vision Impairment

- Encourage the use of eyeglasses or contact lenses (contacts) if worn.
- If the resident has eyeglasses, make sure they are clean. Clean glass lenses with water and a soft tissue. Clean plastic lenses with cleaning fluid and/or a lens cloth. Make sure that eyeglasses are in good condition and fit well. Report to the nurse if they do not.
- Contact lenses are made of many types of plastic. Some can be worn and disposed of daily; others are worn for longer periods. If the resident is able, it is best to leave contact lens care to him.
- Knock on the door and identify yourself as soon as you enter the room. Do not touch the resident until you have said your name. Explain why you are there and what you would like to do. Let the resident know when you are leaving the room.
- Make sure there is proper lighting in the room. Face the resident when speaking.
- When you enter a new room with the resident, orient him to where things are. Describe the things you see around you. Try not to use words such as "see," "look," or "watch."
- Always tell the resident what you are doing while caring for him. Give specific directions, such as "on your right" or "in front of you." Talk directly to the resident whom you are

assisting. Do not talk to other residents or staff members.

- Use the face of an imaginary clock as a guide to explain the position of objects that are in front of the resident. An example is "There is a sofa at 7 o'clock" (Fig. 2-7).

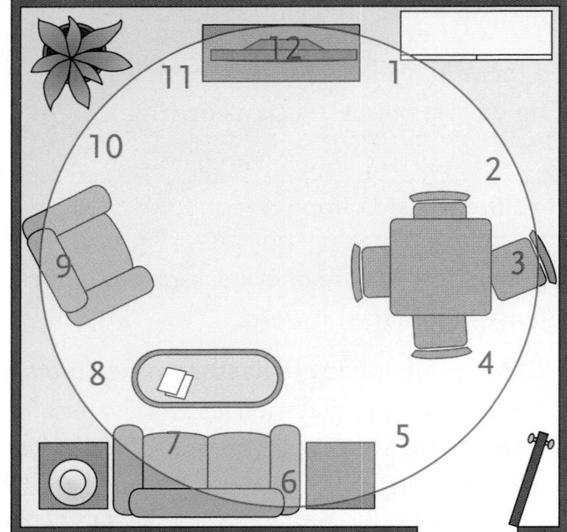

Fig. 2-7. *Using the face of an imaginary clock to explain the position of objects can be helpful.*

- Do not move personal items, furniture, or other objects. Put everything back where you found it.
- Tell the resident where the call light is. Make sure it is within the resident's reach.
- Leave doors completely open or completely closed, never partly open.
- If the resident needs guidance in getting around, walk slightly ahead. Let the resident touch or grasp your arm lightly. Walk at the resident's pace, not yours.
- Give assistance with cutting food and opening containers as needed.
- Use large clocks, clocks that chime, and radios to help keep track of time.
- Large-print books, audiobooks, digital books, and Braille books are available. Learning to read Braille, however, takes a long time and requires training.
- If the resident has a guide dog, do not play with, distract, or feed it.
- Encourage the use of the other senses, such as hearing, touch, and smell. Encourage the resident to feel and touch things, such as clothing, furniture, or items in the room.

Mental Health Disorder

Mental health is the normal functioning of emotional and intellectual abilities. A person who is mentally healthy is able to

- Get along with others (Fig. 2-8)
- Adapt to change
- Care for himself and others
- Give and accept love
- Deal with situations that cause anxiety, disappointment, and frustration
- Take responsibility for decisions, feelings, and actions
- Control and fulfill desires and impulses appropriately

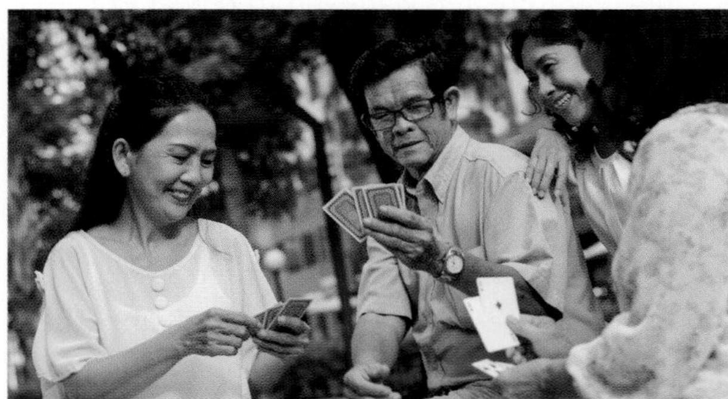

Fig. 2-8. *The ability to interact well with other people is a characteristic of mental health.*

Although it involves emotions and mental functions, a **mental health disorder** is like any physical disorder. It is a condition that produces signs and symptoms and affects the body's ability to function. It responds to proper treatment and care. A mental health disorder disrupts a person's ability to function in the family, home, or community. It often causes inappropriate behavior. Some signs and symptoms of a mental health disorder are confusion, disorientation, agitation, and anxiety.

People who have a mental health disorder cannot simply choose to be well. People who are mentally healthy are usually able to control their emotions and actions. People who have a mental health disorder may not have this control.

Different types of mental health disorders affect how well residents communicate. Nursing assistants should treat each resident as an individual. They should tailor their approach to the situation.

Guidelines: Communication and Mental Health Disorders

- G Do not talk to adults as if they were children.
- G Use simple, clear statements and a normal tone of voice.
- G Be sure that what you say and how you say it show respect and concern.
- G Sit or stand at a normal distance from the resident. Be aware of your body language.
- G Be honest and direct, as you would with any resident.
- G Avoid arguments.
- G Maintain eye contact and listen carefully (Fig. 2-9).

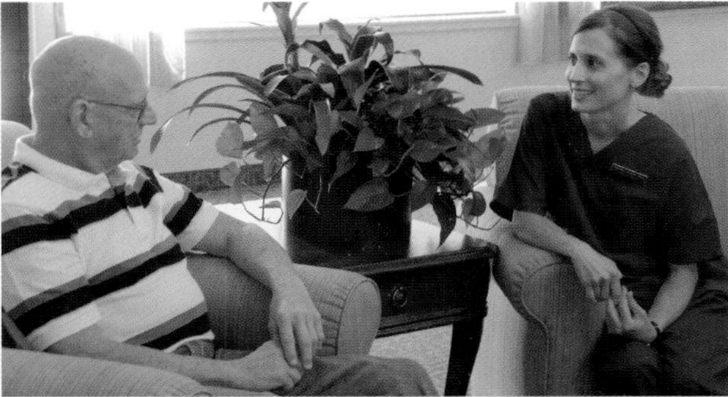

Fig. 2-9. *Nursing assistants should maintain eye contact and sit at a normal distance when communicating with a resident who has a mental health disorder.*

Learning Objective 9 in Chapter 3 has more information about mental health disorders.

Combative Behavior

Residents may display **combative**, meaning violent or hostile, behavior. Such behavior may include hitting, pushing, kicking, or verbal attacks. It may be the result of a disease affecting the brain. It may also be due to frustration. Or it may just be part of someone's personality. In general, combative behavior is not a reaction to the caregiver and should not be taken personally. NAs should always report and document combative behavior. Even if an NA does not find the behavior upsetting, the care team needs to be aware of it.

Guidelines: Combative Behavior

- G Block physical blows or step out of the way, but never hit back (Fig. 2-10). No matter how much a resident hurts you, or how angry or afraid you are, never hit or threaten a resident.

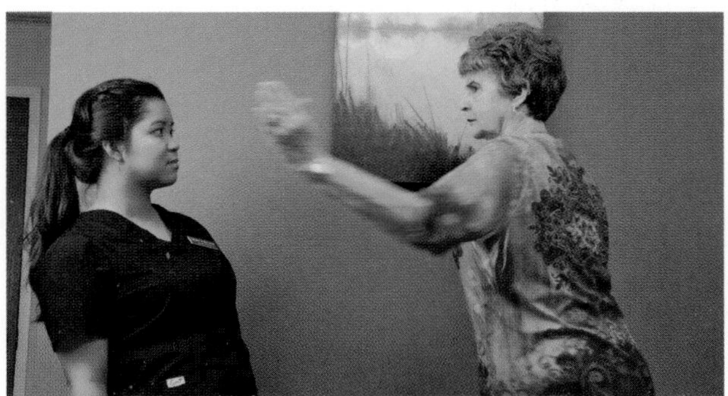

Fig. 2-10. *When dealing with combative residents, step out of the way, but never hit back.*

- G Allow the resident time to calm down before the next interaction.
- G Ensure the resident is safe and give him or her space. When possible, stand at least an arm's length away.
- G Remain calm. Lower the tone of your voice.
- G Be flexible and patient.
- G Stay neutral. Do not respond to verbal attacks. Do not argue or accuse the resident of wrongdoing. If you must respond, say something

like "I understand that you're angry and frustrated. How can I make things better?"

- G Do not use gestures that could frighten or startle the resident. Try to keep your hands open and in front of you.
- G Be reassuring and supportive.
- G Consider what provoked the resident. Sometimes something as simple as a change in caregiver or routine can be very upsetting to a resident. Get help to take the resident to a quieter place if needed.
- G Report inappropriate behavior to the nurse.

Anger

Anger is a natural emotion that has many causes. These include disease, fear, pain, loneliness, and loss of independence. Anger may also just be a part of someone's personality. Some people get angry more easily than others.

People express anger in different ways. Some may shout, yell, threaten, throw things, or pace. Others express their anger by withdrawing, being silent, or sulking. Angry behavior should always be reported to the nurse.

Guidelines: Angry Behavior

- G Stay calm. Do not argue or respond to verbal attacks.
- G Empathize with the resident. Try to understand what he or she is feeling.
- G Try to find out what caused the resident's anger. Listen attentively as the resident speaks. Remain silent. This may help the resident explain.
- G Treat the resident with dignity and respect. Explain what you are going to do and when you will do it.
- G Answer call lights promptly.
- G Stay at a safe distance if the resident becomes combative.

Inappropriate Behavior

Inappropriate behavior from a resident includes trying to establish a personal, rather than a professional, relationship with an NA. Examples include asking personal questions, requesting visits on personal time, asking for or doing favors, giving tips or gifts, and lending or borrowing money.

Inappropriate behavior also includes making sexual advances and comments. Sexual advances include any sexual words, comments, or behavior that makes the person to whom the advances are directed feel uncomfortable.

Inappropriate behavior may include residents removing their clothes or touching themselves in public. Illness, dementia, confusion, or medication may cause this behavior.

Confused residents may have problems that mimic inappropriate sexual behavior. They may have an uncomfortable rash, clothes that are too tight, too hot, or too scratchy, or they may need to go to the bathroom. NAs need to observe for these problems.

The NA can address inappropriate behavior directly, saying something like "That makes me uncomfortable." Appropriate responses to personal questions include "I really can't talk about my personal life on the job." If an NA encounters a resident in any embarrassing situation, she should remain professional and not overreact. Trying to distract the resident may help. If it does not, the resident should be taken to a private area. The nurse should be notified. When residents act inappropriately, NAs should report the behavior, even if they think it was harmless.

Residents' Rights

Communicating with Residents

Nursing assistants' interactions with residents are important. Residents' physical and psychological health can depend a great deal on how NAs communicate. This is especially true for residents who are cognitively impaired, lonely, helpless, or bored. NAs should be comforting and kind with residents. They should listen if residents want to talk. Just the presence of a caring person can reassure residents that they are not alone.

4. Identify ways to promote safety and handle non-medical emergencies

Safety

All staff members, including nursing assistants, are responsible for safety in a facility. It is very important to try to prevent accidents *before* they occur. Prevention is the key to safety. As NAs work, they should watch for safety hazards. They should report unsafe conditions to the supervisor promptly. Before leaving a resident's room, an NA should do a final check and ask himself:

- Is the call light within reach of the resident's stronger hand?
- Is the room tidy? Are the resident's items in their proper places?
- Is the furniture in the same place as I found it? Is the bed in its lowest position?
- Does the resident have a clear walkway around the room and into the bathroom?

Principles of Body Mechanics

Back strain or injury can be a serious problem for nursing assistants. **Body mechanics** is the way the parts of the body work together when a person moves. Using proper body mechanics helps save energy and prevent injury.

Alignment. Whether standing, sitting, or lying down, the body should be in alignment and should have good posture. This means that the two sides of the body are mirror images of each other, with body parts lined up naturally. **Posture** is the way a person holds and positions his body. A person can maintain correct body alignment when lifting or carrying an object by keeping it close to his body (Fig. 2-11). His feet and body should be pointed in the direction he is moving. He should avoid twisting at the waist.

Base of support. The base of support is the foundation that supports an object. The feet are the body's base of support. The wider the support, the more stable a person is. Standing with the feet shoulder-width apart allows for a greater base of support. This is more stable than standing with the feet together.

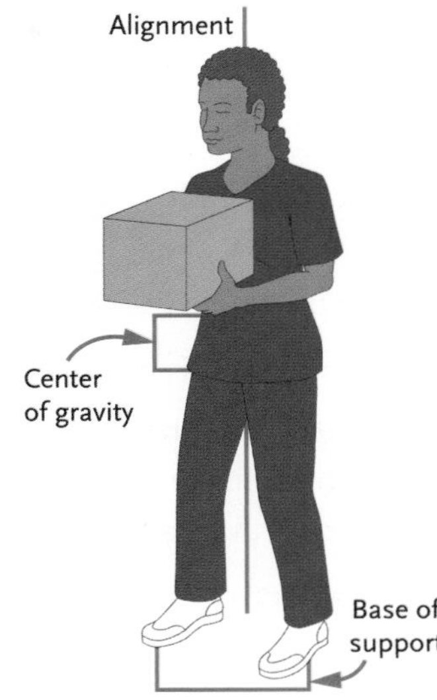

***Fig. 2-11.** Proper body alignment is important when standing and when sitting.*

Center of gravity. The center of gravity in the body is the point where the most weight is concentrated. This point will depend on the position of the body. When a person stands, weight is centered in the pelvis. A low center of gravity gives a more stable base of support. Bending the knees when lifting an object lowers the pelvis and, therefore, lowers a person's center of gravity. This gives the person more stability. It makes him less likely to fall or strain the working muscles.

Guidelines: Using Proper Body Mechanics

- G Assess the situation first. Clear the path. Remove any obstacles.
- G Use both arms and hands to lift, push, or carry objects.
- G When lifting a heavy object from the floor, spread your feet shoulder-width apart. Bend your knees. Use the strong, large muscles in your thighs, upper arms, and shoulders to lift the object. Raise your body and the object together (Fig. 2-12).

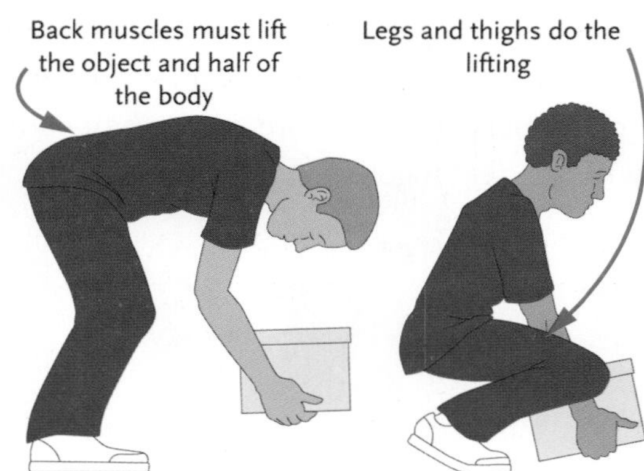

Fig. 2-12. In this illustration, which person is lifting correctly?

- **G** Hold objects close to you when you are lifting or carrying them. This keeps the object closer to your center of gravity and base of support.
- **G** Push or slide objects rather than lifting them.
- **G** Avoid bending and reaching as much as possible. Move or position furniture so that you do not have to bend or reach.
- **G** If you are making a bed, adjust the height to a safe working level, usually waist high. Avoid bending at the waist.
- **G** When a task requires bending, use a good stance. Bend your knees to lower yourself (squat), rather than bending from the waist. This uses the big muscles in your legs and thighs rather than the smaller muscles in your back.
- **G** Do not twist when you are lifting or moving an object. Instead, turn your whole body. Pivot your feet instead of twisting at the waist. Your feet should point toward what you are lifting or moving.
- **G** Get help from coworkers when possible for lifting or helping residents.
- **G** Talk to residents before moving them. Let them know what you will do so they can help if possible. Agree on a signal, such as counting to three. Lift or move on three so that everyone moves together.
- **G** To help a resident sit up, stand up, or walk, place your feet shoulder-width apart. Put one foot in front of the other and bend your knees. Your upper body should stay upright and in alignment. Do this whenever you have to support a resident's weight.
- **G** Never try to catch a falling resident. If the resident falls, assist her to the floor. If you try to reverse a fall in progress, you could injure yourself and/or the resident.
- **G** Report to the nurse any task that you cannot safely do. Never try to lift an object or a resident that you feel you cannot handle.

Accident Prevention

Falls

A fall is any sudden, uncontrollable descent from a higher to a lower level, with or without injury resulting. Falls make up most of the accidents that occur in care facilities. They can be caused by an unsafe environment, loss of abilities, diseases, and medications. Problems resulting from falls range from minor bruises to fractures and life-threatening injuries. A **fracture** is a broken bone. Falls are particularly common among the elderly. Older people are often more seriously injured by falls because their bones are more fragile. NAs should be especially alert to the risk of falls. All falls must be reported to the supervisor. These factors increase the risk of falls:

- Clutter
- Throw rugs
- Exposed electrical cords
- Slippery or wet floors
- Uneven floors or stairs
- Poor lighting
- Call lights that are out of reach or not promptly answered

Personal conditions that increase the risk of falls include medications, loss of vision, gait (walking) or balance problems, weakness, paralysis, and disorientation. **Disorientation** means confusion about person, place, or time.

Guidelines: Preventing Falls

- **G** Clear all walkways of clutter, trash, throw rugs, and cords.
- **G** Use rugs with a nonslip backing.
- **G** Have residents wear nonskid, sturdy shoes. Make sure shoelaces are tied.
- **G** Residents should not wear clothing that is too long or drags on the floor.
- **G** Keep items that are used often close to residents, including call lights.
- **G** Answer call lights right away.
- **G** Immediately clean up spills on the floor.
- **G** Report loose handrails immediately.
- **G** Mark uneven flooring or stairs with tape of a contrasting color to indicate a hazard.
- **G** Improve lighting where needed.
- **G** Lock wheels and move footrests out of the way before helping residents into or out of wheelchairs.
- **G** Lock bed wheels before helping a resident into and out of bed or when giving care.
- **G** After completing care, return beds to their lowest position.
- **G** Get help when moving residents. Do not assume you can do it alone. Keep residents' walking aids, such as canes or walkers, within their reach.
- **G** Offer help with elimination needs often. Respond to requests for help immediately. Think about how you would feel if you had to wait for help to go to the bathroom.
- **G** Leave furniture in the same place as you found it.
- **G** Know which residents are at risk for falls. Pay attention so that you can give help often.
- **G** If a resident starts to fall, be in a good position to help support her. Never try to catch a falling resident. Use your body to slide her to the floor. If you try to reverse a fall, you may hurt yourself and/or the resident.
- **G** Whenever a resident falls, it must be reported to the nurse. Always complete an incident report, even if the resident says he or she feels fine.

Burns/Scalds

Burns can be caused by dry heat (e.g., a hot iron, stove, other electrical appliances), wet heat (e.g., hot water or other liquids, steam), or chemicals (e.g., lye, acids). Small children, older adults, or people with loss of sensation (such as from paralysis or diabetes) are at greatest risk of burns. **Scalds** are burns caused by hot liquids. It takes five seconds or less for a serious burn to occur when the temperature of liquid is 140°F. Coffee, tea, and other hot drinks are usually served at 160°F to 180°F. These temperatures can cause almost instant burns that require surgery. Preventing burns is very important.

Guidelines: Preventing Burns and Scalds

- **G** Always check water temperature with a water thermometer or on the inside of your wrist before using.
- **G** Immediately report frayed electrical cords or appliances that look unsafe. Do not use them. Remove them from the room.
- **G** Let residents know when you are about to pour or set down a hot liquid.
- **G** Pour hot drinks away from residents. Keep hot drinks and liquids away from edges of tables. Put lids on them.
- **G** Make sure residents are sitting down before serving hot drinks.
- **G** If plate warmers or other equipment that produces heat are used, monitor them carefully.

Resident Identification

Residents must always be identified before giving care or serving food. Failure to identify residents can cause serious problems, even death. Facilities have different methods of identification. Some have pictures to identify residents. Others have signs outside residents' doors (Fig. 2-13). NAs must identify each resident before beginning any procedure or giving any care. They should identify residents before placing meal trays or helping with eating. The diet card should be checked against the resident's identification to make sure they match. The resident should be called by name and asked to state her name if able.

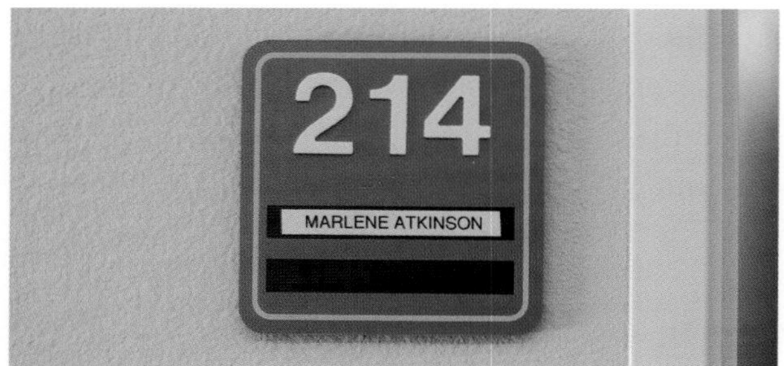

Fig. 2-13. *A resident's name may be displayed outside the room to identify who is living in that room. Before giving any care, nursing assistants must always identify residents.*

Choking

Choking can occur when eating, drinking, or taking medication. People who are weak, ill, or unconscious can choke on their own saliva. A person's tongue can also become swollen and obstruct the airway. To guard against choking, residents should eat in as upright a position as possible. Residents with swallowing problems may need to have liquids thickened to the consistency of nectar, honey, or pudding. Thickened liquids are easier to swallow. Chapter 8 contains more information about thickened liquids.

Poisoning

There are many harmful substances in facilities that should not be swallowed. These include cleaning products, paints, medicines, toiletries, and glues. These products should be stored or locked away from confused residents or those with limited vision. Cleaning products should not be left in residents' rooms. Residents with dementia may hide food and let it spoil in closets, drawers, or other places. NAs should investigate any odors they notice. The number for the Poison Control Center should be posted near all telephones.

Cuts/Abrasions

Cuts or abrasions typically occur in the bathroom at a facility. An **abrasion** is an injury that rubs off the surface of the skin. Sharp objects, such as scissors, nail clippers, and razors, should be put away after use. NAs should take care when transferring residents into and out of beds, chairs, and wheelchairs. When moving residents in wheelchairs, NAs should push the wheelchair forward. Wheelchairs should not be pulled from behind. When using elevators, wheelchairs should be turned around before entering, so that residents are facing forward.

Safety Data Sheet (SDS)

The Occupational Safety and Health Administration (**OSHA**, osha.gov) is a federal government agency that makes rules to protect workers from hazards on the job. OSHA requires that all hazardous chemicals have a Safety Data Sheet (SDS) (formerly called *Material Safety Data Sheet*, or *MSDS*). This sheet details the chemical ingredients, chemical dangers, and safe handling, storage, and disposal procedures for the product. Information about emergency response actions to be taken are also included. Some facilities use a toll-free number to access SDS information. These sheets must be accessible in work areas for all employees. Important information about the SDS includes the following:

- Employers must have an SDS for every chemical used.

- Employers must provide easy access to the SDS.
- Staff members must know where these sheets are kept and how to read them. They should ask for help if they do not know how to do this.

The list of hazardous chemicals that must have an SDS will be updated as new chemicals are purchased.

Fire

All facilities have a fire safety plan, and all workers need to know this plan. Guidelines regarding fires and evacuations will be explained to all employees. Evacuation routes are posted in facilities. NAs should read and review them often. They should attend fire and disaster training when it is offered. A fast, calm, and confident response by the staff saves lives.

Guidelines: Reducing Fire Hazards and Responding to Fires

G Some facilities are nonsmoking, while others allow smoking. If residents smoke, make sure they are in the proper area for smoking. Be sure that cigarettes are extinguished. Empty ashtrays often. Before emptying ashtrays, make sure there are no hot ashes or hot matches in the ashtray. Burn-resistant aprons for smokers may be available. These aprons help protect a person from burns from hot ashes and lit cigarettes if they are dropped. If a resident wears this apron when smoking, make sure the buckles and snaps are properly fastened and that the apron covers his torso and lap. Never leave any smoker unattended.

G Residents may use electronic cigarettes (e-cigarettes, e-cigs). Matches or lighters are not needed to light this type of cigarette; they use a battery to turn the liquid nicotine into vapor. To reduce the risk of fire, e-cigarettes should only be charged using the appliance supplied by the manufacturer. Batteries may need to be turned off manually and may need to be removed from chargers after they are fully charged. Follow instructions.

G Report frayed or damaged electrical cords immediately. Report electrical equipment in need of repair immediately.

G Fire alarms and exit doors should not be blocked. If they are, report this to the nurse.

G Every facility will have multiple fire extinguishers (Fig. 2-14). The PASS acronym will help you understand how to use one:

Pull the pin.

Aim at the base of the fire when spraying.

Squeeze the handle.

Sweep back and forth at the base of the fire.

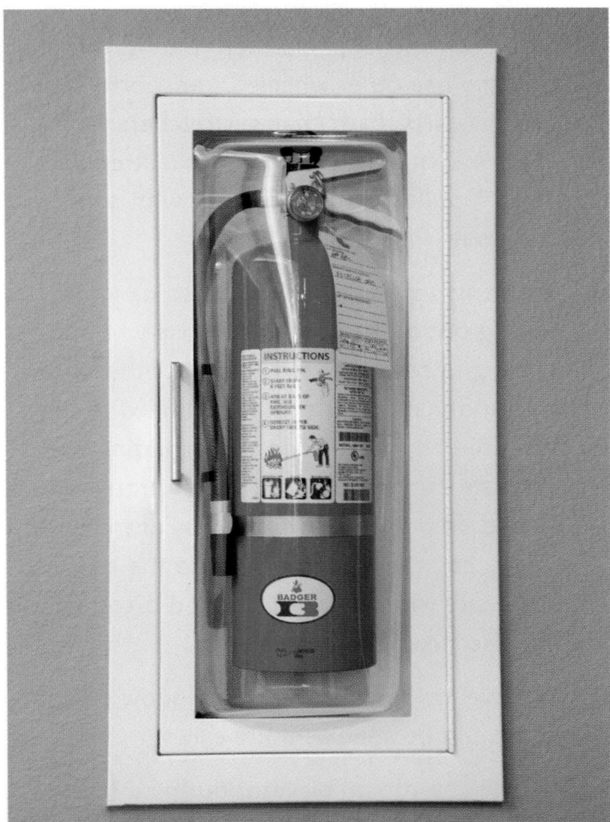

Fig. 2-14. *Nursing assistants should know where the extinguishers are stored and how to use them.*

- In case of fire, the RACE acronym is a good rule to follow:

  Remove anyone in danger if you are not in danger.

  Activate alarm or call 911.

  Contain fire if possible by closing all doors and windows.

  Extinguish the fire, or the fire department will extinguish it. Evacuate the area if instructed to do so.

Follow these guidelines for helping residents exit the building safely:

- Know the facility's fire evacuation plan.
- Stay calm. Do not panic.
- Follow the directions of the fire department.
- Know which residents need one-on-one help or assistive devices. Immobile residents can be moved in several ways. If they have a wheelchair, help them into it. You can also use other wheeled transporters, such as carts, bath chairs, stretchers, or beds. A blanket can be used as a stretcher or even pulled across the floor with someone on it.
- Residents who can walk will also need help getting out of the building. Those who have a hearing impairment may not hear the warnings and instructions. Staff will need to tell them directly what to do while guiding them to a safe exit. People with vision problems should be moved out of the way of the wheelchairs, carts, etc., and helped to the exit. Residents who are confused and disoriented will also need guidance.
- Remove anything blocking a window or door that could be used as a fire exit.
- Do not get into an elevator during a fire unless directed to do so by the fire department.
- Stay low in a room to escape a fire.
- If a door is closed, check for heat coming from it before opening it. If the door or doorknob feels hot, stay in the room if there is no safe exit. Plug the doorway (use wet towels or clothing) to prevent smoke from entering. Stay in the room until help arrives.
- Use the *stop, drop, and roll* fire safety technique to extinguish a fire on clothing or hair. Stop running or stay still. Drop to the ground, lying down if possible. Roll on the ground to try to extinguish the flames.
- Use a damp covering over the mouth and nose to reduce smoke inhalation.
- After leaving the building, move away from it.

Disaster Guidelines

Disasters can include fire, flood, earthquake, hurricane, tornado, or severe weather. Man-made dangers, such as acts of terrorism or bomb threats, are also considered disasters.

Nursing assistants should know the appropriate action to take when disasters occur. Each facility has a local and area-specific disaster plan, and NAs will be trained on these plans. Annual in-services and disaster drills are often held at facilities. NAs should take advantage of these sessions and pay close attention to instructions.

During disasters, a nurse or the administrator will give directions. NAs should listen carefully and follow instructions. Facilities may rely on local or state groups and the American Red Cross to assume responsibility for people who are ill and disabled. The following guidelines apply in any disaster situation:

- Remain calm.
- Know the locations of all exits and stairways.
- Know where the fire alarms and extinguishers are located.
- Know the appropriate action to take in any situation.

- Use the internet to stay informed, or keep the television or radio tuned to a local station to get the latest information.

In addition, NAs will be required to know specific guidelines for the area in which they work. The instructor's teaching material has more information on specific disasters and response guidelines.

5. Demonstrate how to recognize and respond to medical emergencies

Medical emergencies may be the result of accidents or sudden illnesses. This section discusses what to do in a medical emergency. Heart attacks, strokes, diabetic emergencies, choking, automobile accidents, and gunshot wounds are all medical emergencies. Falls, burns, and cuts can also be emergencies. In an emergency, responders should remain calm, act quickly, and communicate clearly. These steps show the correct response to emergencies:

Assess the situation. The responder should try to find out what has happened. She must make sure she is not in danger and notice the time.

Assess the victim. The responder should ask the injured or ill person what has happened. If the person is unable to respond, he may be unconscious. Being **conscious** means being mentally alert and having awareness of surroundings, sensations, and thoughts. Tapping the person and asking if he is all right helps to determine if a person is conscious. The responder should speak loudly and use the person's name if she knows it. If there is no response, she should assume the person is unconscious. This is an emergency situation. She should call for help right away or send someone else to call.

If a person is conscious and able to speak, then he is breathing and has a pulse. The responder should talk with him about what happened. She should get the person's permission to touch him. Anyone who is unable to give consent for treatment, such as a child with no parent near or an unconscious or seriously injured person, may be treated with *implied consent*. This means that if the person were able or the parents were present, they would have given consent. The person should be checked for the following:

- Severe bleeding
- Changes in consciousness
- Irregular breathing
- Unusual color or feel to the skin
- Swollen places on the body
- Medical alert tags
- Pain

If any of these exists, professional medical help may be needed. An NA should always get help. She should call the nurse before doing anything else. If the injured or ill person is conscious, he may be frightened. The responder should listen to the person and tell him what is being done to help him. A calm and confident response will help reassure him.

After an emergency is over, the NA will need to document the emergency and complete an incident report. It is important to include as many details as possible and report only facts.

First aid is emergency care given immediately to an injured person by the first people to respond to an emergency. **Cardiopulmonary resuscitation** (**CPR**) refers to medical procedures used when a person's heart or lungs have stopped working. CPR is used until medical help arrives.

Quick action is necessary. CPR must be started immediately to prevent or lessen brain damage. Brain damage can occur within four to six minutes after the heart stops beating and breathing stops. The person can die within 10 minutes.

Employers often arrange for NAs to be trained in CPR. If not, the American Heart Association

(AHA, heart.org) and American Red Cross (ARC, redcross.org) have more information about training. CPR is an important skill to learn.

Nursing assistants need to know their facility's policies on initiating CPR. Some employers do not allow NAs to begin CPR without direction of the nurse.

Choking

When something is blocking the tube through which air enters the lungs, the person has an **obstructed airway**. When people are choking, they usually put their hands to their throats (Fig. 2-15). An NA may encounter residents who are choking or seem to be choking. As long as the resident can speak, breathe, or cough, the NA should only encourage her to cough as forcefully as possible to get the object out. The NA should stay with the resident until she stops choking or can no longer speak, breathe, or cough.

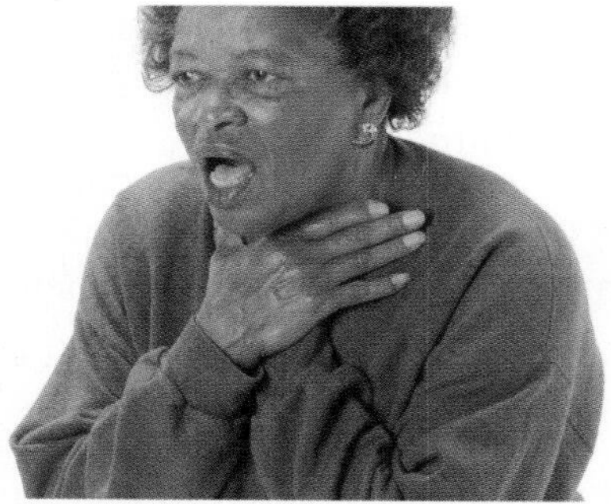

Fig. 2-15. *People who are choking usually put their hands to their throats.*

If a resident can no longer speak, breathe, or cough, the NA should call for help immediately by using the call light or emergency cord. The choking victim should not be left alone.

Abdominal thrusts are a method of attempting to remove an object from the airway of someone who is choking. These thrusts work to remove the blockage upward, out of the throat. The NA should make sure the resident needs help before starting to give abdominal thrusts. The resident must show signs of a severely obstructed airway. These signs include poor air exchange, an increase in trouble breathing, silent coughing, blue-tinged (**cyanotic**) skin, and an inability to speak, breathe, or cough. The NA should ask, "Are you choking? I know what to do. Can I help you?" If the resident nods her head yes, she has a severe airway obstruction and needs immediate help. The NA should begin giving abdominal thrusts. This procedure should never be performed on a person who is not choking. Abdominal thrusts risk injury to the ribs and internal organs.

Performing abdominal thrusts for the conscious person

1. Stand behind the person and bring your arms under her arms. Wrap your arms around the person's waist.
2. Make a fist with one hand. Place the flat, thumb side of the fist against the person's abdomen, above the navel but below the breastbone (Fig. 2-16).

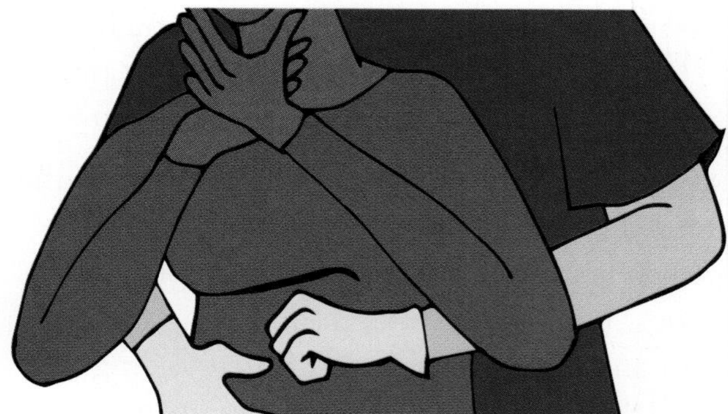

Fig. 2-16. *Place the flat, thumb side of your fist against the person's abdomen, above the navel but below the breastbone.*

3. Grasp the fist with your other hand. Pull both hands toward you and up, quickly and forcefully.
4. Repeat until the object is pushed out or the person loses consciousness.
5. Report and document the incident properly.

If the resident becomes unconscious while choking, she should be helped to the floor gently. She should be lying on her back on a hard surface with her face up. The NA should begin CPR for an unconscious person if trained and allowed to do so. The NA should make sure help is on the way. The resident may have a completely blocked airway and needs medical help immediately. The NA should stay with the victim until help arrives.

Shock

Shock occurs when organs and tissues in the body do not receive an adequate blood supply. Bleeding, heart attack, severe infection, and falling blood pressure can lead to shock. Shock can become worse when the person is very frightened or in severe pain.

Shock is a dangerous, life-threatening situation. Signs of shock include pale or bluish skin, staring, increased pulse and respiration rates, low blood pressure, and extreme thirst. An NA should always call for help if she suspects a resident is in shock.

Responding to shock

1. Notify the nurse immediately. Victims of shock should always receive medical care as soon as possible.
2. If you need to control bleeding, put on gloves first. This procedure is described later in the chapter.
3. Have the person lie down on her back. If the person is bleeding from the mouth or vomiting, place her on her side. Elevate the legs about eight to 12 inches unless the person has a head, neck, back, spinal, or abdominal injury; breathing difficulties; or fractures (Fig. 2-17). Elevating the legs allows blood to flow back to the brain (and other vital areas). Elevate the head and shoulders if a head wound or breathing difficulties are present. Never elevate a body part if the person has a broken bone or if it causes pain.

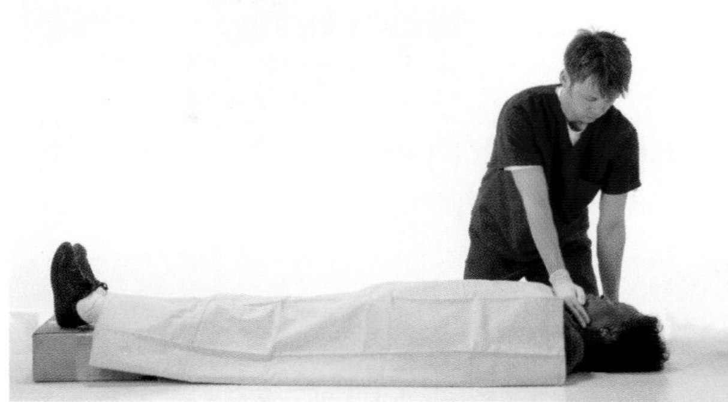

Fig. 2-17. *If a person is in shock, elevate the legs, unless she has a head, neck, back, spinal, or abdominal injury; breathing difficulties; or fractures.*

4. Check pulse and respirations if possible (Chapter 7). If the person stops breathing or has no pulse, begin CPR if trained and allowed to do so.
5. Keep the person as calm and comfortable as possible.
6. Maintain normal body temperature. If the weather is cold, place a blanket around the person. If the weather is hot, provide shade.
7. Do not give the person food or liquids.
8. Report and document the incident properly.

Myocardial Infarction or Heart Attack

Myocardial infarction (**MI**), or heart attack, occurs when the heart muscle itself does not receive enough oxygen because blood vessels are blocked. A myocardial infarction is an emergency that can result in serious heart damage or death. The following are signs and symptoms of MI:

- Sudden, severe pain in the chest, usually on the left side or in the center, behind the breastbone
- Pain or discomfort in other areas of the body, such as one or both arms, the back, neck, jaw, or stomach

- Indigestion or heartburn
- Nausea and vomiting
- **Dyspnea**, or difficulty breathing
- Dizziness
- Pale or bluish (cyanotic) skin color, indicating lack of oxygen
- Perspiration
- Cold and clammy skin
- Weak and irregular pulse rate
- Low blood pressure
- Anxiety and a sense of doom
- Denial of a heart problem

The pain of a heart attack is commonly described as a crushing, pressing, squeezing, stabbing, piercing pain, or "like someone is sitting on my chest." The pain may go down the inside of the left arm. A person may also feel it in the neck and/or in the jaw. The pain usually does not go away.

As with men, women may experience chest pain or pressure. Women, though, can have heart attacks without chest pressure. Women are more likely to have shortness of breath, nausea, lightheadedness, stomach pain, sweating, fatigue, and back, neck, or jaw pain. Some women's symptoms seem more flu-like, and women are more likely to deny that they are having a heart attack. An NA must take immediate action if a resident has any of these symptoms.

Responding to a myocardial infarction

1. Notify the nurse immediately.
2. Place the person in a comfortable position. Encourage him to rest. Reassure him that you will not leave him alone.
3. Loosen clothing around the person's neck (Fig. 2-18).
4. Do not give the person food or liquids.

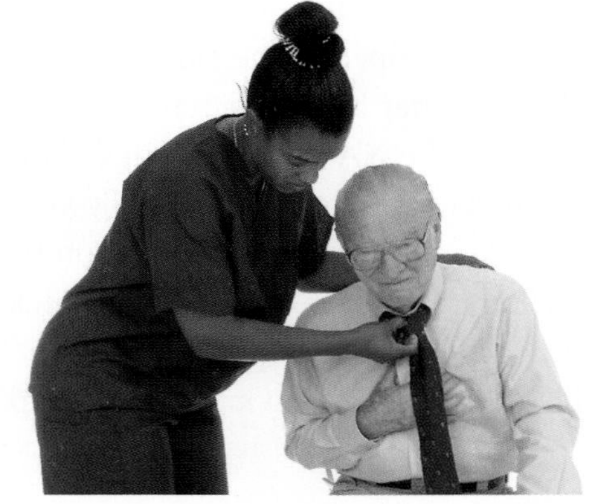

Fig. 2-18. *Loosen clothing around the person's neck if you suspect he is having an MI.*

5. Monitor the person's breathing and pulse. If the person stops breathing or has no pulse, begin CPR if trained and allowed to do so.
6. Stay with the person until help arrives.
7. Report and document the incident properly.

Some states allow nursing assistants to offer heart medication, such as nitroglycerin, to a resident having a heart attack. If allowed to do this, the NA can only offer the medication. She cannot place it in the resident's mouth.

Bleeding

Severe bleeding can cause death quickly and must be controlled.

Controlling bleeding

1. Notify the nurse immediately.
2. Put on gloves. Take time to do this. If the resident is able, he can hold his bare hand over the wound until you can put on gloves.
3. Hold a thick sterile pad, clean cloth, or clean towel against the wound.
4. Press down hard directly on the bleeding wound until help arrives. Do not decrease pressure (Fig. 2-19). Put additional pads or cloths over the first pad if blood seeps through. Do not remove the first pad.

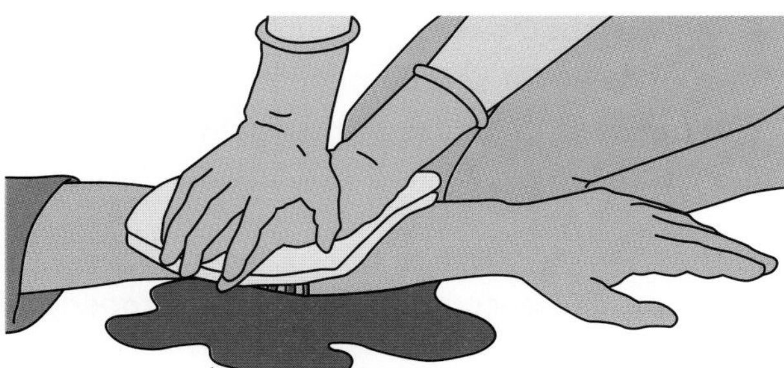

Fig. 2-19. Press down hard directly on the bleeding wound; do not decrease pressure.

5. If you can, raise the wound above the level of the heart to slow the bleeding. Prop up the limb if the wound is on an arm, leg, hand, or foot and there are no broken bones. Use towels or other absorbent material.
6. When bleeding is under control, secure the dressing to keep it in place. Check for symptoms of shock (pale skin, increased pulse and respiration rates, low blood pressure, and extreme thirst). Stay with the person until help arrives.
7. Remove and discard gloves. Wash hands thoroughly.
8. Report and document the incident properly.

Burns

Care of a burn depends on its depth, size, and location. Burns may require emergency help.

Treating burns

To treat a minor burn:

1. Notify the nurse immediately. Put on gloves.
2. Use cool, clean water to decrease the skin temperature and prevent further injury. Do not use ice or ice water, as ice may cause further skin damage. Dampen a clean cloth with cool water. Place it over the burn.
3. Once the pain has eased, you may cover the area with a dry, clean dressing or nonadhesive sterile bandage.
4. Remove and discard gloves. Wash your hands.
5. Never use any kind of ointment, salve, or grease on a burn.

For more serious burns:

1. Remove the person from the source of the burn. If clothing has caught fire, have the person stop, drop, and roll, or smother the fire with a blanket or towel to put out flames. Protect yourself from the source of the burn.
2. Notify the nurse immediately. Put on gloves.
3. Check for breathing, pulse, and severe bleeding. If the person is not breathing and has no pulse, begin CPR if trained and allowed to do so.
4. Do not use any type of ointment, water, salve, or grease on the burn.
5. Do not try to pull away any clothing from burned areas. Cover the burn with sterile gauze or a clean sheet. Apply the gauze or sheet lightly. Take care not to rub the burned area.
6. Monitor vital signs and wait for emergency medical help.
7. Remove and discard gloves. Wash your hands.
8. Report and document the incident properly.

Fainting

Fainting, called **syncope**, occurs as a result of decreased blood flow to the brain, causing a loss of consciousness. Fainting may be the result of hunger, hypoglycemia (low blood glucose), dehydration, fear, pain, fatigue, standing for a long time, poor ventilation, certain medications, pregnancy, or overheating. Signs and symptoms of fainting include dizziness, nausea, perspiration, pale skin, weak pulse, shallow respirations, and blackness in the visual field.

Responding to fainting

1. Notify the nurse immediately.
2. Have the person lie down or sit down before fainting occurs.
3. If the person is in a sitting position, have him bend forward (Fig. 2-20). He can place his head between his knees if he is able. If the person is lying flat on his back, elevate his legs about 12 inches.

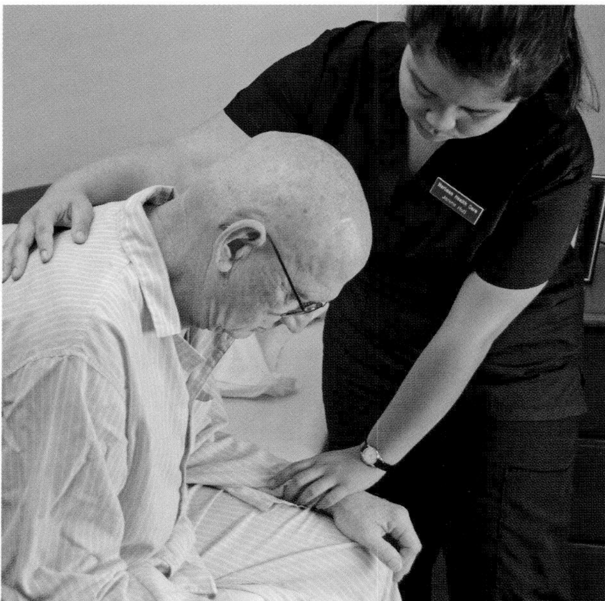

Fig. 2-20. *Have the person bend forward if he is sitting.*

4. Loosen any tight clothing.
5. Have the person stay in position for at least five minutes after symptoms disappear.
6. Help the person get up slowly. Continue to observe him for symptoms of fainting. Stay with him until he feels better. If you need help but cannot leave him, use the call light.
7. If a person does faint, lower him to the floor or other flat surface. Position him on his back. If he has no head, neck, back, spinal, or abdominal injuries, elevate his legs eight to 12 inches. If unsure about injuries, leave him flat on his back. Loosen any tight clothing. Check to make sure the person is breathing. He should recover quickly, but keep him lying down for several minutes. Report the incident to the nurse immediately. Fainting may be a sign of a more serious medical condition.
8. Report and document the incident properly.

Insulin Reaction and Diabetic Ketoacidosis

Insulin reaction and diabetic ketoacidosis are problems of diabetes that can be life-threatening. **Insulin reaction**, or hypoglycemia, can result from either too much insulin or too little food. It occurs when insulin is given and the person skips a meal or does not eat all the food required. Even when a regular amount of food is eaten, physical activity may rapidly metabolize the food. This causes too much insulin to be in the body. Vomiting and diarrhea may also lead to insulin reaction in people who have diabetes.

The first signs of insulin reaction include feeling weak or different, nervousness, dizziness, and perspiration. The NA should immediately report these signs to the nurse. These signal that the resident needs food in a form that can be rapidly absorbed. A glass of milk, fruit juice, or water with sugar dissolved in it should be consumed right away. A glucose tablet is another quick source of sugar. A fingerstick blood glucose test may need to be done right away. Other signs and symptoms include the following:

- Hunger
- Headache
- Rapid pulse
- Low blood pressure
- Cold, clammy skin
- Confusion
- Trembling
- Nervousness
- Blurred vision

- Numbness of the lips and tongue
- Unconsciousness

Diabetic ketoacidosis (**DKA**) is caused by having too little insulin. It can result from undiagnosed diabetes, infection, going without insulin or not taking enough, eating too much, not getting enough exercise, or physical or emotional stress. The signs of the onset of diabetic ketoacidosis include increased hunger, thirst, or urination; abdominal pain; deep or labored breathing; and breath that smells sweet or fruity. The nurse should be notified immediately if the resident has shown signs of DKA. Other signs and symptoms include the following:

- Headache
- Weakness
- Rapid, weak pulse
- Low blood pressure
- Dry skin
- Flushed cheeks
- Drowsiness
- Nausea and vomiting
- Shortness of breath or air hunger (person gasping for air and being unable to catch his breath)
- Unconsciousness

Chapter 4 has more information about diabetes.

Seizures

Seizures are involuntary, often violent, contractions of muscles. They can involve a small area or the entire body. Seizures are caused by abnormalities in the brain. They can occur in young children who have a high fever. Older children and adults who have a serious illness, fever, head injury, or a seizure disorder such as epilepsy may also have seizures.

The main goal during a seizure is to make sure the resident is safe. During a seizure, a person may shake severely and thrust arms and legs uncontrollably. He may clench his jaw, drool, and be unable to swallow. Most seizures only last a short time.

Responding to seizures

1. Note the time. Put on gloves.
2. Lower the person to the floor. Cradle the head to protect it. If a pillow is nearby, place it under the person's head. Loosen clothing to help with breathing. Try to turn the person's head to one side to help lower the risk of choking. This may not be possible during a violent seizure.
3. Have someone call the nurse immediately or use the call light. Do not leave the person unless you must do so to get medical help.
4. Move furniture away to prevent injury.
5. Do not try to restrain the person or stop the seizure.
6. Do not force anything between the person's teeth. Do not place your hands in the person's mouth for any reason. You could be bitten.
7. Do not give the person food or liquids.
8. When the seizure is over, note the time. Gently turn the person to his left side if you do not suspect head, neck, back, spinal, or abdominal injuries. Turning the person reduces the risk of choking on vomit or saliva. If the person begins to choke, get help immediately. Check for adequate breathing and pulse. Begin CPR if breathing and pulse are absent and if you are allowed and trained to do so. Do not begin CPR during a seizure.
9. Remove and discard gloves. Wash your hands.
10. Report and document the incident properly, including how long the seizure lasted.

CVA or Stroke

Cerebrovascular accident (**CVA**), or stroke, occurs when blood supply to a part of the brain is blocked or a blood vessel leaks or ruptures within the brain. A quick response to a suspected stroke is critical. Tests and treatment need to be given within a short time of the stroke's onset. Early treatment may be able to reduce the severity of the stroke.

A **transient ischemic attack** (**TIA**) is a warning sign of a CVA. It is the result of a temporary lack of blood supply to the brain. Symptoms may last up to 24 hours. They include difficulty speaking, weakness on one side of the body, temporary loss of vision, and numbness or tingling. These symptoms should not be ignored. They should be reported to the nurse immediately. These are also signs that a TIA or CVA is occurring:

- Facial numbness, weakness, or drooping, especially on one side
- Paralysis on one side of the body (**hemiplegia**)
- Arm numbness or weakness, especially on one side (**hemiparesis**)
- Slurred speech or inability to speak (**expressive aphasia**)
- Inability to understand spoken or written words (**receptive aphasia**)
- Use of inappropriate words
- Severe headache
- Blurred vision
- Ringing in the ears
- Redness in the face
- Noisy breathing
- Elevated blood pressure
- Slow pulse rate
- Nausea or vomiting
- Loss of bowel and bladder control
- Seizures
- Dizziness
- Loss of consciousness

In addition to the symptoms listed above, women may have these symptoms:

- Pain in the face, arms, and legs
- Hiccups
- Weakness
- Chest pain
- Shortness of breath
- Palpitations

F.A.S.T.

The acronym F.A.S.T. can be used as a way to remember the sudden signs that a stroke is occurring.

(F)ace: Is one side of the face drooping? Is it numb? Ask the person to smile. Is the smile uneven?

(A)rms: Is one arm numb or weak? Ask the person to raise both arms. Check to see if one arm drifts downward.

(S)peech: Is the person's speech slurred? Is the person unable to speak? Can the person be understood? Ask the person to repeat a simple sentence and see if the sentence is repeated correctly.

(T)ime: Time is of the utmost importance when responding to a stroke. If the person shows any of the symptoms listed above, report to the nurse immediately.

Websites for the American Stroke Association (strokeassociation.org) and The National Stroke Association (stroke.org) have more information.

Chapter 4 has more information about CVAs.

Vomiting

Vomiting, or **emesis**, is the act of ejecting stomach contents through the mouth and/or nose. It can be a sign of a serious illness or injury. Some residents, such as those with cancer who are undergoing chemotherapy, may vomit frequently as a result of treatment. Because an NA may not know when a resident is going to vomit, he may not have time to explain what he will do and assemble supplies ahead of time. The NA should talk to the resident soothingly as he helps him clean up. He should tell the resident what he is doing to help him.

Responding to vomiting

1. Notify the nurse immediately.
2. Put on gloves.
3. Make sure the head is up or turned to one side. Place an emesis basin under the chin. Remove it when vomiting has stopped.
4. Remove soiled linens or clothes and set aside. Replace with fresh linens or clothes.
5. If the resident's intake and output (I&O) is being monitored (Chapter 7), measure and note the amount of vomitus.
6. Flush the vomit down the toilet unless the vomit is red, has blood in it, or looks like wet coffee grounds, or if medication/pills are in the vomit. If these signs are observed, show this to the nurse before discarding the vomit. After disposing of the vomit, wash, dry, and store the basin.
7. Remove and discard gloves.
8. Wash your hands.
9. Put on fresh gloves.
10. Provide comfort to the resident. Wipe his face and mouth (Fig. 2-21). Position him comfortably. Offer a drink of water or oral care. Oral care helps get rid of the taste of vomit in the mouth.
11. Put soiled linen in the proper containers.
12. Remove and discard gloves.
13. Wash your hands again.

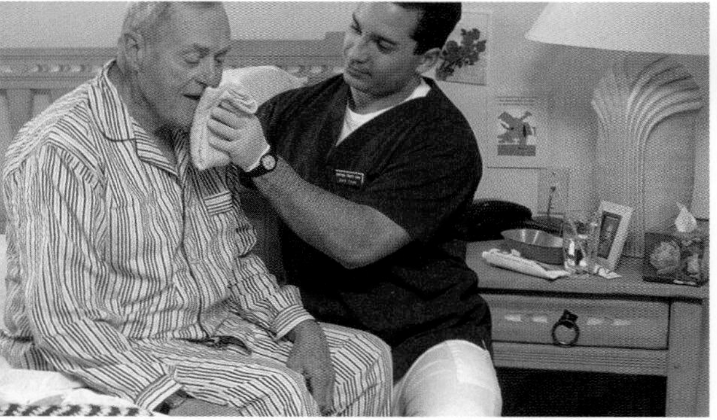

Fig. 2-21. *Be calm and comforting when helping a resident who has vomited.*

14. Report and document the incident properly. Document the time, amount, color, odor, and consistency of vomitus.

6. Describe and demonstrate infection prevention and control practices

Infection prevention is the set of methods practiced in healthcare facilities to prevent and control the spread of disease. Preventing the spread of infection is the responsibility of all care team members. NAs must know and follow their facility's infection prevention policies. These policies help protect staff members, residents, and others from disease.

A **microorganism** (**MO**) is a living thing that is so small that it can be seen only under a microscope. A **microbe** is another name for a microorganism. Microorganisms are always present in the environment. **Infections** occur when harmful microorganisms, called **pathogens**, invade the body and multiply.

There are two main types of infections: localized and systemic. A **localized infection** is limited to a specific location in the body. It has local symptoms, which means the symptoms are near the site of infection. For example, if a wound becomes infected, the area around it may become red, swollen, warm, and painful. A **systemic infection** affects the entire body. This type of infection travels through the bloodstream and is spread throughout the body. It causes general symptoms, such as fever, chills, mental confusion, or lower than normal blood pressure.

A type of infection that can be localized or systemic is a healthcare-associated infection. A **healthcare-associated infection** (**HAI**) is an infection acquired in a healthcare setting during the delivery of medical care. Healthcare settings include hospitals, long-term care facilities, and outpatient surgery centers, among others.

Preventing the spread of infection is important. To understand how to prevent disease, it is helpful to first understand how it is spread. The **chain of infection** is a way of describing how disease is transmitted from one human being to another (Fig. 2-22). Definitions and examples of each of the six links in the chain of infection follow.

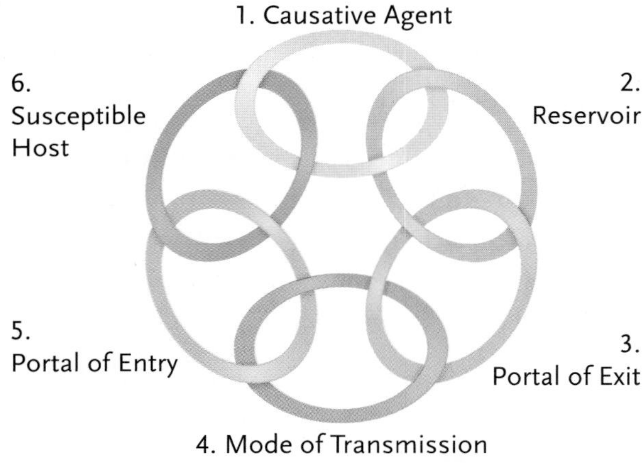

Fig. 2-22. The chain of infection.

Link 1: The **causative agent** is a pathogenic microorganism that causes disease. Causative agents include bacteria, viruses, fungi, and parasites. Normal flora are the microorganisms that live in and on the body. They normally do not cause harm to a healthy person as long as the flora remain in that particular area. When they enter a different part of the body, they may cause an infection.

Link 2: A **reservoir** is where the pathogen lives and multiplies. A reservoir can be a human, animal, plant, soil, or a substance. Warm, dark, and moist places are the ideal environments for microorganisms to live, grow, and multiply. Some microorganisms need oxygen to survive; others do not. Examples of reservoirs include the lungs, blood, and the large intestine.

Link 3: The **portal of exit** is any body opening on an infected person that allows pathogens to leave (Fig. 2-23). These include the nose, mouth, eyes, or a cut in the skin.

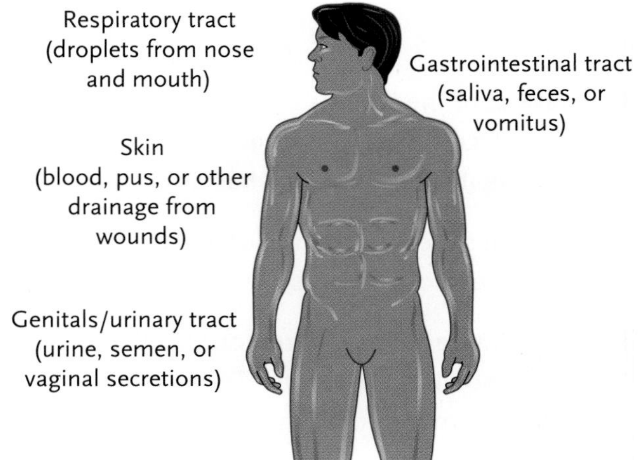

Fig. 2-23. Portals of exit.

Link 4: The **mode of transmission** describes how the pathogen travels. Transmission can occur through the air or through direct or indirect contact. **Direct contact** happens by touching the infected person or his secretions. **Indirect contact** results from touching an object contaminated by the infected person, such as a needle, dressing, or tissue. The primary route of disease transmission within the healthcare setting is via the hands of healthcare workers.

Link 5: The **portal of entry** is any body opening on an uninfected person that allows pathogens to enter (Fig. 2-24). These include the nose, mouth, eyes, and other mucous membranes, cuts in the skin, and cracked skin. **Mucous membranes** are the membranes that line body cavities that open to the outside of the body.

These include the linings of the mouth, nose, eyes, rectum, and genitals.

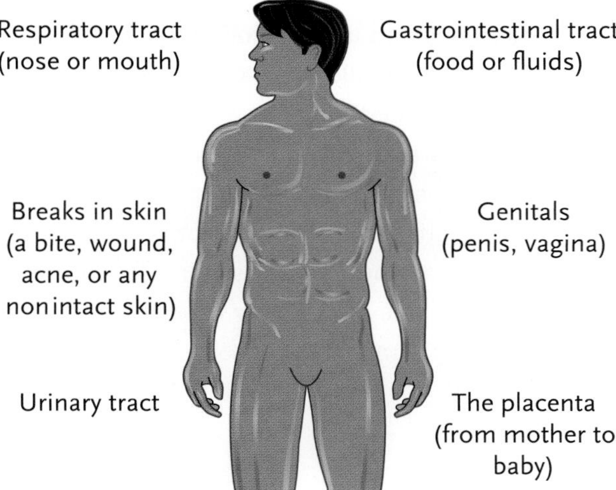

Fig. 2-24. *Portals of entry.*

Link 6: A **susceptible host** is an uninfected person who could get sick. Examples include all healthcare workers and anyone in their care who is not already infected with that particular disease.

If one of the links in the chain of infection is broken, then the spread of infection is stopped. Infection prevention practices help stop pathogens from traveling (Link 4) and from getting on a person's hands, nose, eyes, mouth, skin, etc. (Link 5). Immunizations (Link 6) reduce a person's chances of getting sick from diseases such as hepatitis B and influenza.

Transmission (passage or transfer) of most **infectious** diseases can be blocked by using proper infection prevention practices, such as handwashing. Handwashing is the most important way to stop the spread of infection. All caregivers should wash their hands often.

Handwashing is a part of medical asepsis. **Medical asepsis** refers to measures used to reduce and prevent the spread of pathogens. Medical asepsis is used in all healthcare settings. **Surgical asepsis**, also known as *sterile technique,* makes an object or area free of all microorganisms (not just pathogens). Surgical asepsis is used for many types of procedures, such as changing catheters.

Standard Precautions and Transmission-Based Precautions

State and federal government agencies have guidelines and laws concerning infection prevention. The **Centers for Disease Control and Prevention** (**CDC**, cdc.gov) is a federal government agency that issues guidelines to protect and improve the health of individuals and communities. Through education, the CDC aims to prevent and control disease, injury, and disability, as well as to promote public health.

In 1996, the CDC created a new infection prevention system to reduce the risk of contracting infectious diseases in healthcare settings. Some changes were made to this system in 2007. There are two levels of precautions within the infection prevention system: Standard Precautions and Transmission-Based Precautions.

Following **Standard Precautions** means treating blood, body fluids, nonintact skin (like abrasions, pimples, or open sores), and mucous membranes as if they were infected. Body fluids include tears, saliva, **sputum** (mucus coughed up), urine, feces, semen, vaginal secretions, pus or other wound drainage, and vomit. They do not include sweat.

Standard Precautions must be used with every resident. This promotes safety. An NA cannot tell by looking at residents or even by reading their medical charts whether residents have a contagious disease such as tuberculosis, hepatitis, or influenza. Many diseases can be spread even before the infected person shows signs or has been diagnosed.

Standard Precautions and Transmission-Based Precautions are ways to stop the spread of infection. They interrupt the mode of transmission. In other words, these guidelines do not stop an infected person from giving off pathogens.

However, the NA helps prevent those pathogens from infecting her or those in her care by following these guidelines:

- Standard Precautions must be practiced with every single person in an NA's care.
- Transmission-Based Precautions vary based on how an infection is transmitted. When indicated, they are used **in addition** to Standard Precautions. More information about these precautions is located later in the chapter.

Guidelines: Standard Precautions

G **Wash your hands** before putting on gloves. Wash your hands immediately after removing your gloves. Be careful not to touch clean objects with your used gloves.

G **Wear gloves** if you may come into contact with blood; body fluids or secretions; broken or open skin, such as abrasions, acne, cuts, stitches, or staples; or mucous membranes. Such contacts occur during mouth care; toilet assistance; perineal care; helping with a bedpan or urinal; ostomy care; cleaning up spills; cleaning basins, urinals, bedpans, and other containers that have held body fluids; and disposing of wastes.

G **Remove gloves** immediately when finished with a procedure and wash your hands.

G **Immediately wash all skin surfaces that have been contaminated** with blood and body fluids.

G **Wear a disposable gown** that is resistant to body fluids if you may come into contact with blood or body fluids or when splashing or spraying of blood or body fluids is likely. If a resident has a contagious illness, wear a gown even if it is not likely you will come into contact with blood or body fluids.

G **Wear a mask and protective goggles and/or a face shield** if you may come into contact with blood or body fluids or when splashing or spraying of blood or body fluids is likely.

G **Wear gloves and use caution when handling razor blades, needles, and other sharps. Sharps** are needles or other sharp objects. Avoid nicks and cuts when shaving residents. Place sharps carefully in a biohazard container for sharps. Biohazard containers used for sharps are puncture-resistant, leakproof containers. They are clearly labeled and warn of the danger of the contents inside (Fig. 2-25).

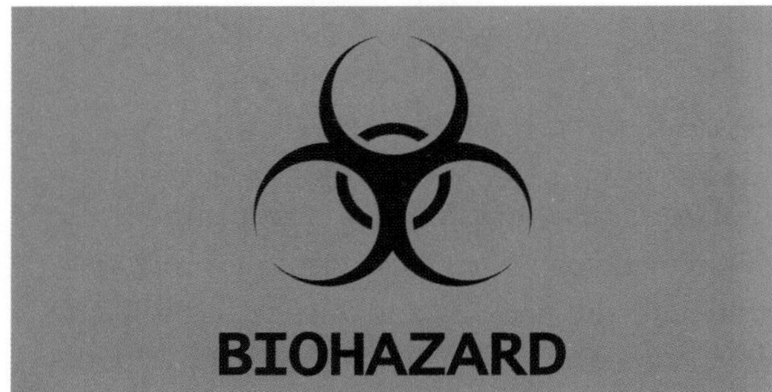

Fig. 2-25. This label indicates that the material is potentially infectious.

G **Never attempt to recap needles or sharps after use.** You might stick yourself. Dispose of them in a biohazard container for sharps.

G **Carefully bag all contaminated supplies.** Dispose of them according to your facility's policy.

G **Clearly label body fluids** that are being saved for a specimen with the resident's name, date of birth, and room number; the date; and a biohazard label. Keep them in a container with a lid. Put in a biohazard specimen bag for transportation if required.

G **Dispose of contaminated wastes** according to your facility's policy. Waste containing blood or body fluids is considered biohazardous waste. Liquid waste can usually be disposed of through the regular sewer system as long as there is no splashing, spraying, or aerosolizing of the waste as it is being disposed. Appropriate personal protective equipment needs to be worn, followed by proper removal and handwashing. Follow instructions.

Standard Precautions should always be practiced on all residents, regardless of their infection status. This greatly reduces the risk of transmitting infection.

Nursing assistants use their hands constantly while they work. Microorganisms are on everything they touch. The single most common way for healthcare-associated infections (HAIs) to be spread is via the hands of healthcare workers. Handwashing is the most important thing NAs can do to prevent the spread of disease.

The CDC has defined **hand hygiene** as washing hands with either plain or antiseptic soap and water or using alcohol-based hand rubs. Alcohol-based hand rubs (often called *hand sanitizers*) include gels, rinses, and foams that do not require the use of water.

Alcohol-based hand rubs have proven effective in reducing bacteria on the skin. However, they are not a substitute for frequent, proper handwashing. When hands are visibly soiled, they should be washed using antimicrobial soap and water. An **antimicrobial** agent destroys, resists, or prevents the development of pathogens. Hand rubs can be used in addition to handwashing any time hands are not visibly soiled. When using a hand rub, the hands must be rubbed together until the product has completely dried. Hand lotion can help prevent dry, cracked skin.

NAs should avoid wearing rings and bracelets while working. They may increase the risk of contamination. Fingernails should be short, smooth, and clean. Artificial nails should not be worn because they harbor bacteria and increase the risk of contamination even if hands are washed often. NAs should wash their hands at these times:

- When first arriving at work
- Whenever hands are visibly soiled
- Before, between, and after all contact with residents
- Before putting on gloves and after removing gloves
- After contact with any body fluids, mucous membranes, nonintact skin, or wound dressings
- After handling contaminated items
- After contact with objects in the resident's room (care environment)
- Before and after touching meal trays and/or handling food
- Before and after helping residents with meals
- Before getting clean linen
- Before and after using the toilet
- After touching garbage or trash
- After picking up anything from the floor
- After blowing the nose, wiping the nose, or coughing or sneezing into the hands
- Before and after eating
- After smoking
- After touching areas on the body, such as the mouth, face, eyes, hair, ears, or nose
- Before and after applying makeup
- After any contact with pets or any pet care items
- Before leaving the facility

Washing hands (hand hygiene)

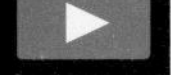

Equipment: soap, paper towels

1. Turn on the water at the sink. Keep your clothes dry.
2. Wet hands and wrists thoroughly (Fig. 2-26).

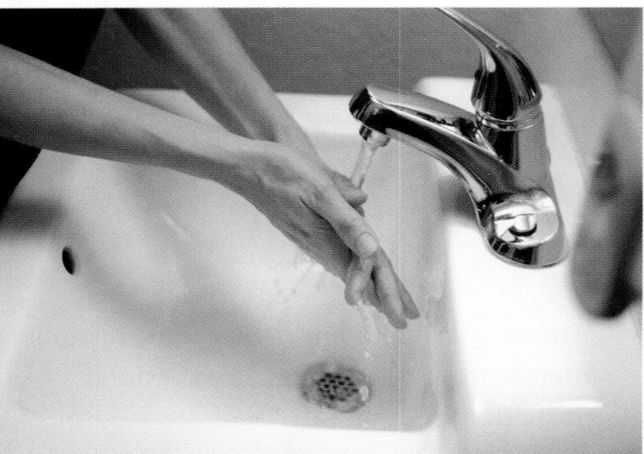

Fig. 2-26. *Keeping arms angled downward, wet hands and wrists thoroughly.*

3. Apply soap to your hands.
4. Keep your hands lower than your elbows and your fingertips down. Rub hands together and fingers between each other to create a lather. Lather all surfaces of wrists, hands, and fingers, using friction for at least 20 seconds (Fig. 2-27).
   Lather and friction loosen skin oils and allow pathogens to be rinsed away.

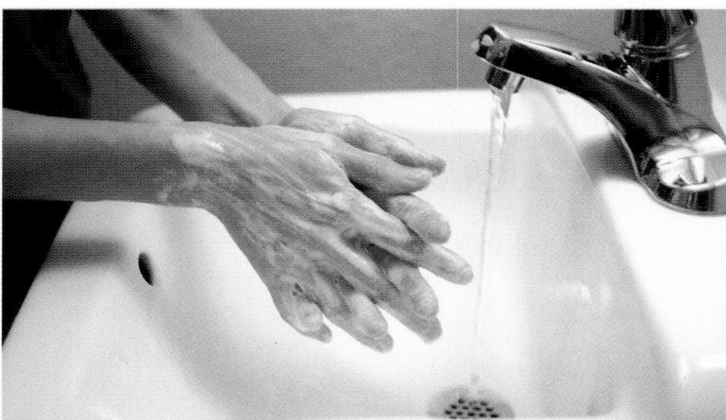

Fig. 2-27. *Using friction for at least 20 seconds, lather all surfaces of your wrists, hands, and fingers.*

5. Clean your nails by rubbing them in the palm of your other hand.
   Most pathogens on hands are under the nails.
6. Keep your hands lower than your elbows and your fingertips down. Being careful not to touch the sink, rinse thoroughly under running water. Rinse all surfaces of your wrists and hands. Run water down from your wrists to your fingertips. Do not run water over unwashed arms down to clean hands.
   Water should run from cleanest to dirtiest. Wrists are cleanest; fingertips are dirtiest.
7. Use a clean, dry paper towel to dry all surfaces of your fingers, hands, and wrists, starting at the fingertips. Do not wipe the towel on unwashed forearms and then wipe your clean hands. Discard the towel in the waste container without touching the container. If your hands touch the sink or wastebasket, start over.
8. Use a clean, dry paper towel to turn off the faucet (Fig. 2-28). Discard the towel in the waste container. Do not contaminate your hands by touching the surface of the sink or faucet.
   Hands will be recontaminated if you touch the dirty faucet or sink with clean hands.

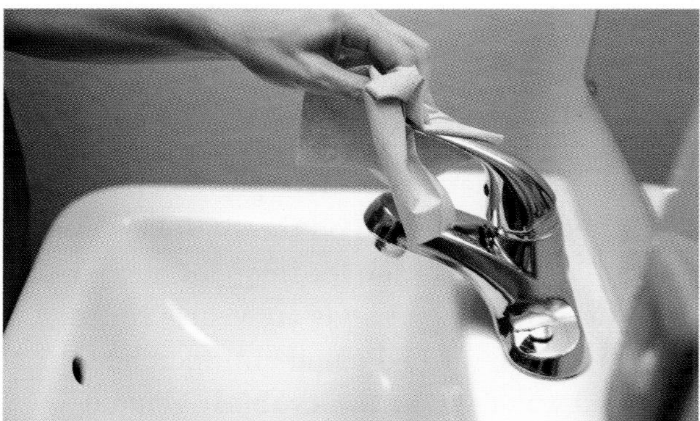

Fig. 2-28. *Use a clean, dry paper towel to turn off the faucet so that you do not contaminate your hands.*

Personal Protective Equipment

Personal protective equipment (PPE) is equipment that helps protect employees from serious injuries or illnesses resulting from contact with workplace hazards. In care facilities, this equipment helps protect nursing assistants from contact with potentially infectious material. Employers are responsible for providing the appropriate PPE to wear. OSHA requires that PPE be readily available in a variety of sizes. It must be easy to access.

Personal protective equipment includes gowns, masks, goggles, face shields, and gloves. Gowns protect the skin and/or clothing. Masks protect the mouth and nose. Goggles protect the eyes. Face shields protect the entire face—the eyes, nose, and mouth. Gloves protect the hands. Gloves are used most often by all caregivers.

NAs must wear personal protective equipment if there is a chance of coming into contact with body fluids, mucous membranes, or open wounds. They must wear, or **don**, gowns, masks, goggles, and face shields when splashing or spraying of body fluids or blood could occur. Hand hygiene should be performed before donning PPE and after removing and discarding PPE.

Clean, non-sterile gowns protect exposed skin. They also prevent soiling of clothing. Gowns should fully cover the torso. They should fit comfortably over the body, and have long sleeves that fit snugly at the wrists.

Gowns can be worn only once before they need to be discarded. OSHA requires fluid-resistant gowns if fluid penetration is likely. If a gown becomes wet or soiled during care, it should be discarded and a new gown should be donned. When finished with a procedure, NAs should remove, or **doff**, the gown as soon as possible and wash their hands.

Putting on (donning) and removing (doffing) gown

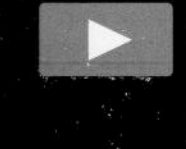

1. Wash your hands.
2. Open the gown. Hold it out in front of you and allow it to open/unfold (Fig. 2-29). Do not shake the gown or touch it to the floor. Facing the back opening of the gown, place your arms through each sleeve.
3. Fasten the neck opening.

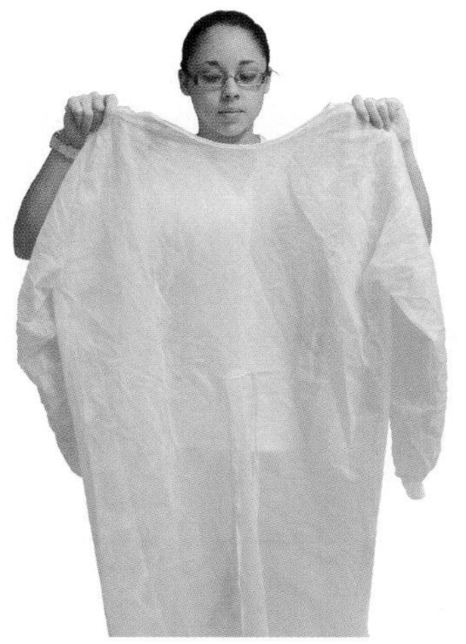

Fig. 2-29. *Let the gown unfold without shaking it.*

4. Reach behind you. Pull the gown until it completely covers your clothing. Secure the gown at your waist (Fig. 2-30).

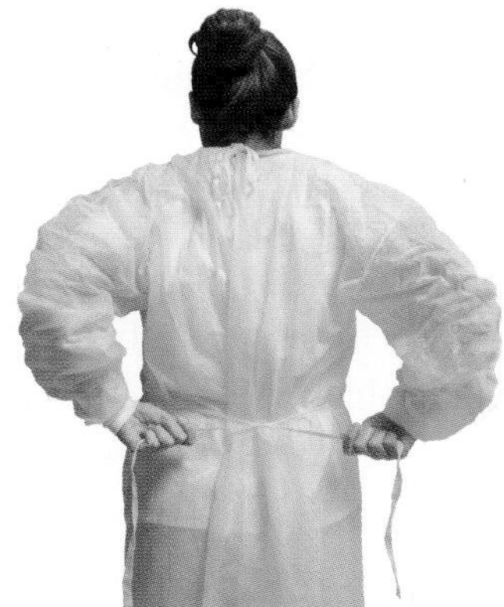

Fig. 2-30. *Reaching behind you, secure the gown at the waist.*

5. Put on your gloves after putting on the gown. The cuffs of the gloves should overlap the cuffs of the gown (Fig. 2-31).

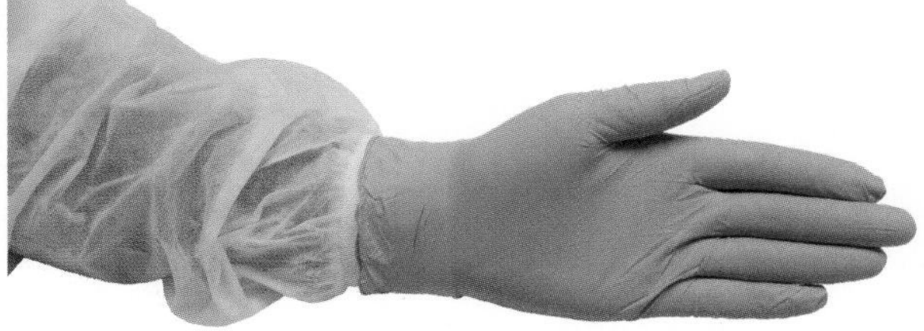

Fig. 2-31. *The cuffs of the gloves should overlap the cuffs of the gown.*

6. When removing a gown, remove and discard gloves properly (see procedure later in the chapter). Unfasten the gown at the waist and neck. Remove the gown without touching the outside of the gown. Roll the dirty side in, while holding the gown away from your body. Dispose of the gown properly and wash your hands.
Rolling puts dirtiest surface inward, lessening the risk of contamination.

Masks can prevent inhalation of microorganisms through the nose or mouth. Masks should be worn when caring for residents with respiratory illnesses. They should also be worn when it is likely that contact with blood or body fluids may occur. Sometimes special masks (respirators) are required for certain diseases, such as tuberculosis (TB). Masks should fully cover the nose and mouth and prevent fluid penetration. Masks should fit snugly over the nose and mouth.

Masks can be worn only once before they need to be discarded. Masks that become wet or soiled must be changed immediately without touching the outside of the soiled mask. NAs must always change their masks when moving between residents. The same mask should not be worn from one resident to another.

Goggles provide protection for the eyes. Goggles are worn with a mask and are used whenever it is likely that blood or body fluids may be splashed or sprayed into the eye area or into the eyes. Eyeglasses alone do not provide proper eye protection. Goggles should fit snugly over and around the eyes or eyeglasses.

Putting on (donning) mask and goggles 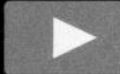

1. Wash your hands.
2. Pick up the mask by the top strings or elastic strap. Do not touch the mask where it touches your face.
3. Pull the elastic strap over your head, or if the mask has strings, tie the top strings first, then the bottom strings. Do not wear a mask hanging from only the bottom ties or straps.
4. Pinch the metal strip at the top of the mask (if part of the mask) tightly around your nose so that it feels snug (Fig. 2-32). Fit the mask snugly around your face and below the chin.

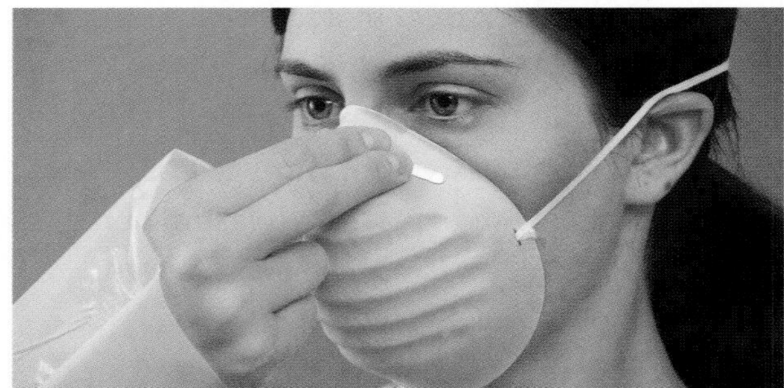

Fig. 2-32. *Adjust the metal strip until the mask fits snugly around your nose.*

5. Place the goggles over your eyes or eyeglasses. Use the headband or earpieces to secure them to your head. Make sure they are on snugly.
6. Put on gloves after putting on the mask and goggles.

Face shields may be worn when blood or body fluids may be splashed or sprayed into the eyes or eye area. A face shield can be substituted for a mask or goggles, or it can be worn with a mask. The face shield should cover the forehead, go below the chin, and wrap around the sides of the face. The headband can secure it to the head.

Non-sterile gloves are used for basic care. They are available in different sizes, and may be made of nitrile, vinyl, or latex. However, due to allergy issues, some facilities have banned the use of latex gloves.

Gloves should fit the hands comfortably and should not be too loose or too tight. Facilities have specific policies and procedures on when to wear gloves. NAs must learn and follow these rules. Gloves must always be worn for the following tasks:

- Anytime an NA might come into contact with blood or any body fluid, open wounds, or mucous membranes
- When performing or helping with mouth care or care of any mucous membrane
- When performing or helping with **perineal care** (care of the genitals and anal area)
- When performing personal care on **nonintact skin**—skin that is broken by abrasions, cuts, rashes, pimples, lesions, surgical incisions, or boils
- When the NA has open sores or cuts on her hands
- When shaving a resident
- When disposing of soiled bed linens, gowns, dressings, and pads
- When touching surfaces or equipment that either is visibly contaminated or may be contaminated

Disposable gloves can only be worn once. They cannot be washed or reused. Gloves should be changed immediately if they become wet, worn, soiled, or torn. Gloves should also be changed before contact with mucous membranes or broken skin. After removing gloves, the NA should wash his hands before donning new gloves. Nonintact areas on the hands should be covered with bandages or gauze before putting on gloves.

Putting on (donning) gloves 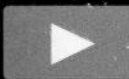

1. Wash your hands.
2. If you are right-handed, slide one glove on your left hand (reverse if left-handed).
3. Using your gloved hand, slide the other hand into the second glove.
4. Interlace your fingers. Smooth out folds and create a comfortable fit.
5. Carefully look for tears, holes, or spots. Replace the glove if needed.
6. Adjust the gloves until they are pulled up over your wrists and fit correctly. If wearing a gown, pull the cuffs of the gloves over the sleeves of the gown (Fig. 2-33).

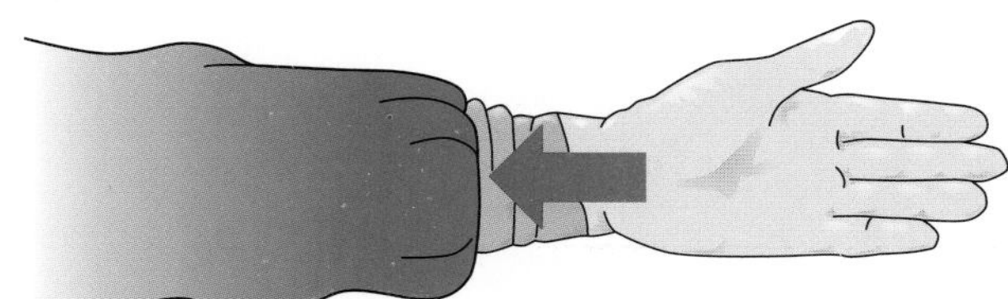

***Fig. 2-33.** Adjust gloves until they are pulled up over the sleeves of the gown.*

Gloves should be removed promptly after use, and the NA should wash his hands directly after removing gloves. He should be careful not to contaminate his skin or clothing when removing gloves. Gloves are worn to protect the skin from becoming contaminated. After giving care, gloves are contaminated. If an NA opens a door with the gloved hand, the doorknob becomes contaminated. Later, anyone who opens the door with an ungloved hand will be touching a contaminated surface. Before touching surfaces or leaving residents' rooms, the NA must remove gloves and wash his hands. Afterward, new gloves can be donned if needed.

Removing (doffing) gloves 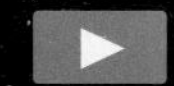

1. Touch only the outside of one glove. With one gloved hand, grasp the other glove at the palm and pull the glove off (Fig. 2-34).

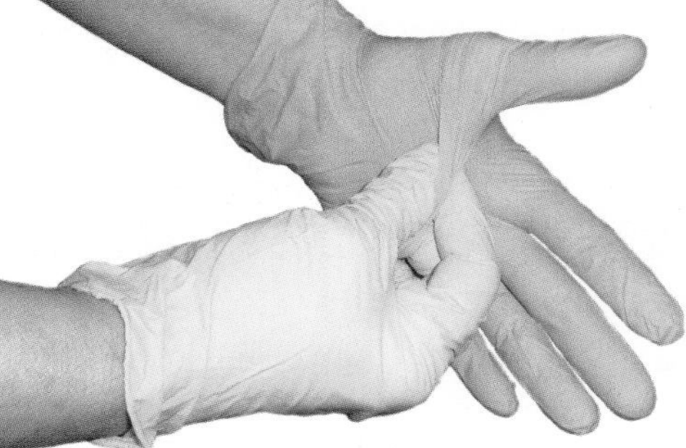

***Fig. 2-34.** Grasp the glove at the palm and pull it off.*

2. With the fingertips of your gloved hand, hold the glove you just removed. With your ungloved hand, slip two fingers underneath the cuff of the remaining glove at the wrist. Do not touch any part of the outside of the glove (Fig. 2-35).
The outside of the glove is contaminated.

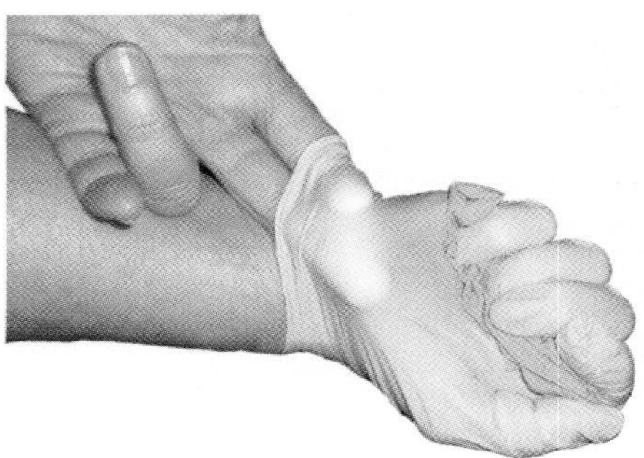

Fig. 2-35. *Reach inside the glove at the wrist, without touching any part of the outside of the glove.*

3. Pull down, turning this glove inside out and over the first glove as you remove it.
4. You should now be holding one glove from its clean inner side. The other glove should be inside it.
5. Drop both gloves into the proper container without contaminating yourself.
6. Wash your hands.

This is the correct order that the NA should follow when donning (putting on) PPE:

1. Wash your hands.
2. Put on gown.
3. Put on mask.
4. Put on goggles or face shield.
5. Put on gloves.

This is the correct order that the NA should follow when doffing (removing) PPE:

1. Remove and discard gloves.
2. Remove goggles or face shield.
3. Remove and discard gown.
4. Remove and discard mask.
5. Wash your hands. Washing hands is always the final step after removing and discarding PPE.

Equipment and Linen Handling

In health care, an object is called **clean** if it has not been contaminated with pathogens. An object that is **dirty** has been contaminated with pathogens. Facilities have special rooms or areas for equipment, linen, and supplies. There are separate rooms for supplies that are considered clean and for supplies that are considered dirty or contaminated. NAs will be told where these rooms are located and what types of equipment and supplies are found in each room. NAs should wash their hands before entering clean rooms and before leaving dirty rooms. This helps prevent the spread of pathogens.

Guidelines: Handling Equipment, Linen, and Clothing

G Handle all equipment in a way that prevents
- Skin/mucous membrane contact
- Contamination of your clothing
- Transfer of disease to other residents or areas

G Do not use reusable equipment again until it has been properly cleaned and reprocessed. **Sterilization** is a cleaning measure that destroys all microorganisms, including pathogens. Sterilization is part of surgical asepsis. It uses steam under pressure, dry heat, or liquid or gas chemicals to sterilize. Items that need to be sterilized are ones that go directly into the bloodstream or into other normally sterile areas of the body (for example, surgical instruments). **Disinfection** is a process that kills pathogens but does not destroy all pathogens. It reduces the pathogen count to a level that is considered not infectious. Disinfection is carried out with pasteurization or chemical germicides. Examples of items that are usually disinfected are reusable oxygen tanks, wall-mounted blood pressure cuffs, and any reusable resident care equipment.

G Dispose of all single-use, or disposable, equipment properly. **Disposable** means it is discarded after one use. Disposable razors and disposable thermometers are examples of disposable equipment.

G Clean and disinfect
- All environmental surfaces
- Beds, bedrails, and all bedside equipment
- All frequently touched surfaces (such as doorknobs and call lights)

G Handle, transport, and process soiled linens and clothing in a way that prevents
- Skin and mucous membrane exposure
- Contamination of clothing (hold linen and clothing away from your uniform)
- Transfer of disease to other residents and areas (do not shake linen or clothes; fold or roll linen so that dirtiest area is inside; do not put soiled linen on floor)

G Bag soiled linen at point of origin.

G Sort soiled linen away from resident care areas.

G Place wet linen in leakproof bags.

More information about cleaning equipment and supplies is in Chapter 7.

Spills

Spills can pose a serious risk of infection and can put residents and staff at risk for falls. The housekeeping department may be responsible for cleaning spills. If NAs must clean spills, there are general guidelines to follow.

Guidelines: Cleaning Spills Involving Blood, Body Fluids, or Glass

G Don gloves before starting. In some cases, special heavy-duty gloves are best.

G First, absorb the spill with whatever product is used by the facility. It may be an absorbing powder.

G Scoop up the absorbed spill, and dispose of it in a designated container.

G Apply the proper disinfectant to the spill area and allow it to stand wet for a minimum of 10 minutes (follow directions on the label).

G Clean up spills immediately with the proper cleaning solution.

G Do not pick up any pieces of broken glass, no matter how large, with your hands. Use a dustpan and broom or other tools.

G Waste containing broken glass, blood, or body fluids should be properly bagged. Waste containing blood or body fluids may need to be placed in a special biohazard waste bag. Follow facility policy.

Transmission-Based Precautions

These precautions are used for persons who are infected or may be infected with certain diseases. These precautions are called **Transmission-Based Precautions**. When ordered, these precautions are used in addition to Standard Precautions. These precautions will always be listed in the care plan and on the assignment sheet. Following these precautions promotes the NA's safety, as well as the safety of others.

There are three categories of Transmission-Based Precautions: Airborne Precautions, Droplet Precautions, and Contact Precautions. The category used depends on the pathogen or disease and how it spreads. They may also be used in combination for diseases that have multiple routes of transmission.

Airborne Precautions prevent the spread of pathogens that can be transmitted through the air after being expelled (Fig. 2-36). The pathogens are able to remain floating for some time. Tuberculosis is an example of an airborne disease. Precautions include wearing special masks, such as N95 or HEPA masks, to avoid being infected.

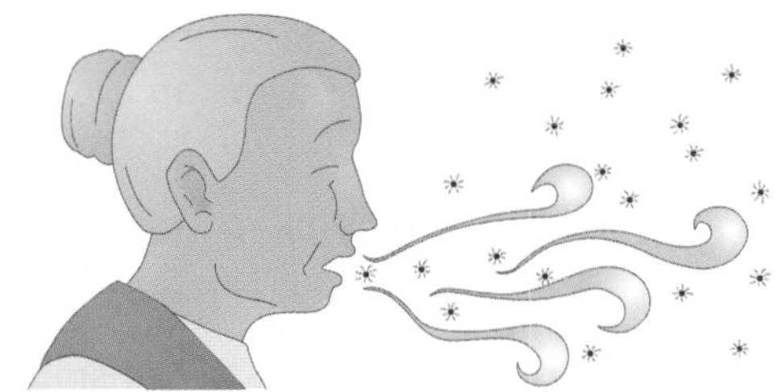

Fig. 2-36. *Airborne Precautions are used for diseases that can be transmitted through the air.*

Droplet Precautions are used for diseases that are spread by droplets in the air. Droplets normally do not travel more than six feet. Coughing, sneezing, talking, laughing, singing, or suctioning can spread droplets (Fig. 2-37). An example of a droplet disease is influenza. Precautions include wearing a face mask during care and restricting visits from uninfected people. NAs should cover their noses and mouths with a tissue when they sneeze or cough. They should ask others to do the same. Used tissues should be disposed of in the nearest waste container. Used tissues should not be placed in a pocket for later use. If a tissue is not available, NAs should cough or sneeze into their upper sleeve or elbow, not their hands. They should wash their hands immediately afterward. Residents should wear masks when being moved from room to room.

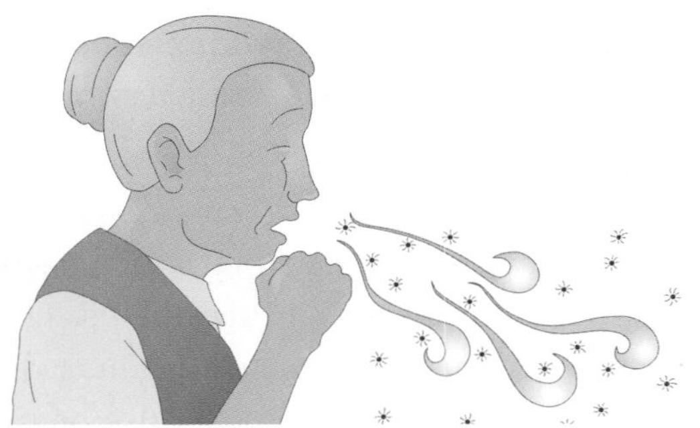

Fig. 2-37. *Droplet Precautions are followed when the disease-causing microorganism does not remain in the air.*

Contact Precautions are used when the resident is at risk of spreading an infection by direct contact with a person or object. The infection can be spread by touching a contaminated area on the resident's body or her blood or body fluids (Fig. 2-38). It may also be spread by touching contaminated items, linen, equipment, or supplies. Conjunctivitis (pink eye) and *Clostridium difficile* infection are examples of situations that require Contact Precautions. Precautions include wearing gloves and a gown and resident isolation. Contact Precautions require washing hands with antimicrobial soap and not touching infected surfaces with ungloved hands or uninfected surfaces with contaminated gloves.

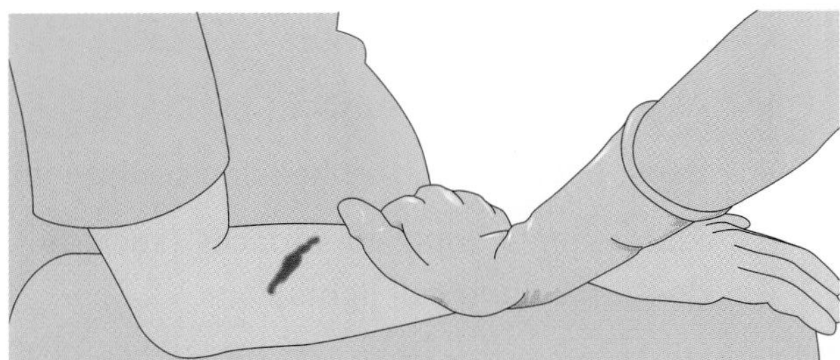

Fig. 2-38. *Contact Precautions are followed when the person is at risk of transmitting a microorganism by touching an object or person.*

Staff often refer to residents who need Transmission-Based Precautions as being "in isolation." A sign should be on the door indicating *Isolation* or *Contact Precautions* and alerting people to see the nurse before entering the room.

Guidelines: Isolation

- When they are indicated, Transmission-Based Precautions are always used **in addition** to Standard Precautions.
- You will be told the proper PPE to wear for care of each resident in isolation. Make sure to put on the PPE properly and remove it safely. Remove PPE and place it in the appropriate container before exiting a resident's room. PPE cannot be worn outside the resident's room. Wash your hands following the removal of PPE and again after exiting the resident's room. In addition to handwashing areas within the resident's room, there may be an alcohol-based hand rub dispenser mounted on the wall inside the room as you exit.
- Do not share equipment between residents. Use disposable supplies that can be discarded

after use whenever possible. Use dedicated (only for use by one resident) equipment when disposable is not an option. When using disposable supplies, discard them in the resident's room before leaving. Be careful not to contaminate reusable equipment by setting it on furniture or counters in the resident's room. When the resident no longer needs the additional precautions, properly dispose of dedicated equipment if required. If the dedicated equipment is to be used for other residents, it should be cleaned and disinfected after use.

- **G** Wear the proper PPE, if indicated, when serving food and drink to residents. Do not leave uneaten food uncovered in the resident's room. When the meal is completed, remove the meal tray. Take it to the proper area.
- **G** Follow Standard Precautions when dealing with body waste removal. Wear gloves when touching or handling waste. Wear gowns and goggles when indicated. The waste must be disposed of in such a manner as to minimize splashing and spraying.
- **G** If required to take a specimen from a resident in isolation, wear the proper PPE. Collect the specimen. Place it in the appropriate container without the outside of the container coming into contact with the specimen. Properly remove your PPE and dispose of it in the room. Perform hand hygiene before leaving the room. Take the specimen to the nurse.
- **G** Residents need to feel that staff understand what they are going through. Listen to what residents are saying. Allow time to talk with them about their concerns. Reassure residents. Explain why these steps are being taken. Relay any requests outside your scope of practice to the nurse.

Common Infectious Diseases

Bloodborne pathogens are microorganisms found in human blood. They can cause infection and disease in humans. They may also be found in certain other body fluids, draining wounds, and mucous membranes. These pathogens are transmitted by infected blood entering the bloodstream, or if infected semen or vaginal secretions contact mucous membranes. Having sexual contact with someone carrying a bloodborne disease can also transmit the disease. Sexual contact includes sexual intercourse (vaginal and anal), contact of the mouth with the genitals or anus, and contact of the hands with the genital area. Sharing infected drug needles can also spread bloodborne diseases. Infected pregnant women may transmit bloodborne diseases to their babies in the womb or at birth.

In health care, contact with infected blood or body fluids is the most common way to be infected with a bloodborne disease. Infections can be spread through contact with contaminated blood or body fluids, needles or other sharp objects, or contaminated supplies or equipment. Standard Precautions, handwashing, isolation, and PPE are all ways to prevent transmission of bloodborne diseases. Employers are required by law to help prevent exposure to bloodborne pathogens. Following Standard Precautions and other procedures helps protect caregivers from bloodborne diseases.

Two major bloodborne diseases in the United States are acquired immunodeficiency syndrome (AIDS) and the viral hepatitis family. Chapter 4 has more information about AIDS.

Hepatitis is inflammation of the liver caused by certain viruses and other factors, such as alcohol abuse, some medications, and trauma. Liver function can be permanently damaged by hepatitis. It can lead to other chronic, lifelong illnesses. Several different viruses can cause hepatitis. The most common types of hepatitis are A, B, and C. Hepatitis B and C are bloodborne diseases that can cause death.

Hepatitis B (HBV) is spread through sexual contact, by sharing infected needles, and from a mother to her baby during delivery. It can be spread through improperly sterilized needles used for tattoos and piercings and through grooming supplies such as razors and toothbrushes. It is also spread by exposure at work from accidental contact with infected needles or other sharps or from splashing blood. HBV is a threat to healthcare workers. Employers must offer NAs a free vaccine to protect them from hepatitis B. The HBV vaccine is usually given as a series of three shots. Prevention is the best option for dealing with this disease. Employees should take the vaccine when it is offered. Hepatitis C (HCV) is also transmitted through blood or body fluids. Hepatitis C can lead to cirrhosis and liver cancer and can even cause death. There is no vaccine for hepatitis C.

Other serious infections include the following:

Tuberculosis, or **TB**, is a highly contagious disease. It is caused by a bacterium that is carried on mucous droplets suspended in the air. The bacteria usually affect the lungs, which is known as pulmonary tuberculosis. TB is an airborne disease. When a person infected with TB talks, coughs, breathes, sings, laughs, or sneezes, he may spread the disease. Tuberculosis causes coughing, trouble breathing, weight loss, and fatigue (Fig. 2-39). Other symptoms include chest pain, coughing up blood, loss of appetite, slight fever, chills, and night sweats. Usually TB can be cured by taking all of the prescribed medication. However, if left untreated, it may cause death.

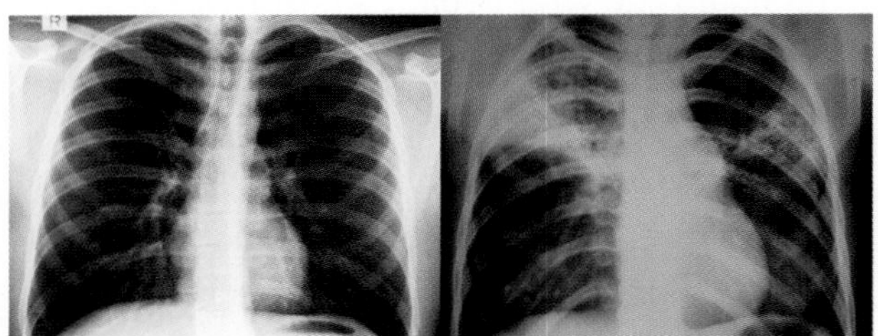

Fig. 2-39. *A normal lung X-ray on the left, and an X-ray of a lung with TB on the right.*

When caring for residents who have TB, NAs should follow Standard Precautions and Airborne Precautions. They should use personal protective equipment as instructed. Special masks, such as N95, high efficiency particulate air (HEPA), or other masks must be used. NAs must take care when handling sputum. Residents will be placed in a special airborne infection isolation room (AIIR). These rooms have a controlled flow of air. The door to this type of room should remain closed except when entering or exiting the room. The door should not be opened or closed quickly. This pulls contaminated room air into the hallway. NAs must follow isolation procedures if directed. They should help the resident remember to take all medication prescribed. Failure to do so is a major factor in the spread of TB.

Staphylococcus aureus is a common type of bacteria that can cause infection. Methicillin is a powerful antibiotic often used in healthcare facilities. **MRSA** (methicillin-resistant *Staphylococcus aureus*) is an infection that is resistant to methicillin. Resistant means that drugs no longer work to kill the specific bacteria. This type of MRSA is also known as *HA-MRSA*, which stands for hospital-associated MRSA. Community-associated methicillin-resistant *Staphylococcus aureus* (CA-MRSA) is a type of MRSA infection that occurs in people who have not recently been admitted to healthcare facilities and who have no past diagnosis of MRSA. Often CA-MRSA manifests as skin infections, such as boils or pimples. This type of infection is becoming more common.

MRSA is almost always spread by direct physical contact with infected people. This means if a person has MRSA on his skin, especially on the hands, and touches another person, he may spread MRSA. Spread also occurs through indirect contact by touching equipment or supplies (for example, sheets or wound dressings) contaminated by a person with MRSA.

NAs can help prevent the spread of MRSA by practicing proper hygiene. Handwashing, using soap and warm water, is the single most important measure to control the spread of MRSA. NAs must always follow Standard Precautions, along with Transmission-Based Precautions as ordered. Cuts and abrasions should be kept clean and covered with a proper dressing (e.g., bandage) until healed. Contact with other people's wounds or material that is contaminated from wounds should be avoided.

Enterococci are bacteria that live in the digestive and genital tracts. Although they normally do not cause problems in healthy people, they can sometimes cause infection. Vancomycin is a powerful antibiotic used to treat infections caused by *enterococci*. If the *enterococci* become resistant to vancomycin, then they are called vancomycin-resistant *Enterococcus*, or **VRE**.

VRE is spread through direct and indirect contact. VRE infections are often difficult to treat and may require several medications. VRE infections can cause life-threatening infections in those with weak immune systems—the very young, the very old, and the very ill. Preventing VRE is much easier than trying to treat it. Proper hand hygiene can help prevent the spread of VRE. NAs should wash their hands often and wear PPE as directed. NAs must always follow Standard Precautions, along with Transmission-Based Precautions as ordered. Items may need to be disinfected. That information should be listed in the care plan.

Clostridium difficile infection is commonly known as ***C. diff*** or ***C. difficile***. It is a spore-forming bacterium which can be part of the normal intestinal flora. When the normal intestinal flora is altered, *C. difficile* can flourish in the intestinal tract and can cause infection. It produces a toxin that causes a watery diarrhea. Enemas, nasogastric tube insertion, and GI tract surgery increase a person's risk of developing the infection. The overuse of antibiotics may also alter the normal intestinal flora and increase the risk of developing *C. difficile*. It can also cause colitis, a more serious intestinal condition.

When released in the environment, *C. difficile* can form a spore that makes it difficult to kill. These spores can be carried on the hands of people who have direct contact with infected residents or with environmental surfaces (floors, bedpans, toilets, etc.) contaminated with *C. difficile*. Touching an object contaminated with *C. difficile* can transmit the infection. Alcohol-based hand sanitizer is not considered effective on *C. difficile*. Soap and water must be used each time hand hygiene is performed.

Proper handwashing with soap and water is vital in preventing the spread of the infection. Handling contaminated wastes properly can help prevent its spread. Cleaning surfaces with a proper disinfectant, such as a bleach solution, can also reduce transmission. Limiting the use of antibiotics helps lower the risk of developing *C. difficile* infection.

Employer-Employee Responsibilities

The **employer's** responsibilities for infection prevention include the following:

- Establish infection prevention procedures and an exposure control plan to protect workers
- Provide continuing in-service education on infection prevention, including bloodborne and airborne pathogens and updates on any new safety standards
- Have written procedures to follow should an exposure occur, including medical treatment and plans to prevent similar exposures
- Provide personal protective equipment (PPE) for employees to use and teach them when and how to properly use it
- Provide free hepatitis B vaccinations for all employees

The **employee's** responsibilities for infection prevention include the following:

- Follow Standard Precautions
- Follow all facility policies and procedures
- Follow care plans and assignments
- Use provided PPE as indicated or as appropriate
- Take advantage of the free hepatitis B vaccination
- Immediately report any exposure to infection, blood, or body fluids
- Participate in annual education programs covering the prevention of infection

3 Understanding Residents

1. Identify basic human needs

People have different genes, physical appearances, cultural backgrounds, ages, and social and financial positions. But all human beings have the same basic physical needs:

- Food and water
- Protection and shelter
- Activity
- Sleep and rest
- Comfort, especially freedom from pain

People also have **psychosocial needs**, which involve social interaction, emotions, intellect, and spirituality. Although they are not as easy to define as physical needs, psychosocial needs include the following:

- Love and affection
- Acceptance by others
- Safety and security
- Self-reliance and independence in daily living
- Contact with others (Fig. 3-1)
- Success and self-esteem

Health and well-being affect how well psychosocial needs are met. Stress and frustration occur when basic needs are not met. This can lead to fear, anxiety, anger, aggression, withdrawal, indifference, and depression. Stress can also cause physical problems that may eventually lead to illness.

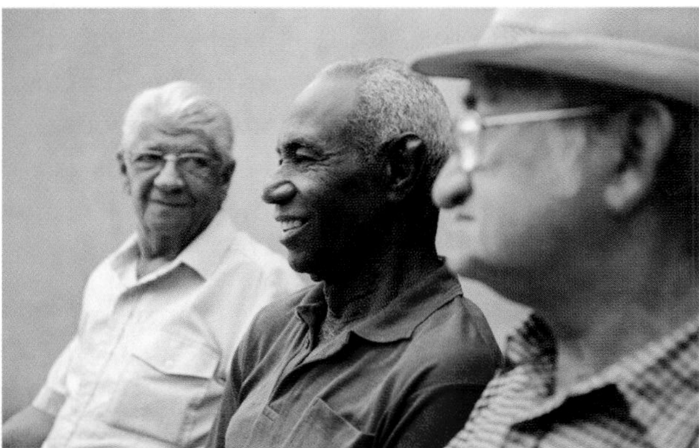

***Fig. 3-1.** Interaction with other people is a basic psychosocial need. Nursing assistants can encourage residents to spend time with others. Social contact is important.*

Abraham Maslow was a researcher of human behavior. He wrote about human physical and psychosocial needs. He arranged these needs by order of importance. He thought that physical needs must be met before psychosocial needs can be met. His theory is called *Maslow's Hierarchy of Needs* (Fig. 3-2).

Human beings also have sexual needs. These needs continue throughout their lives. Sexual urges do not end due to age or admission to a care facility. The ability to engage in sexual activity, such as intercourse and masturbation, continues unless disease or injury occurs to prevent it. **Masturbation** means to touch or rub sexual organs in order to give oneself or another person sexual pleasure. Residents have the right to choose how they express their sexuality. In all age groups, there is a variety of sexual behavior. This is also true of residents.

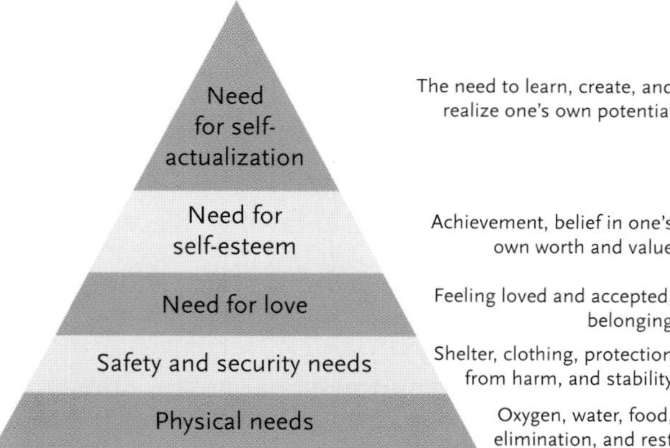

Fig. 3-2. *Maslow's Hierarchy of Needs is a model developed by Abraham Maslow to show how physical and psychosocial needs are arranged in order of importance.*

Guidelines: Respecting Sexual Needs

- **G** Always knock or announce yourself before entering residents' rooms. Listen and wait for a response before entering.
- **G** If you encounter a sexual situation between consenting adult residents, provide privacy and leave the room.
- **G** Be open and nonjudgmental about residents' sexual attitudes. Respect residents' sexual orientation and gender identity. No matter what your personal or religious feelings regarding sexuality may be, always treat residents with respect.
- **G** When possible, ask transgender residents which pronouns they would like you to use, and use them (using "she," for example, to refer to a resident who has a penis but identifies as female). Always use a transgender person's chosen name.
- **G** Honor *Do Not Disturb* signs.
- **G** Do not view expression of sexuality by the elderly as disgusting or cute. That attitude is inappropriate. It deprives residents of their right to dignity and respect.

Residents' Rights

Sexual Abuse

Residents must be protected from unwanted sexual advances. If an NA sees sexual abuse happening, he should remove the resident from the situation and take the resident to a safe place. The NA should then report to the nurse immediately.

Helping residents meet their spiritual needs can help them cope with illness or disability. Spirituality is a sensitive area. NAs must never make judgments about residents' spiritual beliefs or try to push their own beliefs on residents.

Guidelines: Respecting Spiritual Needs

- **G** Learn about residents' religions or beliefs. Listen carefully to what residents say.
- **G** Respect residents' decisions to participate in, or refrain from, food-related rituals.
- **G** If residents are religious, encourage participation in religious services.
- **G** Respect all religious items.
- **G** Report to the nurse (or social worker) if a resident expresses the desire to see clergy.
- **G** Allow privacy for clergy visits.
- **G** If asked, read religious materials aloud. If you are uncomfortable doing this, find another staff member who is not.
- **G** If a resident asks you, help find spiritual resources in the area. Check the internet for churches, synagogues, mosques, and other houses of worship. You can also refer this request to the nurse or social worker.
- **G** You should never do any of the following:
    - Try to change someone's religion
    - Tell residents their belief or religion is wrong
    - Express judgments about a religious group
    - Insist residents join religious activities

- Interfere with religious practices
- Discuss your personal beliefs or opinions, either directly or indirectly

2. Define *holistic care*

Holistic means considering a whole system, such as a whole person, rather than dividing the system up into parts. **Holistic care** means caring for the whole person—the mind as well as the body. This is the approach NAs should use when caring for residents. Caring for a person holistically is part of providing person-centered care. Person-centered care revolves around the resident and promotes his or her individual preferences, choices, dignity, and interests. A simple example of holistic care is taking time to talk with residents while helping them bathe. The NA is meeting the physical need with the bath and meeting the psychosocial need for interaction with others at the same time.

3. Explain why promoting independence and self-care is important

Any big change in lifestyle, such as moving into a long-term care facility, requires a huge emotional adjustment. Residents may be experiencing fear, loss, and uncertainty, along with their decline in health and independence. Other common reactions to illness are denial, withdrawal, anger, and depression. All of these feelings may cause residents to behave differently than they have before. Each person adjusts to illness and change in his or her own way and in his or her own time. It is important for NAs to be supportive and encouraging. NAs should be patient, understanding, and empathetic.

Moving to a care facility represents a tremendous loss of independence for a resident. Somebody else must now do what residents did for themselves all of their lives. It is also difficult for residents' friends and family members. For example, a resident may have been the main provider for his or her family. A resident may have been the person who did all of the cooking for the family. Other losses residents may be experiencing include the following:

- Loss of spouse, family members, or friends due to death
- Loss of workplace and its relationships due to retirement
- Loss of ability to go to favorite places
- Loss of ability to attend services and meetings at their faith communities
- Loss of home and personal possessions (Fig. 3-3)
- Loss of health and ability to care for themselves
- Loss of ability to move freely
- Loss of pets
- Lesbian, gay, bisexual, transgender, or queer (LGBTQ) residents may fear the loss of a comfortable and accepting environment.

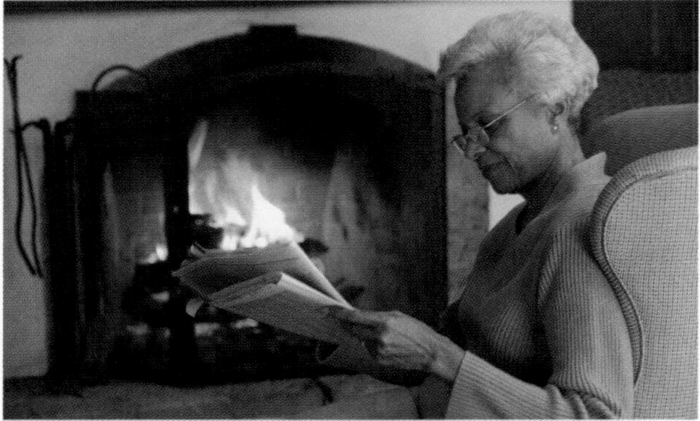

Fig. 3-3. *Nursing assistants should understand and be sympathetic to the fact that many residents had to leave familiar places.*

Independence often means not having to rely on others for money, daily care, or participation in social activities. Activities of daily living (ADLs) are the personal care tasks a person does every day to care for himself. People may take these activities for granted until they can no longer do them for themselves. ADLs include bathing or showering, dressing, caring for teeth and hair, eliminating, eating and drinking, and moving from place to place. When a person loses independence, these problems can result:

- Poor self-image
- Anger toward caregivers, others, and self
- Feelings of helplessness, sadness, and hopelessness
- Feelings of being useless
- Increased dependence
- Depression

To prevent these feelings, NAs should encourage residents to do as much as possible for themselves. Even if it seems easier for the NA to do a task for a resident, the resident should be allowed to do it independently. NAs must be patient and encourage self-care, regardless of how long it takes or how well residents are able to do it (Fig. 3-4).

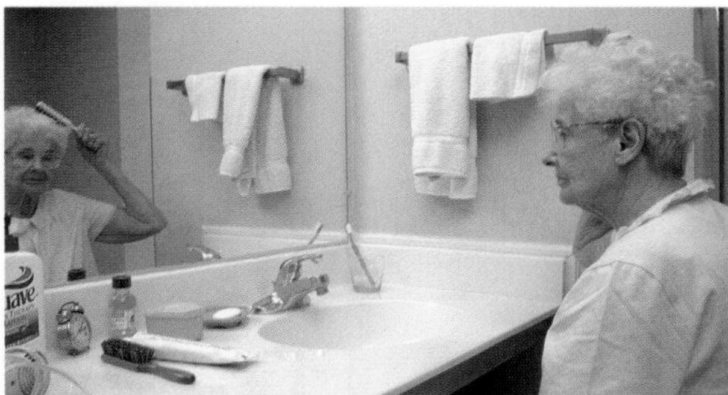

Fig. 3-4. *Even if tasks take a long time, residents should be encouraged to do what they can for themselves.*

Allowing residents to make choices is another way to promote independence and person-centered care. For example, residents can choose where to sit while they eat. They can choose what they eat and in what order. NAs must respect a resident's right to make choices.

Residents' Rights

Dignity and Independence

Residents are adults; they should not be treated like children. NAs should encourage residents to do self-care without rushing them. Residents have the right to refuse care and to make their own choices. Promoting dignity and independence is part of protecting their legal rights. It is also the proper and ethical way for NAs to work.

4. Identify ways to accommodate cultural differences

The term **cultural diversity** refers to different groups of people with varied backgrounds and experiences living together in the world. Positive responses to cultural diversity include acceptance and knowledge, not prejudice. Each culture may have different knowledge, behaviors, beliefs, values, attitudes, religions, and customs. Nursing assistants will take care of residents with backgrounds and traditions different from their own. It is important that NAs respect and value each person as an individual. They should respond to differences and new experiences with acceptance.

There are so many different cultures that they cannot all be listed here. One might talk about American culture being different from Japanese culture. But within American culture there are thousands of different groups with their own cultures. Japanese Americans, African Americans, and Native Americans are just a few. Even people from a particular region, state, or city can be said to have a different culture (Fig. 3-5). The culture of the South is not the same as the culture of New York City.

Cultural background affects how friendly people are to strangers. It can affect how close they want others to stand to them when talking. It can affect how they feel about NAs performing care for them or discussing their health with them. NAs should be sensitive to residents' backgrounds. They may have to adjust their behavior around some residents. Regardless of background, all residents must be treated with respect and professionalism. NAs should expect to be treated respectfully as well.

A resident's primary language may be different from the NA's. If the resident speaks a different language, an interpreter may be necessary. It can be helpful if staff learn a few common phrases in a resident's language. Picture cards and flash cards can assist with communication.

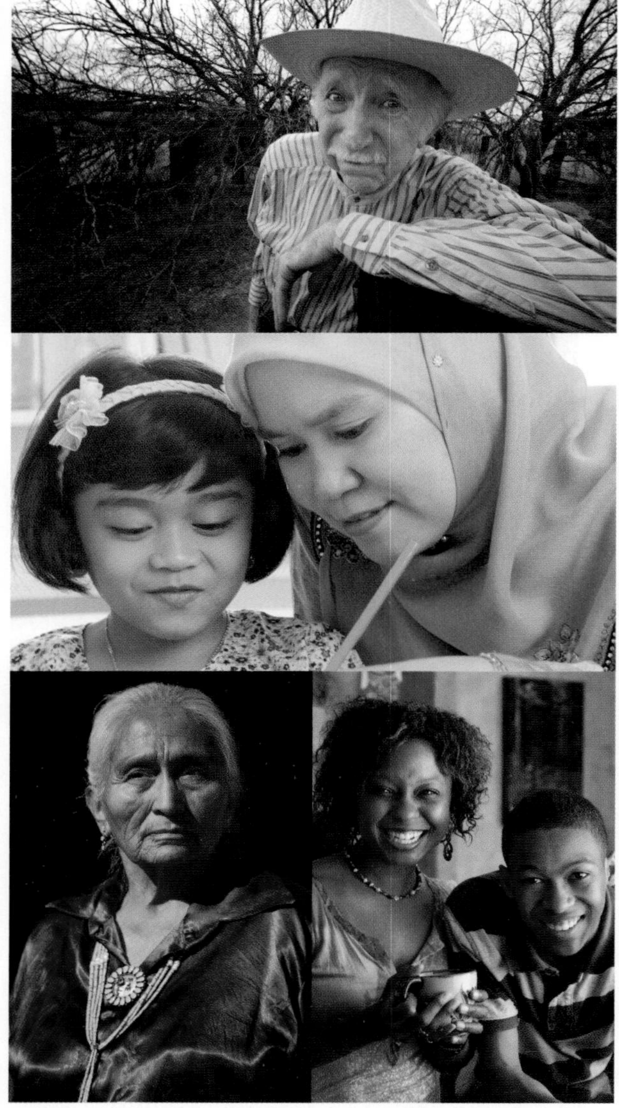

Fig. 3-5. There are many different cultures in the United States.

Religious differences also influence the way people behave. Religion may be very important in people's lives, particularly when they are ill or dying. Nursing assistants must respect the religious beliefs and practices of residents. Respect for residents' beliefs regarding religion and spirituality is a way in which NAs provide person-centered care. NAs should not question residents' beliefs or discuss their beliefs with residents.

Some specific practices affect an NA's work. Many religious beliefs include dietary restrictions. These are rules about what and when followers can eat and drink. For example, many Jewish people do not eat pork. (Chapter 8 has more information about food preferences and special diets.)

Some people's backgrounds may make them less comfortable being touched. The NA should ask permission before touching residents. He should be sensitive to their feelings. NAs must touch residents in order to do their jobs. However, they should recognize that some residents feel more comfortable when there is little physical contact. The NA should learn about his residents and adjust care to their needs.

Residents' Rights

Culturally Sensitive Care

Nursing assistants should focus on compassionate, respectful, and culturally sensitive care. An NA should treat residents as residents wish to be treated, not as the NA would want to be treated. This is part of person-centered care. Culture, age, family, and background shape each person's way of thinking. It is important for the NA to ask questions to find out what is appropriate and to always respect residents' choices, beliefs, and behaviors.

5. Describe the need for activity

Activity is an essential part of a person's life; it improves and maintains physical and mental health. Meaningful activities help promote independence, memory, self-esteem, and quality of life. In addition, physical activity can help manage illnesses, such as diabetes, high blood pressure, or high cholesterol. Regular physical activity can also help in these ways:

- Lessening the risk of heart disease, colon cancer, diabetes, and obesity
- Relieving symptoms of anxiety and depression
- Improving mood and concentration
- Improving body function
- Lowering the risk of falls

- Improving sleep quality
- Improving the ability to cope with stress
- Increasing energy
- Increasing appetite and promoting better eating habits

Inactivity and immobility can result in physical and mental problems, such as the following:

- Loss of self-esteem
- Anxiety
- Depression
- Boredom
- Pneumonia
- Urinary tract infection
- Skin breakdown and pressure injuries
- Constipation
- Blood clots
- Dulling of the senses

OBRA requires that facilities provide an activities program designed to meet the interests and the physical and psychosocial well-being of each resident. The activities are created to help residents socialize and keep them physically and mentally active. Daily schedules are normally posted with activities for that particular day. Activities include exercise, arts and crafts, board games, newspapers, magazines, books, music, TV and radio, pet therapy, gardening, and group religious events. When activities are scheduled, NAs should help residents with grooming beforehand, as needed and requested. They should assist with any personal care that residents require. NAs may need to help residents with walking and wheelchairs as well.

6. Discuss family roles and their significance in health care

Families play an important part in most people's lives. Often a family is defined by the level of support people have rather than by biological relationships. There are many different kinds of families (Fig. 3-6):

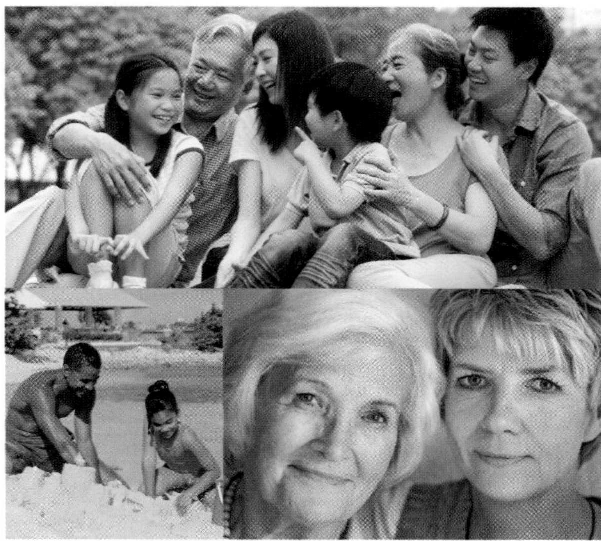

Fig. 3-6. *Families come in all shapes and sizes.*

- Nuclear families (two parents and one or more children)
- Single-parent families (one parent and one or more children)
- Married or committed couples of the same sex or opposite sex, with or without children
- Extended families (parents, children, grandparents, aunts, uncles, cousins, other relatives, and even friends)
- Blended families (divorced or widowed parents who have remarried and have children from previous relationships and/or the current marriage)

Whatever kinds of families residents have, they have an important role to play. Family members help in many ways:

- Helping residents make care decisions
- Communicating with the care team
- Giving support and encouragement
- Connecting the resident to the outside world
- Offering assurance to dying residents that family memories and traditions will be valued and carried on

NAs should be respectful to friends and family members and allow privacy for visits. After any visitor leaves, the NA should observe the effect the visit had on the resident. Any noticeable effects should be reported to the nurse. Some residents have good relationships with their families. Others do not. Any abusive behavior from a visitor toward a resident should be reported immediately to the charge nurse.

Families are great sources of information for residents' personal preferences, history, diet, habits, and routines. The NA should ask them questions. Families often seek out nursing assistants because they are closest to the residents. This is an important responsibility. NAs should show families that they have time for them. They can communicate with family members but cannot discuss a resident's care. Any questions about care should be reported to the nurse.

7. Describe the stages of human growth and development

Throughout their lives, people change physically and psychologically. These changes are called human growth and development. Everyone will go through the same stages of development. However, no two people will follow the exact pattern or rate of development. Each resident must be treated as an individual and a whole person who is growing and developing. He or she should not be treated as someone who is merely ill or disabled.

Infancy (Birth to 12 Months)

Infants grow and develop very quickly. In one year, a baby moves from total dependence to the relative independence of moving around, communicating basic needs, and feeding himself. Physical development in infancy moves from the head down. For example, infants gain control over the muscles of the neck before the muscles in their shoulders. Control over muscles in the trunk area, such as the shoulders, develops before control of the arms and legs (Fig. 3-7).

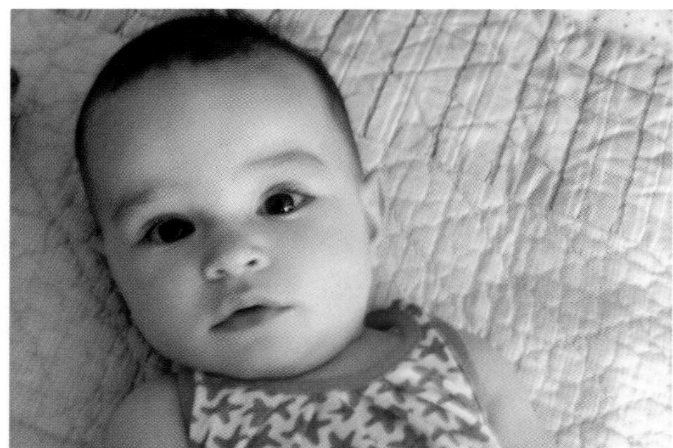

Fig. 3-7. *An infant's physical development moves from the head down.*

Toddler (Ages 1 to 3)

During the toddler years, children gain independence. One part of this independence is new control over their bodies. Toddlers learn to speak, gain coordination of their limbs, and learn to control their bladders and bowels (Fig. 3-8). Toddlers assert their new independence by exploring. Poisons and other hazards, such as sharp objects, must be locked away. Psychologically, toddlers learn that they are individuals, separate from their parents. Children of this age may try to control their parents. They may try to get what they want by throwing tantrums, whining, or refusing to cooperate. This is a key time for parents to set rules and standards.

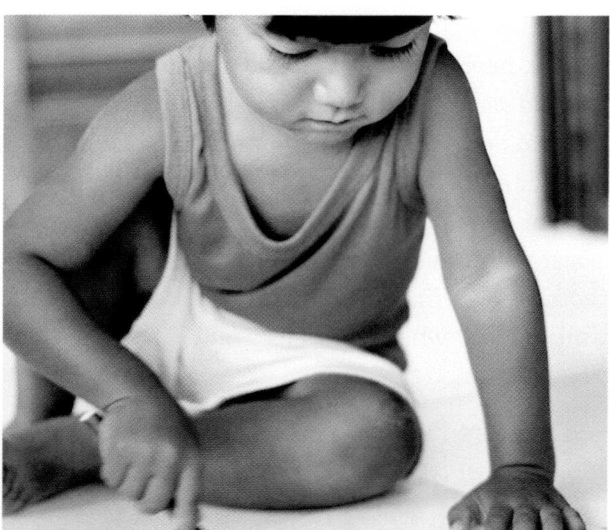

Fig. 3-8. *Toddlers gain coordination of their limbs.*

Preschool (Ages 3 to 6)

Children in their preschool years develop skills that help them become more independent and have social relationships (Fig. 3-9). They learn new words and language skills. They learn to play in groups. They become more physically coordinated and learn to care for themselves. Preschoolers also develop ways of relating to family members. They begin to learn right from wrong.

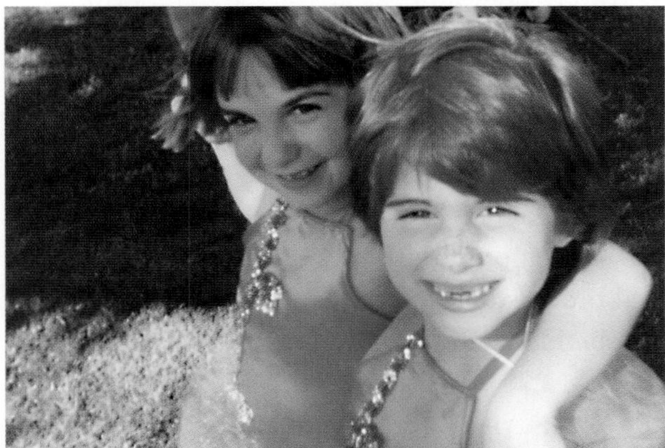

Fig. 3-9. *Children in preschool years develop social relationships.*

School-Age (Ages 6 to 10)

From ages 6 to about 10 years, children's development is centered on **cognitive** (related to thinking and learning) and social development. As children enter school, they also explore the world around them. They relate to other children through games, peer groups, and classroom activities. In these years, children learn to get along with each other. They also begin to behave in ways common to their gender. They begin to develop a conscience, morals, and self-esteem.

Preadolescence (Ages 10 to 13)

During the years between 10 and 13, children enjoy a growing sense of self-identity and a strong sense of identity with their peers. They tend to be very social. This is usually a relatively calm period, and preadolescents are often easy to get along with and able to handle more responsibility at home and school. Childhood fears of ghosts or monsters will give way to fears based in the real world. It is important that preadolescents feel able to trust in the attention and care of parents or other adults. Girls may reach puberty in the later years of this stage. During puberty, a person develops secondary sex characteristics, such as body hair.

Adolescence (Ages 13 to 19)

During adolescence, genders become sexually mature. Boys usually reach puberty during this stage. If girls did not reach puberty during the previous stage, it will start here. Many teenagers have a hard time adapting to the changes that occur in their bodies during puberty. Peer acceptance is important to them. Adolescents may be afraid that they are unattractive or abnormal. This concern for body image and acceptance, combined with changing hormones that influence moods, can cause rapid mood swings. Pressures develop as they remain dependent on their parents and yet need to express themselves socially and sexually (Fig. 3-10). This can cause conflict and stress.

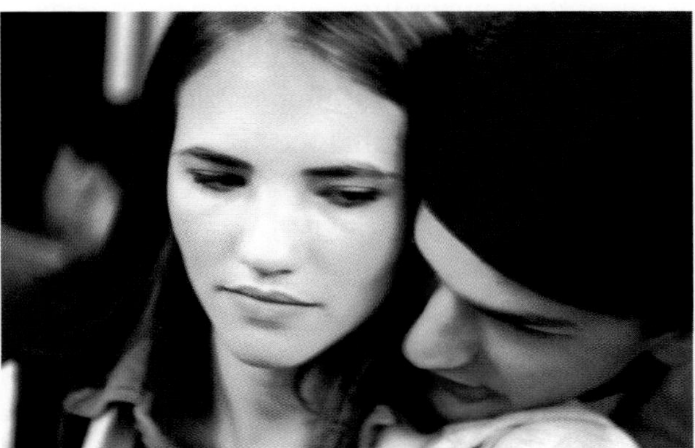

Fig. 3-10. *Adolescence is a time of adapting to change.*

Young Adulthood (Ages 19 to 40)

Physical growth has usually been completed by this time. Adopting a healthy lifestyle in these years can make life better now and prevent health problems in later adulthood. Psychological and social development continues, however. The tasks of these years include the following:

- Selecting an appropriate education
- Selecting an occupation or career
- Selecting a mate (Fig. 3-11)
- Learning to live with a mate or others
- Raising children
- Developing a satisfying sex life

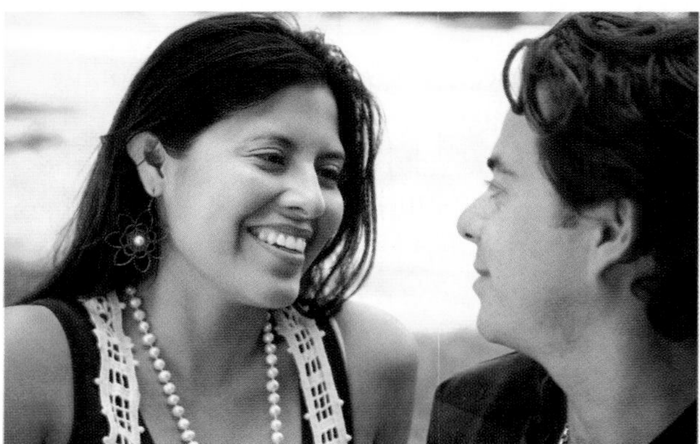

Fig. 3-11. *Young adulthood often involves finding mates.*

Middle Adulthood (Ages 40 to 65)

In general, people in middle adulthood are more comfortable and stable than they were before. Many of their major life decisions have already been made. Physical changes related to aging also occur in middle adulthood. Adults in this age group may notice that they have difficulty maintaining their weight or notice a decrease in strength and energy. Metabolism and other body functions slow down. Wrinkles and gray hair appear. Many diseases and illnesses can develop in these years. These disorders can become chronic and life-threatening.

Late Adulthood (65 years and older)

Persons in late adulthood must adjust to the effects of aging. These changes can include the loss of strength and health, the death of loved ones, retirement, and preparation for their own death. The developmental tasks of this age may seem to deal entirely with loss. But solutions to these problems often involve new relationships, friendships, and interests.

Later adulthood covers an age range of as many as 25 to 35 years. People in this age category can have very different abilities, depending on their health. Some 70-year-old people enjoy active sports, while others are not active. Many 85-year-old people can still live alone. Others may live with family members or in skilled care facilities.

Ideas about older people are often false. They create prejudices against the elderly. These are as unfair as prejudices against racial, ethnic, or religious groups. In movies, older people are often shown as helpless, lonely, disabled, slow, forgetful, dependent, or inactive. However, research shows that most older people are active and engaged in work, volunteer activities, and learning and exercise programs. Aging is a normal process, not a disease. Most older people live independent lives and do not need assistance (Fig. 3-12). Prejudice toward, stereotyping of, and/or discrimination against older persons or the elderly is called **ageism**.

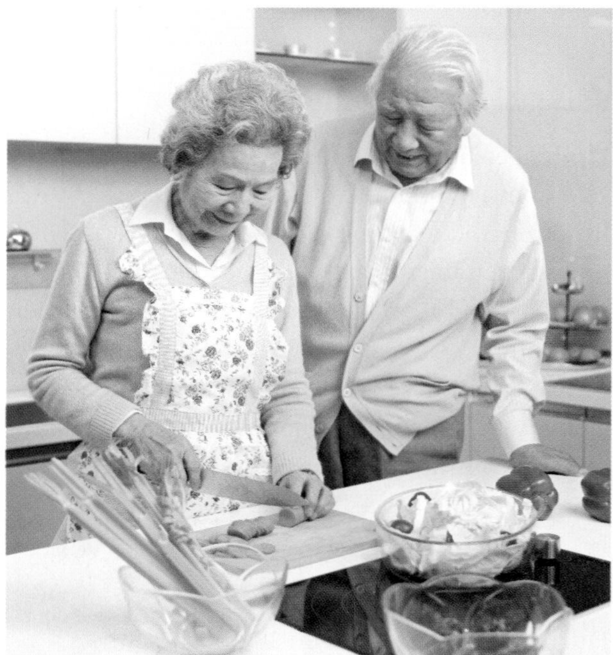

Fig. 3-12. *Most older people lead active lives.*

Nursing assistants are likely to spend much of their time working with residents who are elderly. They must be able to know what is true about aging and what is not true. Aging causes many changes. However, normal changes of aging do not mean an older person must become dependent, ill, or inactive. Knowing normal changes of aging from signs of illness or disability will allow NAs to better help residents. Normal changes of aging include the following:

- Skin is thinner, drier, more fragile, and less elastic.
- Muscles weaken and lose tone.
- Bones lose density and become more brittle.
- Sensitivity of nerve endings in the skin decreases.
- Responses and reflexes slow.
- Short-term memory loss occurs.
- Senses of vision, hearing, taste, touch, and smell weaken.
- Heart pumps less efficiently.
- Lung strength and lung capacity decrease.
- Oxygen in the blood decreases.
- Appetite decreases.
- Urinary elimination is more frequent.
- Digestion takes longer and is less efficient.
- Levels of hormones decrease.
- Immunity weakens.
- Lifestyle changes occur.

There are also changes that are NOT considered normal changes of aging and should be reported to the nurse. These include the following:

- Signs of depression
- Suicidal thoughts
- Loss of ability to think logically
- Poor nutrition
- Shortness of breath
- Incontinence

This is not a complete list. An NA's job includes reporting any change, normal or not.

8. Discuss developmental disabilities

Developmental disabilities are disabilities that are present at birth or emerge during childhood. A developmental disability is a chronic condition. It restricts physical and/or mental ability. These disabilities prevent a child from developing at a normal rate. Language, mobility, learning, and the ability to perform self-care may be affected. The care residents need will depend on the type and the extent of their disability.

An intellectual disability (formerly called *mental retardation*) is a type of developmental disability. It is neither a disease nor a mental illness. People with an intellectual disability develop at a below-average rate. They have below-average mental functioning. They have difficulty learning, communicating, moving, and may have problems adjusting socially. Their ability to care for themselves may be affected.

Despite their special needs, residents who have an intellectual disability have the same emotional and physical needs that others have. They experience the same emotions, such as anger, sadness, love, and joy, as others do, but their ability to express their emotions may be limited.

Guidelines: Intellectual Disability

- **G** Treat adult residents as adults, regardless of their intellectual abilities.
- **G** Praise and encourage often, especially positive behavior.
- **G** Help teach activities of daily living by dividing a task into smaller units.
- **G** Promote independence. Assist residents with activities and motor functions that are difficult.
- **G** Encourage social interaction.
- **G** Repeat what you say to make sure they understand.
- **G** Be patient.

9. Describe some types of mental health disorders

Mental health disorders were first discussed in Chapter 2. There are different degrees of these disorders; they can range from mild to severe.

Mood Disorders: Mood disorders are marked by changes in mood. Depression (sometimes called **major depressive disorder** or *clinical depression*) is a type of mood disorder. Depression is characterized by a loss of interest in everything a person once cared about, and may interfere with the person's ability to work, sleep, and eat. It may cause intense mental, emotional, and physical pain and disability. Depression also makes other illnesses worse. If left untreated, it may result in suicide. Clinical depression is not a normal reaction to stress. Sadness is only one symptom of this illness. Not all people who have depression complain of sadness or appear sad. Other common symptoms of clinical depression include the following:

- Pain, including headaches, stomach pain, and other body aches
- Low energy or fatigue
- **Apathy**, or lack of interest in activities
- Irritability
- Anxiety
- Loss of appetite or overeating
- Problems with sexual functioning and desire
- Sleeplessness, trouble sleeping, or excessive sleeping
- Lack of attention to basic personal care tasks (e.g., bathing, combing hair, changing clothes)
- Intense feelings of despair
- Guilt
- Trouble concentrating
- Withdrawal and isolation
- Repeated thoughts of suicide and death

People cannot overcome depression through sheer will. It is a disorder like any physical illness. It can be treated successfully. People who suffer from depression need compassion and support. An NA should know the symptoms so she can recognize the beginning or worsening of depression. Any suicide threat should be taken seriously and reported immediately. It should not be dismissed as an attempt to get attention.

Bipolar disorder causes a person to have mood swings and changes in energy levels and the ability to function. A person may swing from periods of extreme activity (a manic episode) to periods of deep depression (a depressive episode). Manic episodes can include high energy, little sleep, big speeches, rapidly changing thoughts and moods, high self-esteem, overspending, and poor judgment. These episodes may last days, weeks, or months.

Anxiety Disorders: **Anxiety** is uneasiness, worry, or fear, often about a situation or condition. When a person who is mentally healthy feels anxiety, he usually knows the cause. The anxiety fades once the cause is removed. A person who has a mental health disorder may feel anxiety all the time. He may not know the reason why. Anxiety causes physical symptoms such as shakiness, muscle aches, sweating, cold and clammy hands, dizziness, chest pain, rapid heartbeat, cold or hot flashes, a choking or smothering sensation, and a dry mouth.

One type of anxiety disorder is **generalized anxiety disorder (GAD)**. GAD is characterized by chronic anxiety and worry, even when there is no reason for concern. A person with GAD may be excessively worried about health, finances, work, or other issues.

A panic attack is an episode of intense fear that occurs along with physical symptoms, such as rapid heartbeat, chest pain, dizziness, and shortness of breath. A person having a panic attack may think he is having a heart attack or dying. Having regular panic attacks or living with constant anxiety about having another attack is classified as **panic disorder**.

Obsessive-compulsive disorder (**OCD**) is an anxiety disorder characterized by obsessive behavior or thoughts. This may cause the person to repeatedly perform a behavior or routine. For example, a person may wash his hands over and over as a way to ease anxiety. **Posttraumatic stress disorder** (**PTSD**) is an anxiety disorder brought on by experiencing a traumatic event, such as being a victim of a violent crime or being involved in combat while in the military.

A **phobia** is an intense, irrational fear of or anxiety about an object, place, or situation. Many people are afraid of some things or situations. Examples are a fear of dogs or a fear of flying. A phobia can be long-lasting. It may prevent the person from doing normal things. For example, the fear of being in a confined space, **claustrophobia**, may make using an elevator terrifying.

Psychotic Disorders: Psychotic disorders are severe mental disorders marked by abnormal thinking and problems with understanding reality. Schizophrenia is one type of psychotic disorder. **Schizophrenia** affects a person's ability to think and communicate clearly. It also affects the ability to manage emotions, make decisions, and understand reality. It affects a person's ability to interact with other people. Treatment makes it possible for many people to lead relatively normal lives.

Hallucinations and delusions are two symptoms of schizophrenia. **Hallucinations** are false or distorted sensory perceptions. A person may see something that is not really there or hear a conversation that is not real. **Delusions** are persistent false beliefs. For example, a person may believe that other people are controlling his thoughts.

Guidelines: Mental Health Disorders

G Observe residents carefully for changes in condition or abilities. Document and report your observations.

G Support the resident and his family and friends. Coping with a mental health disorder can be frustrating. Your positive, professional attitude can help the resident and his family.

G Encourage residents to do as much as possible for themselves. Progress may be very slow. Be patient, supportive, and positive.

G Mental health disorders can be treated. Medication and psychotherapy are common methods. Medication must be taken properly to promote benefits and reduce side effects. **Psychotherapy** involves talking about one's problems with mental health professionals. **Cognitive behavioral therapy** (**CBT**) is a type of psychotherapy that is often used to treat anxiety and depression. This type of therapy is usually short-term and focuses on skills and solutions that a person can use to modify negative thinking and behavior patterns.

Observing and Reporting: Mental Health Disorders

O/R Changes in ability

O/R Positive or negative mood changes, especially withdrawal (Fig. 3-13)

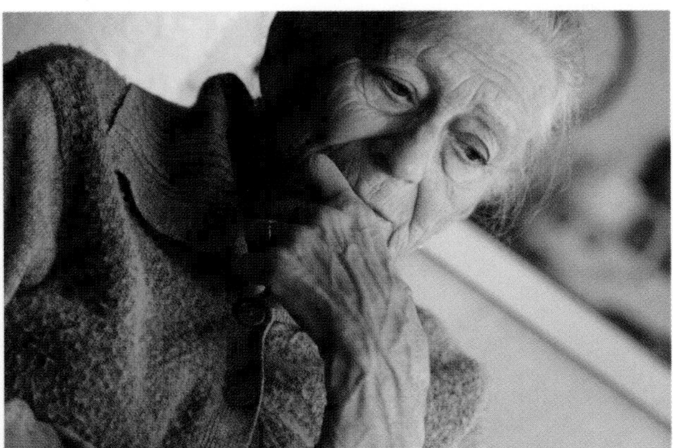

Fig. 3-13. *Withdrawal is an important change to report.*

O/R Behavior changes, including changes in personality, extreme behavior, and behavior that does not seem to fit the situation

- O/R Comments, even jokes, about hurting oneself or others
- O/R Failure to take medicine or improper use of medicine
- O/R Real or imagined physical symptoms
- O/R Events, situations, or people that seem to upset or excite residents

Intellectual Disabilities and Mental Health Disorders

People may confuse the terms *intellectual disability* and *mental health disorder*. They are not the same. An intellectual disability is a developmental disability that causes below-average mental functioning. It may affect a person's ability to care for himself, as well as to live independently. It is not a type of mental health disorder.

An intellectual disability affects mental ability. A mental health disorder may or may not affect mental ability. There is no cure for an intellectual disability, although persons who have an intellectual disability can be helped. Many mental health disorders can be cured with treatment, such as medications and therapy.

Although they are different conditions, persons who have either condition need emotional support, as well as care and treatment.

10. Explain how to care for residents who are dying

Death can occur suddenly without warning, or it can be expected. Older people or those with terminal illnesses may have time to prepare for death. A **terminal illness** is a disease or condition that will eventually cause death. Preparing for death is a process. It affects the dying person's emotions and behavior.

Grief is deep distress or sorrow over a loss. It is an adaptive, or changing process, and usually involves healing. Dr. Elisabeth Kübler-Ross studied and wrote about the grief process. Her book, *On Death and Dying*, describes five stages that dying people and their loved ones may reach before death. These five stages are listed below.

Not all people go through all the stages. Some may stay in one stage until death occurs. Others may move back and forth between stages during the process.

Denial: People in the denial stage may refuse to believe they are dying. They often believe a mistake has been made. They may avoid discussion about their illness. They may simply act like it is not happening.

Anger: Once people start to face the possibility of their death, they may become angry. They may be angry because they think they are too young to die. They may be angry because they feel they have always taken care of themselves.

Bargaining: Once people have begun to believe that they are dying, they may make promises to God, care providers, or others. They may somehow try to bargain for their recovery.

Depression: As dying people get weaker and symptoms get worse, they may become deeply sad or depressed. They may cry or withdraw or be unable to do even simple things.

Acceptance: Peace or acceptance may or may not come before death. Some people who are dying are eventually able to accept death and prepare for it. They may arrange with loved ones for the care of important people or things. They may make plans for their last days or for the ceremonies that may follow their death.

Advance directives are legal documents that allow people to decide what kind of medical care they wish to have if they are unable to make those decisions themselves. An advance directive can also name someone else to make medical decisions for a person if that person becomes ill or disabled. A living will and a durable power of attorney for health care are examples of advance directives.

A **living will** outlines the medical care a person wants, or does not want, in case he or she becomes unable to make those decisions. It is called a *living will* because it takes effect while the person is still alive. It may also be called a *directive to physicians, health care declaration,* or *medical directive.* A living will is not the same thing as a will. A will is a legal declaration of how a person wishes his or her possessions to be distributed after death.

A **durable power of attorney for health care** (sometimes called *health care proxy*) is a signed, dated, and witnessed legal document that appoints someone else to make medical decisions for a person in the event he or she becomes unable to do so. This can include instructions about medical treatment that the person does not want.

A **do-not-resuscitate** (**DNR**) order is another tool that helps medical providers honor wishes about care. A DNR is a medical order that tells medical professionals not to perform CPR. A DNR order means that medical personnel will not attempt emergency CPR if the person's heartbeat or breathing stops.

> Residents' Rights
>
> **Advance Directives**
>
> By law, advance directives and DNR orders must be honored. Nursing assistants should respect each resident's decisions about advance directives. This is a very personal and private matter. NAs should not make comments about residents' choices to anyone, including family members, other residents, or staff.

Death is a very sensitive topic. Many people find it hard to discuss death. Feelings and attitudes about death can be formed by many factors:

- Experiences with death
- Personality type
- Religious beliefs
- Cultural background

Guidelines: Caring for the Dying Resident

G **Diminished senses**: Vision may begin to fail. Reduce glare and keep room lighting low (Fig. 3-14). Hearing is usually the last sense to leave the body. Speak in a normal tone. Tell the resident about care that is being done or what is happening in the room. Do not expect an answer. Ask few questions. Observe body language to anticipate a resident's needs.

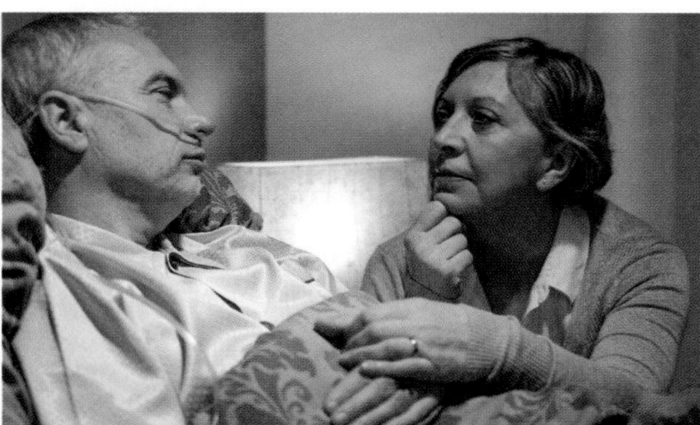

Fig. 3-14. *Keep a resident's room softly lit without glare.*

G **Care of the mouth and nose**: Give mouth care often. If the resident is unconscious, give mouth care every two hours. The lips and nostrils may be dry and cracked. Apply lubricant, such as lip balm, to the lips and nose.

G **Skin care**: Give bed baths and incontinence care as needed. Bathe perspiring residents often. Skin should be kept clean and dry. Change sheets and clothes for comfort. Keep sheets wrinkle-free. Careful skin care to prevent pressure injuries is important. (Chapter 6 has information about pressure injuries.)

G **Pain control and comfort**: Pain relief is critical. Residents may not be able to tell you that they are in pain. Observe body language and watch for other signs of pain. Report them. Frequent changes of position, back massage, skin care, mouth care, and proper body alignment may help.

G **Environment**: Put favorite objects and photographs where the resident can easily see them. Make sure the room is comfortable, appropriately lit, and well-ventilated. When leaving the room, place the call light within reach. Do this even if the resident is unaware of his surroundings.

G **Emotional and spiritual support**: Listening may be one of the most important things you can do for a resident who is dying. Pay attention to these conversations. Report any comments about fear to the nurse. Touch can also be important. Holding the resident's hand as you sit quietly can be very comforting. Do not avoid the dying person or his family. Do not deny that death is approaching. Do not tell the resident that anyone knows how or when it will happen. Do give accurate information in a reassuring way. If other residents ask for information about the dying resident, refer their questions to the nurse.

Some residents may seek spiritual comfort from clergy. Give privacy for visits from clergy, family, and friends. Do not discuss your religious or spiritual beliefs with residents or their families or make recommendations.

NAs can treat residents with dignity when they are approaching death by respecting their rights and their preferences. There are some legal rights to remember when caring for people who are dying:

The right to refuse treatment. NAs must remember that whether they agree or disagree with a resident's decisions, the choice is not theirs. It belongs to the person involved and/or his family. NAs should be supportive of family members and not judge them. They are most likely following the resident's wishes.

The right to have visitors. When death is close, it is an emotional time for all those involved. Saying goodbye can be a very important part of dealing with a loved one's death. It may also be reassuring to the person who is dying to have someone in the room, even if the person does not seem to be aware of his surroundings.

The right to privacy. Privacy is a basic legal right, but privacy for visiting, or even when the person is alone, may be even more important now.

Other rights of a dying person are listed below in *The Dying Person's Bill of Rights*. This was created at a workshop, *The Terminally Ill Patient and the Helping Person*, sponsored by the Southwestern Michigan In-Service Education Council, and appeared in the *American Journal of Nursing*, Vol. 75, January 1975, p. 99.

I have the right to:

- Be treated as a living human being until I die.
- Maintain a sense of hopefulness, however changing its focus may be.
- Be cared for by those who can maintain a sense of hopefulness, however changing this might be.
- Express my feelings and emotions about my approaching death in my own way.
- Participate in decisions concerning my care.
- Expect continuing medical and nursing attentions even though "cure" goals must be changed to "comfort" goals.
- Not die alone.
- Be free from pain.
- Have my questions answered honestly.
- Not be deceived.
- Have help from and for my family in accepting my death.
- Die in peace and dignity.
- Retain my individuality and not be judged for my decisions, which may be contrary to the beliefs of others.
- Discuss and enlarge my religious and/or spiritual experiences, whatever these may mean to others.
- Expect that the sanctity of the human body will be respected after death.

- Be cared for by caring, sensitive, knowledgeable people who will attempt to understand my needs and will be able to gain some satisfaction in helping me face my death.

Guidelines: Treating Residents Who Are Dying with Dignity

G Respect the resident's wishes in all possible ways. Communication is extremely important at this time so that everyone understands what the resident's wishes are. Listen carefully for ideas on how to provide simple gestures that may be special and appreciated.

G Do not isolate or avoid a resident who is dying. Enter his room regularly.

G Be careful not to make promises that cannot or should not be kept.

G Continue to involve the resident in his care and in facility activities. Be person-centered. Do not talk with other staff members about your personal life when caring for a resident.

G Listen if a resident wants to talk but do not offer advice. Do not make judgmental comments.

G Do not babble or act especially cheerful or sad. Be professional.

G Keep the resident as comfortable as possible. The nurse needs to know immediately if pain medication is requested. Keep the resident clean and dry.

G Assure privacy when it is desired.

G Respect the privacy of the family and other visitors. They may be upset and not want to be social at this time. They may welcome a friendly smile, however, and should not be isolated, either.

G Help with the family's physical comfort. If requested, get them coffee, water, chairs, blankets, etc.

Common signs of approaching death include the following:

- Blurred and failing vision
- Unfocused eyes
- Impaired speech
- Diminished sense of touch
- Loss of movement, muscle tone, and feeling
- A rising or below-normal body temperature
- Decreasing blood pressure
- Weak pulse that is abnormally slow or rapid
- Alternating periods of slow, irregular respirations and rapid, shallow respirations, along with short periods of not breathing, called **Cheyne-Stokes** respirations
- A rattling or gurgling sound as the person breathes (which does not cause discomfort for the dying person)
- Cold, pale skin
- Mottling (bruised appearance), spotting, or blotching of skin caused by poor circulation
- Perspiration
- Incontinence (both urine and stool)
- Disorientation or confusion

When death occurs, the body will not have a heartbeat, pulse, respiration, or blood pressure. The eyelids may remain open or partially open with the eyes in a fixed stare. The mouth may remain open. The body may be incontinent of urine and stool. Between two to six hours after death, the muscles in the body become stiff and rigid. This is a temporary condition called *rigor mortis,* which is Latin for *stiffness of death.* Though these things are a normal part of death, they can be frightening. NAs should inform the nurse immediately to help confirm the death.

Postmortem care is care of the body after death. It takes place after the resident has been declared dead by a nurse or doctor. NAs must be sensitive to the needs of the family and friends after death. Family members may wish to sit by the bed to say goodbye. They may wish to stay with the body for a while. They should be allowed to do these things. NAs should be aware of religious and cultural practices that the family wants to observe. NAs should follow their facility's policies and only perform assigned tasks.

Guidelines: Postmortem Care

- **G** Bathe the body. Be gentle to avoid bruising. Place drainage pads where needed. This is most often under the head and/or under the perineum (the genital and anal area). Follow Standard Precautions.
- **G** Do not remove any tubes or other equipment attached to the body. A nurse or someone at the funeral home will do this.
- **G** If instructed, put dentures back in the mouth. Close the mouth. If not possible, place dentures in a denture cup near the resident's head.
- **G** Close the eyes carefully.
- **G** Position the body on the back with legs straight and arms folded across the abdomen. Put a small pillow under the head.
- **G** Follow facility policy about personal items. Check to see if you should remove jewelry. Always have a witness if personal items are removed or given to a family member. Document what was given to whom.
- **G** Strip the bed after the body has been removed. Open windows to air the room as needed. Straighten up.
- **G** Document according to your facility's policy.

Dealing with grief after the death of a loved one is an individual process. No two people will grieve in exactly the same way. It is also a changing or adaptive process. Feelings may change from day to day, or even hour to hour. This is normal. Clergy, counselors, or social workers can help people who are grieving (Fig. 3-15). Family members or friends may have any of these reactions to the death of a loved one:

- Shock
- Denial
- Anger
- Guilt
- Regret
- Relief
- Sadness
- Loneliness

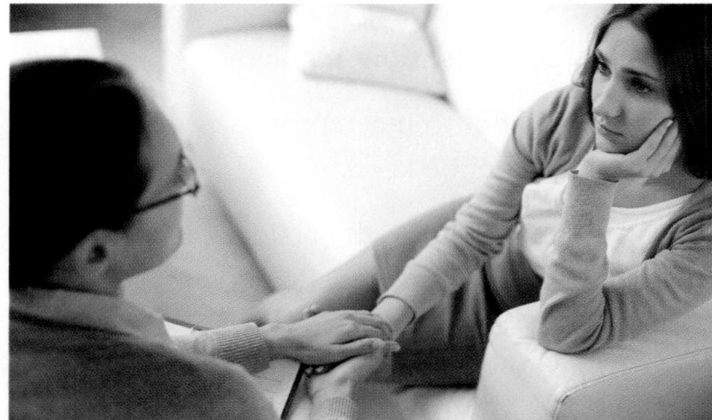

Fig. 3-15. *Some people will speak with counselors to help them deal with their grief.*

11. Define the goals of a hospice program

Hospice care is the term for the special care that a dying person needs. It is a compassionate way to care for dying people and their families. Hospice care uses a holistic, person-centered approach. It treats the person's physical, emotional, spiritual, and social needs.

Hospice care can be given seven days a week, 24 hours a day. It is available with a doctor's order. Hospice care may be given in a hospital, at a care facility, or in the home. A hospice can be any location where a person who is dying is treated with dignity by caregivers. Any caregiver may give hospice care, but often specially trained nurses and volunteers provide it.

Hospice care helps to meet all needs of the resident who is dying. The resident, as well as family and friends, are directly involved in care decisions. The resident is encouraged to participate in family life and decision-making as long as possible.

In long-term care, goals focus on recovery or on the resident's ability to care for herself as much as possible. In hospice care, however, the goals are the comfort and dignity of the resident. This type of care is called **palliative care**. This is an important difference. NAs will need to change their focus when caring for residents in hospice. The focus should be on pain relief, comfort, and managing symptoms, rather than on teaching residents to care for themselves. Residents who are dying need to feel independent for as long as possible. Caregivers should allow residents to have as much control over their lives as possible. Eventually, caregivers may have to meet all of the person's basic needs.

Guidelines: Hospice Care

- **G** Be a good listener. Some people, however, will not want to confide in their caregivers. Never push someone to talk.
- **G** Respect privacy and independence.
- **G** Be sensitive to individual needs. Ask family members or friends how you can help.
- **G** Be aware of your own feelings. Know your limits and respect them.
- **G** Recognize the stress. Talking with a counselor or support group may help. Remember, however, that specific information must be kept confidential.
- **G** Take good care of yourself. Eating right, exercising, and getting enough rest are ways of taking care of yourself. Talk about and acknowledge your feelings. Take time to do things for yourself. Take a break when you need to.
- **G** Allow yourself to grieve. You will develop close relationships with some residents. Know that it is normal to feel sad, angry, or lonely when residents die.

Community Resources

Here are a few of the many community resources available to help residents meet different needs:

- Eldercare Locator, a public service of the US Administration on Aging (eldercare.gov, 800-677-1116)
- Ombudsman program (ltcombudsman.org, 202-332-2275)
- National Resource Center on LGBT Aging (lgbtagingcenter.org, 212-741-2247)
- Alzheimer's Association (alz.org, 800-272-3900)
- American Cancer Society (cancer.org, 800-227-2345)
- AIDSinfo, a service of the US Department of Health and Human Services (aidsinfo.nih.gov, 800-448-0440)
- Meals on Wheels Association of America (mealsonwheelsamerica.org, 888-998-6325)
- American Association on Intellectual and Developmental Disabilities (aaidd.org, 202-387-1968)
- National Institute of Mental Health (nimh.nih.gov, 866-615-6464)
- National Hospice and Palliative Care Organization (nhpco.org, 800-658-8898)

4 Body Systems and Related Conditions

Bodies are organized into body systems. Each system has a condition under which it works best. **Homeostasis** is the name for the condition in which all of the body's systems are working at their best. To be in homeostasis, the body's **metabolism**, or physical and chemical processes, must be working at a steady level. When disease or injury occurs, the body's metabolism is disturbed. Homeostasis is lost.

Each system in the body has its own unique structure and function. There are also normal, age-related changes for each body system. Knowing normal changes of aging will help nursing assistants better recognize any abnormal changes in residents. This chapter also includes tips on how NAs can help residents with their normal changes of aging.

The body's systems can be organized in different ways. In this book the human body is divided into ten systems:

1. Integumentary (skin)
2. Musculoskeletal
3. Nervous
4. Circulatory
5. Respiratory
6. Urinary
7. Gastrointestinal
8. Endocrine
9. Reproductive
10. Immune and Lymphatic

Body systems are made up of organs. An organ has a specific function. Organs are made up of tissues. Tissues are made up of groups of cells that perform a similar task. For example, in the circulatory system, the heart is one of the organs. It is made up of tissues and cells. Cells are the building blocks of the body. Living cells divide, grow, and die, renewing the tissues and organs of the body.

Anatomical Terms of Location

Anatomical terms of location are terms to help identify positions or directions of the body. Here are some anatomical terms used to describe location in the human body:

- Anterior or ventral: the front of the body or body part
- Posterior or dorsal: the back of the body or body part
- Superior: toward the head
- Inferior: away from the head
- Medial: toward the midline of the body
- Lateral: to the side, away from the midline of the body
- Proximal: closer to the torso
- Distal: farther away from the torso

This chapter discusses the structure and function, age-related changes, and common diseases of each body system. Dementia and Alzheimer's disease, common diseases of the nervous system, will be discussed in Chapter 5.

1. Describe the integumentary system

The largest organ and system in the body is the skin. Skin is a natural protective covering, or integument. Skin prevents injury to internal organs. It protects the body against entry of bacteria. Skin also prevents the loss of too much water, which is essential to life. Skin is made up of layers of tissues. Within these layers are sweat glands, which secrete sweat to help cool the body when needed, and sebaceous glands, which secrete oil (sebum) to keep the skin lubricated. There are also hair follicles, many tiny blood vessels (capillaries), and tiny nerve endings (Fig. 4-1).

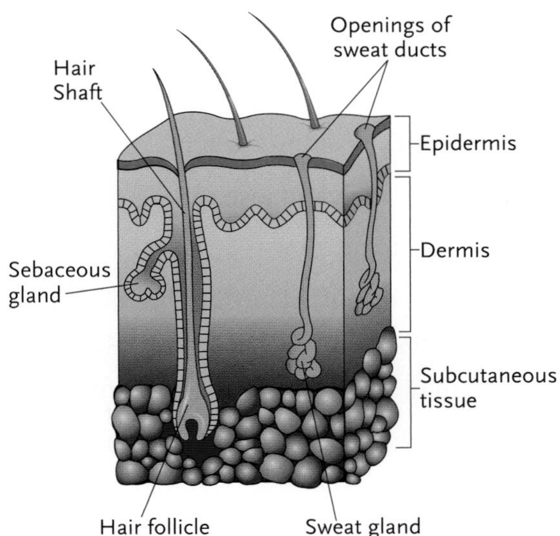

Fig. 4-1. *Cross-section showing details of the integumentary system.*

The skin is also a *sense organ*. It feels heat, cold, pain, touch, and pressure. It then tells the brain what it is feeling. Body temperature is regulated in the skin. Blood vessels **dilate**, or widen, when the outside temperature is too high. This brings more blood to the body's surface to cool it off. The same blood vessels **constrict**, or narrow, when the outside temperature is too cold. By restricting the amount of blood reaching the skin, the blood vessels help the body retain heat.

Normal changes of aging include the following:

- Skin is thinner, drier, and more fragile. It is more easily damaged.
- Skin is less elastic.
- Protective fatty tissue is lost, so the person may feel colder.
- Hair thins and may turn gray.
- Wrinkles and brown spots, or "liver spots," appear.
- Nails are harder and more brittle.
- Dry, itchy skin may result from lack of oil from the sebaceous glands.

How the NA Can Help

Older adults perspire less and do not need to bathe as often. Most elderly people generally need a complete bath only twice a week, with sponge baths every day. Using lotions as ordered helps to relieve dry skin. The NA should be gentle; elderly skin may be fragile and can tear easily. Hair also becomes drier and needs to be shampooed less often. Gently brushing dry hair stimulates and distributes the natural oils. Clothing and bed covers can be layered for additional warmth. Bed linens should be kept wrinkle-free. The NA should not cut residents' toenails. Fluid intake should be encouraged.

Observing and Reporting: Integumentary System

During daily care, a resident's skin should be observed for changes that may indicate injury or disease:

- O/R Pale, white, reddened, or purple areas
- O/R Blisters or bruises
- O/R Complaints of tingling, warmth, or burning
- O/R Dry or flaking skin
- O/R Itching or scratching
- O/R Rash or any skin discoloration
- O/R Swelling
- O/R Cuts, boils, sores, wounds, or abrasions
- O/R Fluid or blood draining from the skin
- O/R Broken skin

- O/R Changes in moistness or dryness
- O/R Changes in an injury or wound (size, depth, drainage, color, odor)
- O/R Redness or broken skin between toes or around toenails
- O/R Scalp or hair changes
- O/R Skin that appears different from normal or that has changed
- O/R In darker complexions, changes in skin tone, skin temperature, and the feel of the tissue as compared to the skin nearby

Pressure injuries, a common disorder of the integumentary system, are covered in Chapter 6.

2. Describe the musculoskeletal system and related conditions

Muscles, bones, ligaments, tendons, and cartilage give the body shape and structure. They work together to move the body. The skeleton, or framework, of the human body has 206 bones (Fig. 4-2). Besides allowing the body to move, bones also protect organs. For example, the skull protects the brain. Two bones meet at a joint. Muscles are connected to bone by tendons. Muscles provide movement of body parts to maintain posture and to produce heat.

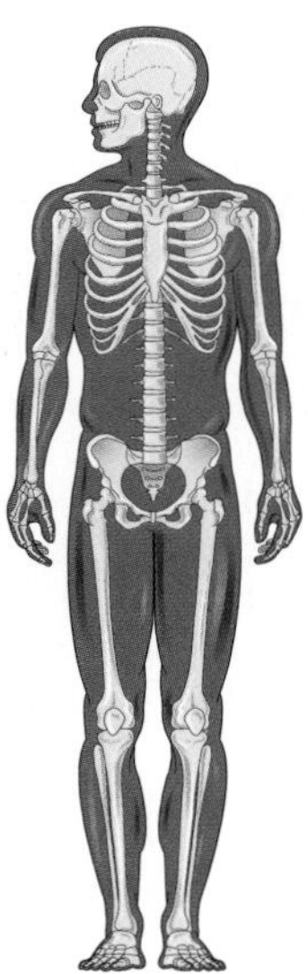

***Fig. 4-2.** The skeleton is composed of 206 bones that aid movement and protect organs.*

Exercise is important for improving and maintaining physical and mental health. Inactivity and immobility can result in a loss of self-esteem, depression, pneumonia, and urinary tract infections. They can also lead to constipation, blood clots, dulling of the senses, and muscle atrophy or contractures. When **atrophy** occurs, the muscle wastes away, decreases in size, and becomes weak. When a **contracture** develops, the muscle or tendon shortens, becomes inflexible, and "freezes" in position. This causes permanent disability of the limb. Range of motion (ROM) exercises can help prevent these conditions. With these exercises, the joints are extended and flexed. Exercise increases circulation of blood, oxygen, and nutrients and improves muscle tone. Chapter 9 has information on ROM exercises.

Normal changes of aging include the following:

- Muscles weaken and lose tone.
- Body movement slows.
- Bones lose density. They become more brittle, making them more susceptible to breaks.
- Joints may stiffen and become painful.
- Height is gradually lost.

How the NA Can Help

Falls can cause life-threatening complications, including fractures. The NA can help prevent falls by answering call lights immediately. She should keep pathways clear, clean up spills, and not move furniture. Walkers or canes need to be placed where residents can easily reach them. Residents should wear nonskid shoes that are securely fastened. The NA should encourage regular movement and self-care. Residents should perform as many activities of daily living as possible. The NA can help with range of motion exercises as needed.

Observing and Reporting: Musculoskeletal System

Observe and report these signs and symptoms:

- O/R Changes in ability to perform routine movements and activities

O/R Any changes in a resident's ability to perform ROM exercises

O/R Pain during movement

O/R Any new or increased swelling of joints

O/R White, shiny, red, or warm areas over a joint

O/R Bruising

O/R Aches and pains reported

Arthritis

Arthritis is a general term. It refers to **inflammation**, or swelling, of the joints. It causes stiffness, pain, and decreased mobility. Arthritis may be the result of aging, injury, or an **autoimmune illness**. An autoimmune illness causes the body's immune system to attack normal tissue in the body. Two common types of arthritis are rheumatoid arthritis and osteoarthritis.

Rheumatoid arthritis can affect people of any ages. Joints become red, swollen, and very painful. Deformities can result and may be severe and disabling (Fig. 4-3). Movement is eventually restricted. Fever, fatigue, and weight loss are also symptoms. Rheumatoid arthritis is considered an autoimmune disease.

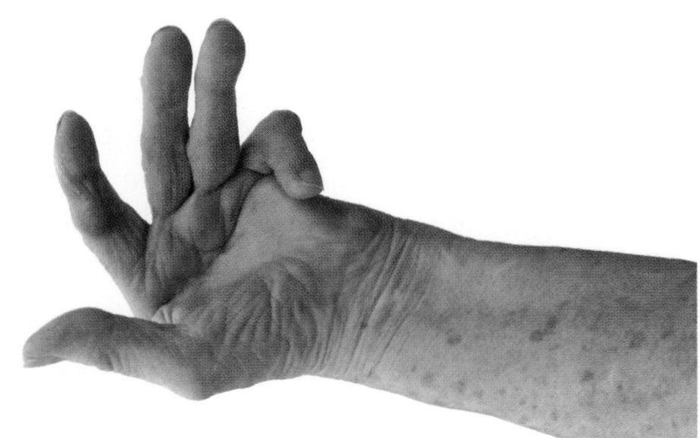

Fig. 4-3. *Rheumatoid arthritis.*

Osteoarthritis, also called *degenerative joint disease* (*DJD*) or *degenerative arthritis,* affects the elderly. It may occur with aging or as the result of joint injury. Hips and knees, which are weight-bearing joints, are usually affected. Joints in the fingers, thumbs, and spine can also be affected. Pain and stiffness seem to increase in cold, damp weather.

Arthritis is often treated with the following:

- Anti-inflammatory medication such as aspirin or ibuprofen, as well as other medication
- Local applications of heat to reduce swelling and pain
- Range of motion exercises (Chapter 9)
- Regular exercise and/or activity routine
- Diet to reduce weight or maintain strength

Guidelines: Arthritis

G Watch for stomach irritation or heartburn caused by aspirin, ibuprofen, or other arthritis medication. Report signs of stomach irritation or heartburn immediately.

G Encourage activity. Gentle activity can help reduce the effects of arthritis. Follow care plan instructions carefully. Use canes or other walking aids as needed.

G Adapt activities of daily living (ADLs) to allow independence. Many devices are available to help residents bathe, dress, and feed themselves when they have arthritis (Chapter 9).

G Choose clothing that is easy to put on and fasten. Encourage use of handrails and safety bars in the bathroom.

G Promote person-centered care. Treat each resident as an individual. Arthritis is very common among older residents. Do not assume that each resident has the same symptoms and needs the same care.

G Help maintain the resident's self-esteem. Encourage self-care. Have a positive attitude. Listen to the resident. You can help him remain independent as long as possible.

Osteoporosis

Osteoporosis is a condition in which bones lose density. This causes them to become porous and brittle. Brittle bones can break easily. Osteoporosis may be caused by a lack of calcium in the diet, the loss of estrogen, a lack of exercise, reduced mobility, or age. It is more common in women after **menopause** (the end of menstruation; occurs when a woman has not had a menstrual period for 12 months). Signs and symptoms of osteoporosis include low back pain, stooped posture, becoming shorter over time, and fractures.

To prevent or slow osteoporosis, NAs should encourage residents to walk and do other light exercise as ordered. Exercise can strengthen bones as well as muscles. NAs must move residents with osteoporosis very carefully. Medication and supplements are also used to treat osteoporosis.

Hip Fracture and Knee Replacement

A fracture is a broken bone. It is caused by an accident or by osteoporosis. Preventing falls, which can lead to fractures, is very important. Fractures of arms, wrists, elbows, legs, and hips are the most common. Signs and symptoms of a fracture are pain, swelling, bruising, changes in skin color at the site, and limited movement.

Weakened bones make hip fractures more common. A sudden fall can result in a fractured hip that takes months to heal. Hip fractures can also occur when weakened bones fracture and then cause a fall. A hip fracture is a serious condition. The elderly heal slowly. They are also at risk for secondary illnesses and disabilities. Most fractured hips require surgery. Total hip replacement (THR) is the surgical replacement of the head of the long bone of the leg (femur) where it joins the hip. This surgery is often done for these reasons:

- Fractured hip from an injury or fall that does not heal properly
- Weakened hip due to aging
- Hip is painful and stiff because the joint is weak and the bones are no longer strong enough to bear the person's weight

After the surgery, the person may not be able to stand on that leg while the hip heals. A physical therapist will assist after surgery. The goals of care include surgical incision healing, strengthening the hip muscles, mobility and gait improvement, and increased endurance.

The resident's care plan will state when the resident may begin putting weight on the leg. It will also give instructions on how much the resident is able to do. NAs should help with personal care and assistive devices, such as walkers or canes.

Guidelines: Hip Replacement

- **G** Keep often-used items, such as medications, phone, tissues, call lights, and water, within easy reach. Avoid placing items in high places.
- **G** Dress the affected (weaker) side first.
- **G** Never rush the resident. Use praise and encouragement often. Do this even for small tasks.
- **G** Ask the nurse to give pain medication prior to moving if needed.
- **G** Have the resident sit to do tasks in order to save energy.
- **G** Follow the care plan exactly, even if the resident wants to do more. Follow orders for bearing weight. After surgery, the doctor's order will be written as *partial weight-bearing (PWB) or non-weight-bearing (NWB)*. **Partial weight-bearing** means the resident is able to support some body weight on one or both legs. **Non-weight-bearing** means the resident is unable to touch the floor or support any weight on one or both legs. Once the resident can bear full weight again, the doctor's order will be written for *full weight-bearing (FWB)*. **Full weight-bearing** means that both legs can bear 100 percent of the body weight on a step. Help as needed with cane, walker, or crutches.

G Never perform ROM exercises on the operative leg unless directed by the nurse.

G Caution the resident not to sit with her legs crossed or turn her toes inward or outward. The hip cannot be bent or flexed more than 90 degrees. It also cannot be turned inward or outward.

G An abduction pillow may be used for six to 12 weeks after surgery while the resident is sleeping in bed. The abduction pillow immobilizes and positions the hips and lower extremities. The pillow is placed in between the legs. The legs are secured to the sides of the pillow using straps (Fig. 4-4). Follow instructions for application and positioning.

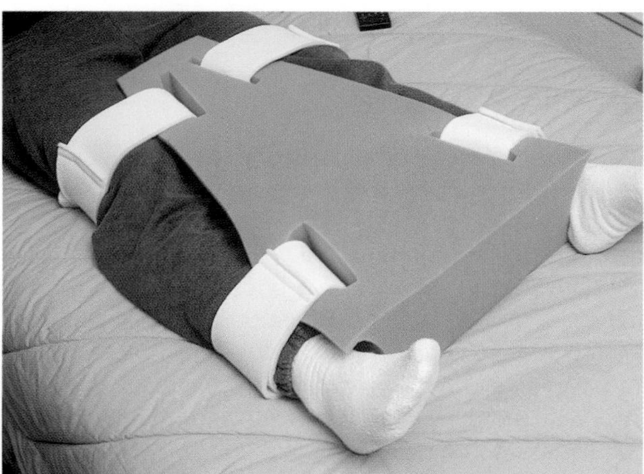

Fig. 4-4. *An abduction pillow is placed in between the legs to immobilize and position the hips and lower extremities.* (PHOTO COURTESY OF NORTH COAST MEDICAL, INC., WWW.NCMEDICAL.COM, 800-821-9319)

G When transferring from the bed, use a pillow between the thighs to keep the legs separated. Raise the head of the bed. This allows the resident to move her legs over the side of the bed with the thighs still separated. Stand on the side of the unaffected hip. The strong side should lead in standing, pivoting, and sitting.

G With chair or toilet transfers, the operative leg should be straightened. The stronger leg should stand first (with a walker or crutches). Then the foot of the affected leg can be brought back to the walking position.

G Report any of these to the nurse:

- Redness, drainage, bleeding, or warmth in incision area
- An increase in pain
- Numbness or tingling
- Tenderness or swelling in the calf of the affected leg
- Shortening and/or external rotation of the affected leg
- Abnormal vital signs, especially a change in temperature
- Resident cannot use equipment properly and safely
- Resident is not following doctor's orders for activity and exercise
- Any problems with appetite
- Any improvements, such as increased strength and improved ability to walk

Total knee replacement (TKR) is the surgical replacement of the knee with a prosthetic knee. This surgery is performed to relieve pain. It also restores motion to a knee damaged by injury or arthritis. It can help stabilize a knee that buckles or gives out repeatedly.

Guidelines: Knee Replacement

G To prevent blood clots, apply special stockings as ordered. One type is a compression stocking. It is a plastic, air-filled, sleeve-like device that is applied to the legs and hooked to a machine. This machine inflates and deflates on its own. It acts in the same way that the muscles usually do during normal activity. The sleeves are normally applied after surgery while the resident is in bed. Anti-embolic stockings are another type of special stocking. They aid circulation.

Chapter 6 has more information on this type of stocking.

- G Perform ankle pumps as ordered. These are simple exercises that promote circulation to the legs. Ankle pumps are done by raising the toes and feet toward the ceiling and lowering them again.
- G Encourage fluids, especially cranberry and orange juices, which contain vitamin C, to prevent urinary tract infections (UTIs).
- G Assist with deep breathing exercises as ordered.
- G Ask the nurse to give pain medication prior to moving and positioning if needed.
- G Report to the nurse if you notice redness, swelling, heat, or deep tenderness in one or both calves.

3. Describe the nervous system and related conditions

The nervous system is the control and message center of the body. It controls and coordinates all body functions. The nervous system also senses and interprets information from outside the human body. The nervous system has two main parts: the central nervous system (CNS) and the peripheral nervous system (PNS). The central nervous system is composed of the brain and spinal cord. The peripheral nervous system deals with the periphery, or outer part, of the body via the nerves that extend throughout the body (Fig. 4-5).

Normal changes of aging include the following:

- Responses and reflexes slow.
- Sensitivity of nerve endings in skin decreases.
- Person may show some memory loss, more often with short-term memory. Long-term memory, or memory for past events, usually remains sharp.

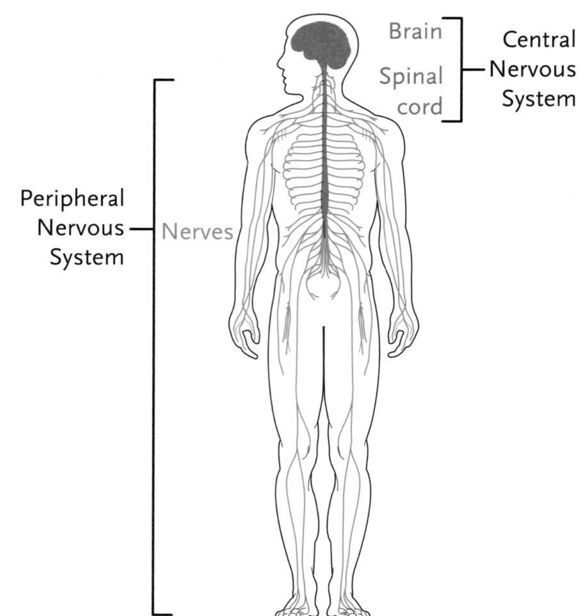

Fig. 4-5. *The nervous system includes the brain, spinal cord, and nerves throughout the body.*

How the NA Can Help

Suggesting residents make lists or write notes about things they want to remember can help with memory loss. Placing a calendar nearby may also help. If residents enjoy reminiscing, the NA can take an interest in their past by asking to see photos or hear stories. The NA should allow time for decision-making and avoid sudden changes in schedule. The NA should allow plenty of time for movement; residents should not be rushed. Reading, thinking, and other mental activities should be encouraged.

Observing and Reporting: Central Nervous System

Observe and report these signs and symptoms:

- O/R Fatigue or any pain with movement or exercise
- O/R Shaking or trembling
- O/R Inability to move one side of the body
- O/R Difficulty speaking or slurring of speech
- O/R Numbness or tingling
- O/R Disturbance or changes in vision or hearing
- O/R Dizziness or loss of balance

- O/R Changes in eating patterns and/or fluid intake
- O/R Difficulty swallowing
- O/R Bowel and bladder changes
- O/R Depression or mood changes
- O/R Memory loss or confusion
- O/R Violent behavior
- O/R Any unusual or unexplained change in behavior
- O/R Decreased ability to perform ADLs

Dementia and Alzheimer's disease are common disorders of the nervous system. Chapter 5 has information on these diseases.

CVA or Stroke

The medical term for a stroke is a cerebrovascular accident (CVA). CVA, or stroke (sometimes called *brain attack*), occurs when blood supply to a part of the brain is blocked or a blood vessel leaks or ruptures within the brain. An ischemic stroke is the most common type of stroke (Fig. 4-6). With this type, the blood supply is blocked. Without blood, part of the brain does not receive oxygen. Brain cells begin to die. Additional damage can occur due to leaking blood, clots, and swelling of the tissues. Swelling can also cause pressure on other areas of the brain. Chapter 2 has information on the warning signs of a CVA.

Strokes can be mild or severe. After a stroke, a resident may experience any of the following:

- Paralysis on one side of the body, called **hemiplegia**
- Weakness on one side of the body, called **hemiparesis**
- Tendency to ignore one side of the body, called *one-sided neglect*
- Loss of ability to tell where affected body parts are

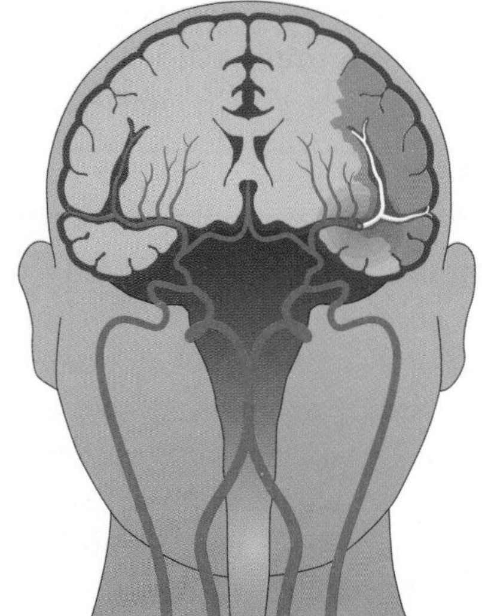

Fig. 4-6. *An ischemic stroke is caused when the blood supply to the brain is blocked.*

- Trouble communicating thoughts through speech or writing, called **expressive aphasia**
- Difficulty understanding spoken or written words, called **receptive aphasia**
- Inappropriate or unprovoked emotional responses, including laughing, crying, and anger, called **emotional lability**
- Loss of sensations such as temperature or touch
- Loss of bowel or bladder control
- Cognitive problems, such as poor judgment, memory loss, loss of problem-solving abilities, and confusion
- Difficulty swallowing, called **dysphagia**

Strokes occur on either the right or left side of the brain. A person's symptoms depend on which side of the brain is affected. Strokes that occur on the right side of the brain affect function on the left side of the body. Strokes that occur on the left side of the brain affect function on the right side of the body.

If the stroke was mild, the resident may experience few, if any, complications. Physical therapy may help restore physical abilities. Speech and occupational therapy can also help with communication and performing ADLs.

Guidelines: CVA/Stroke

- **G** Residents with paralysis, weakness, or loss of movement will usually have physical or occupational therapy. Range of motion exercises will help strengthen muscles and keep joints mobile. Residents may also need to perform leg exercises to aid circulation. Safety is always important when residents are exercising. Assist carefully with exercises as ordered.
- **G** Never refer to the weaker side as the "bad side." Do not talk about the "bad" leg or arm. Use the terms *weaker* or *involved* to refer to the side with paralysis.
- **G** Residents with speech loss or communication problems may receive speech therapy. You may be asked to help. This includes helping residents recognize written or spoken words. Speech-language pathologists will also evaluate a resident's swallowing ability. They will decide if swallowing therapy or thickened liquids are needed.
- **G** Being confused or having memory loss is upsetting. People often cry for no apparent reason after suffering a stroke. Be patient and understanding. Your positive attitude will be important. Keep a routine of care. This may help residents feel more secure.
- **G** Encourage independence and self-esteem. Let the resident do things for himself whenever possible, even if you could do a better or faster job. Make tasks less difficult for the resident to do. Notice and praise residents' efforts to do things for themselves even when they are unsuccessful. Praise even the smallest successes to build confidence.
- **G** Always check on the resident's body alignment. Sometimes an arm or leg can be caught and the resident is unaware.
- **G** Pay special attention to skin care and observe for changes in the skin if a resident is unable to move.
- **G** If residents have a loss of touch or sensation, check for potentially harmful situations (for example, heat and sharp objects). If residents are unable to sense or move part of the body, check and change positioning often to prevent pressure injuries.
- **G** Adapt procedures when caring for residents with one-sided paralysis or weakness. Carefully assist with shaving, grooming, and bathing.
- **G** When helping with transfers or walking, always use a gait belt for safety. Stand on the weaker side. Support the weaker side. Lead with the stronger side (Fig. 4-7).

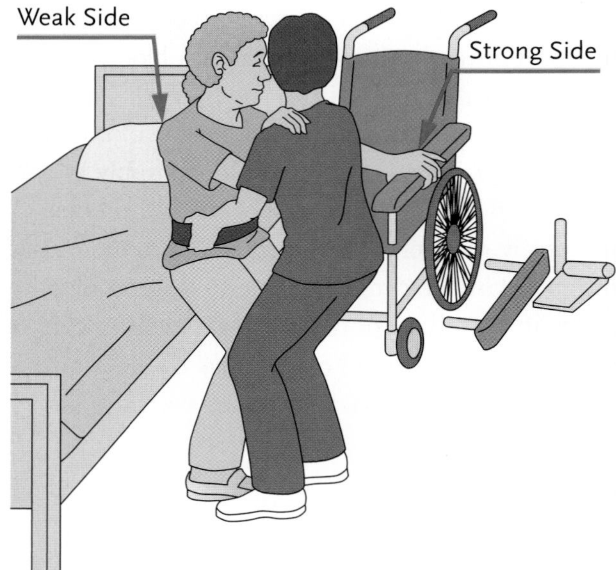

Fig. 4-7. *When helping a resident transfer, support the weaker side while leading with the stronger side.*

When assisting with dressing, remember to

- **G** Dress the weaker side first. Place the weaker arm or leg into clothing first. This prevents unnecessary bending and stretching of the limb. Undress the stronger side first. Then remove the weaker arm or leg from clothing to prevent the limb from being stretched and twisted.

- Use assistive equipment to help the resident dress himself. Encourage self-care.

When assisting with communication, remember to

- Keep questions and directions simple.
- Phrase questions so they can be answered with a "yes" or "no." For example, when helping a resident with eating, ask, "Would you like to start with a drink of milk?"
- Agree on signals, such as shaking or nodding the head or raising a hand or finger for "yes" or "no."
- Give residents time to respond. Listen attentively.
- Use a pencil and paper if the resident can write. A thick handle or tape around the pencil may help the resident hold it more easily.
- Keep the call signal within reach of residents. They can let you know when you are needed.
- Use verbal and nonverbal communication to express your positive attitude. Let the resident know you have confidence in his abilities through smiles, touches, and gestures. Gestures and pointing can also help give information or allow the resident to communicate with you.
- Use communication boards or special cards to aid communication (Fig. 4-8).

Guidelines for helping with eating for a person recovering from CVA are in Chapter 8.

Residents' Rights

Speech Impairment

Nursing assistants should never talk about residents as if they were not there. Even if residents cannot speak, it does not mean they cannot hear. All residents should be treated with respect.

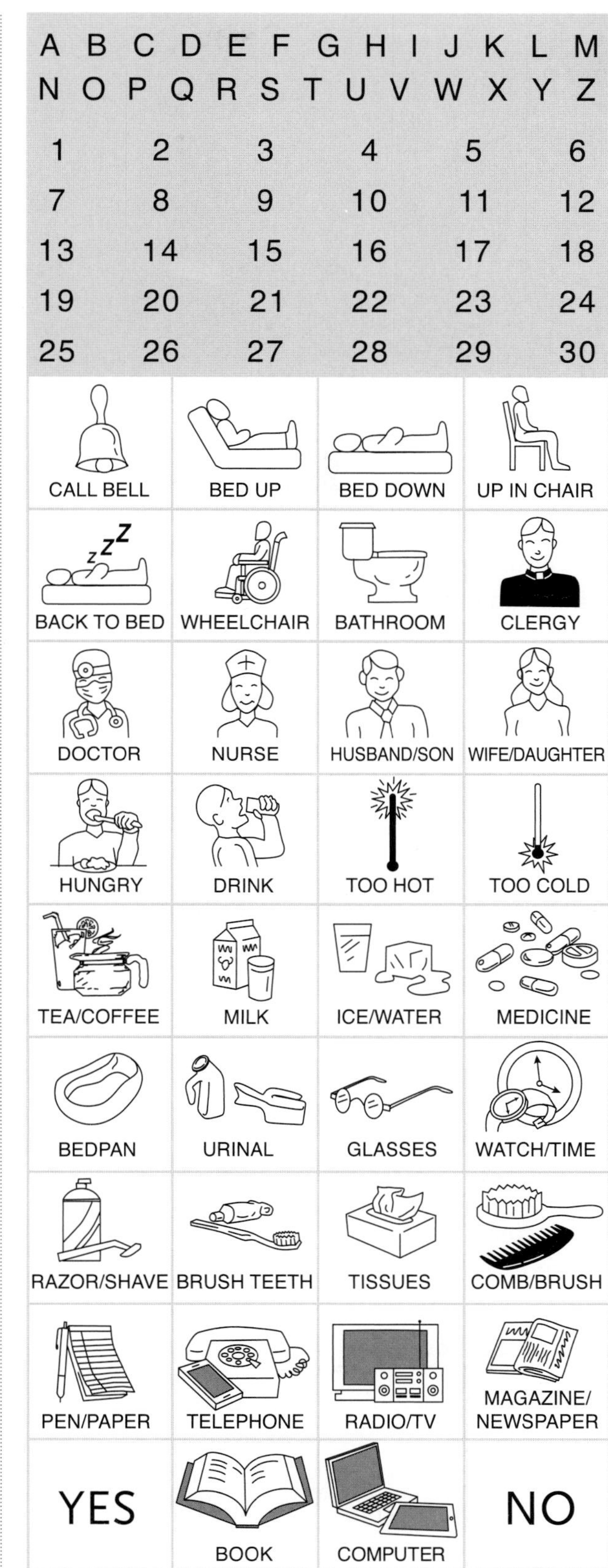

Fig. 4-8. A sample communication board.

Parkinson's Disease

Parkinson's disease is a progressive, incurable disease. Progressive means the disease gets worse with time. Parkinson's disease causes a section of the brain to degenerate. It affects the muscles, causing them to become stiff. It causes stooped posture and a shuffling **gait**, or walk. It can also cause pill-rolling. This is a circular movement of the tips of the thumb and the index finger when brought together, which looks like rolling a pill. Tremors or shaking make it hard for a person to perform ADLs such as eating and bathing. A person with Parkinson's may have a mask-like facial expression. Medications are commonly used to treat this disease. Surgery may be an option for some people.

Guidelines: Parkinson's Disease

- **G** Residents are at a high risk for falls. Visual and spatial impairments may occur, causing problems with bumping into doorways and navigating areas. Protect residents from any unsafe areas and conditions. Help with ambulation as needed.
- **G** Help with ADLs as needed.
- **G** Assist with range of motion exercises to prevent contractures and to strengthen muscles.
- **G** Observe for any swallowing problems and report them to the nurse.
- **G** Encourage self-care. Be patient with self-care and communication.

Multiple Sclerosis (MS)

Multiple sclerosis (MS) is a progressive disease. It affects the central nervous system. When a person has MS, the myelin sheath that covers the nerves, spinal cord, and white matter of the brain breaks down over time. Without this covering, or sheath, nerves cannot send messages to and from the brain in a normal way. MS progresses slowly and unpredictably. Residents who have this disease will have widely varying abilities. Symptoms include blurred vision, fatigue, tremors, poor balance, and trouble walking. Weakness, numbness, tingling, incontinence, and behavior changes are also symptoms. MS can cause blindness, contractures, and loss of function in the arms and legs. MS is often diagnosed in early adulthood. The exact cause is not known, but it may be an autoimmune disease. There is no cure for this disease; it is mostly treated with medication.

Guidelines: Multiple Sclerosis

- **G** Assist with ADLs as needed. Be patient with self-care and movement. Allow enough time for tasks. Offer rest periods as necessary.
- **G** Give the resident plenty of time to communicate. People with MS may have trouble forming their thoughts. Be patient. Do not rush them.
- **G** Prevent falls, which may be due to fatigue, vision problems, or a lack of coordination.
- **G** Stress can worsen the effects of MS. Be calm. Listen to residents when they want to talk.
- **G** Symptoms of MS can sometimes change daily; offer support and encouragement, and adapt care to the symptoms reported.
- **G** Encourage a healthy diet with plenty of fluids.
- **G** Give regular skin care to prevent pressure injuries.
- **G** Assist with range of motion exercises to prevent contractures and to strengthen muscles.

Head and Spinal Cord Injuries

Diving, sports injuries, falls, car and motorcycle accidents, industrial accidents, war, and criminal violence are common causes of head and spinal cord injuries. Problems from these injuries range from mild confusion or memory loss to coma, paralysis, and death.

Head injuries can cause permanent brain damage. Residents who have had a head injury may have the following problems: intellectual disabilities; personality changes; breathing problems; seizures; coma; memory loss; loss of consciousness; paresis; and paralysis. *Paresis* is paralysis, or loss of muscle function, that affects only part of the body. Often, paresis describes a weakness or loss of ability on one side of the body.

The effects of spinal cord injuries depend on the force of impact and location of the injury. The higher the injury on the spinal cord, the greater the loss of function. People with head and spinal cord injuries may have **paraplegia**. This is a loss of function of the lower body and legs. These injuries may also cause **quadriplegia**. This is a loss of function in the legs, trunk, and arms (Fig. 4-9).

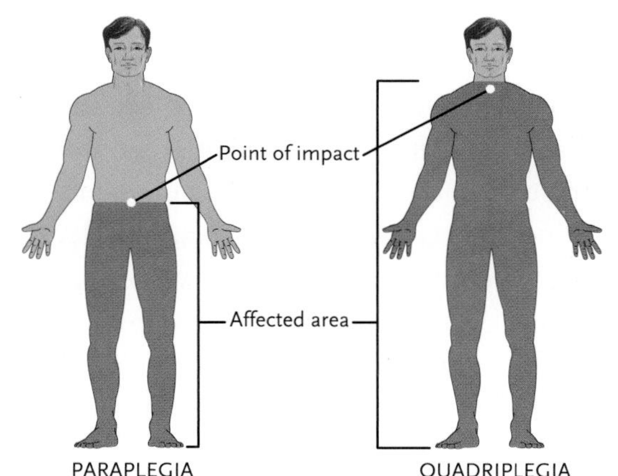

Fig. 4-9. *Loss of function depends on where the spine is injured.*

Guidelines: Head or Spinal Cord Injury

- **G** Give emotional support, as well as physical help.
- **G** Safety is very important. Be very careful that residents do not fall or burn themselves. Because residents who are paralyzed have no sensation, they are unable to feel a burn.
- **G** Be patient with self-care. Allow as much independence as possible with ADLs.
- **G** Give careful skin care. It is important to prevent pressure injuries.
- **G** Assist residents to change positions at least every two hours to prevent pressure injuries. Be gentle when repositioning.
- **G** Perform range of motion exercises as ordered to prevent contractures and to strengthen muscles.
- **G** Immobility leads to constipation. Encourage fluids and a high-fiber diet if ordered.
- **G** Loss of ability to empty the bladder may lead to the need for a urinary catheter. Urinary tract infections are common. Encourage high intake of fluids. Give extra catheter care as needed.
- **G** Lack of activity leads to poor circulation and fatigue. Offer rest periods as necessary. Special stockings to help increase circulation may be ordered.
- **G** Difficulty coughing and shallow breathing can lead to pneumonia. Encourage deep breathing exercises as ordered.
- **G** Male residents may have involuntary erections. Provide for privacy and be sensitive if this happens. Be professional.
- **G** Assist with bowel and bladder training if needed.

The Nervous System: Sense Organs

The eyes, ears, nose, tongue, and skin are the body's major sense organs (Fig. 4-10 and Fig. 4-11). They are part of the central nervous system because they receive impulses from the environment. They relay these impulses to the nerves.

Normal changes of aging include

- Vision and hearing decrease. Sense of balance may be affected.
- Senses of taste, smell, and touch decrease.

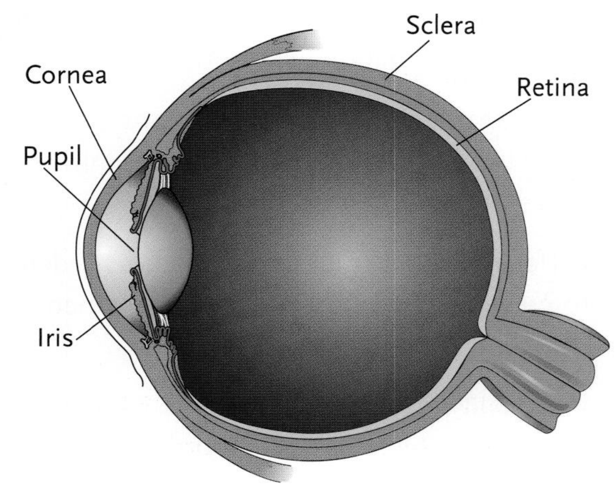

Fig. 4-10. The parts of the eye.

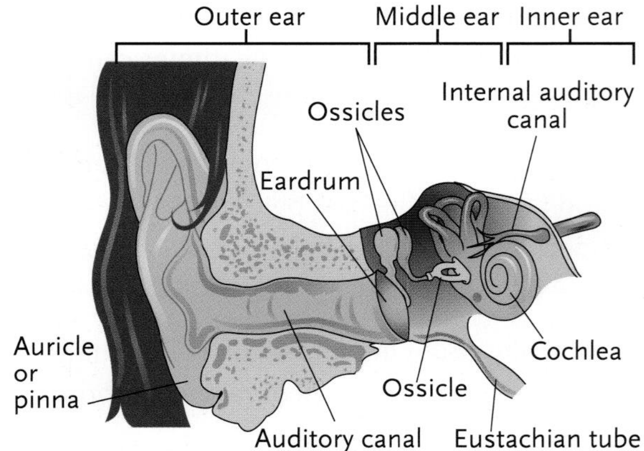

***Fig. 4-11.** The outer ear, middle ear, and inner ear are the three main divisions of the ear.*

How the NA Can Help

Residents should use their eyeglasses. The NA can help by keeping them clean. Bright colors and proper lighting will also help. Hearing aids should be worn, and they should be kept clean. The NA should face the resident when speaking and speak slowly and clearly. Shouting should be avoided. The loss of senses of taste and smell may lead to decreased appetite. Providing oral care often and offering foods with a variety of tastes and textures may help. The loss of smell may make residents unaware of increased body odor. The NA should help as needed with regular bathing. Due to decreased sense of touch, residents may not be able to tell if something is too hot for them. The NA should be careful with hot drinks and hot bath water.

Observing and Reporting: Eyes and Ears

Observe and report these signs and symptoms:

- O/R Changes in vision or hearing
- O/R Signs of infection
- O/R Dizziness
- O/R Complaints of pain in eyes or ears

Vision Impairment

People over the age of 40 are at risk for developing certain serious vision problems. These include cataracts, glaucoma, and blindness. When a cataract develops, the lens of the eye, which is normally clear, becomes cloudy. This prevents light from entering the eye. Vision blurs and dims initially. Vision is eventually lost entirely. This disease can occur in one or both eyes. It is corrected with surgery, in which a permanent lens implant is usually performed.

With glaucoma, the pressure in the eye increases. This eventually damages the retina and the optic nerve. It causes loss of vision and blindness. Glaucoma can occur suddenly, causing severe pain, nausea, and vomiting. It can also occur gradually, with symptoms that include blurred vision, tunnel vision, and blue-green halos around lights. Glaucoma is treated with eye drops and other medication and sometimes with surgery. More information about vision impairment is located in Chapter 2.

4. Describe the circulatory system and related conditions

The circulatory system is made up of the heart, blood vessels, and blood (Fig. 4-12). The heart pumps blood through the blood vessels to the cells. The blood carries food, oxygen, and other substances cells need to function properly.

The circulatory system supplies food, oxygen, and hormones to cells. It supplies the body with infection-fighting blood cells. The circulatory system removes waste products from cells and also helps control body temperature.

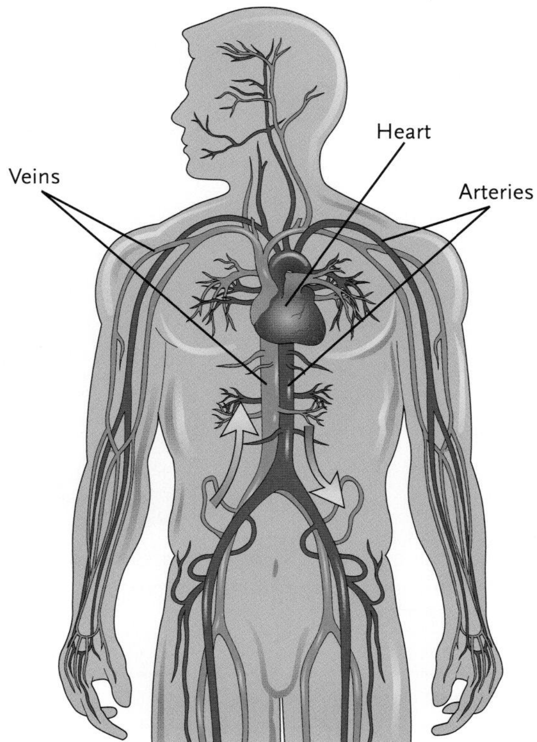

Fig. 4-12. The heart, blood vessels, and blood are the main parts of the circulatory system.

Normal changes of aging include the following:

- The heart pumps less efficiently.
- Blood flow decreases.
- Blood vessels narrow.

How the NA Can Help

Movement and exercise should be encouraged. Walking, stretching, and even lifting light weights can help maintain strength and promote circulation. ROM exercises are important for residents who cannot get out of bed. The NA should allow time to complete activities and try to prevent residents from tiring. Layering clothing helps keep residents warm. Socks, slippers, or shoes help keep the feet warm.

Observing and Reporting: Circulatory System

Observe and report these signs and symptoms:

- O/R Changes in pulse rate
- O/R Weakness, fatigue
- O/R Loss of ability to perform ADLs
- O/R Swelling of ankles, feet, fingers, or hands (edema)
- O/R Pale or bluish hands, feet, or lips
- O/R Chest pain
- O/R Weight gain
- O/R Shortness of breath, changes in breathing patterns, inability to catch breath
- O/R Severe headache
- O/R Inactivity (which can lead to circulatory problems)

Hypertension (HTN) or High Blood Pressure

When blood pressure is consistently 130/80 or higher, a person is diagnosed as having **hypertension** (**HTN**), or high blood pressure. In late 2017, the American Heart Association and American College of Cardiology released new joint guidelines for blood pressure. A systolic reading of 130 mm Hg or higher or a diastolic reading of 80 mm Hg or higher is now considered high blood pressure. More information about this may be found in Chapter 7.

The major cause of hypertension is *atherosclerosis*, or a hardening and narrowing of the blood vessels (Fig. 4-13). It can also result from kidney disease, tumors of the adrenal gland, pregnancy, and certain medications.

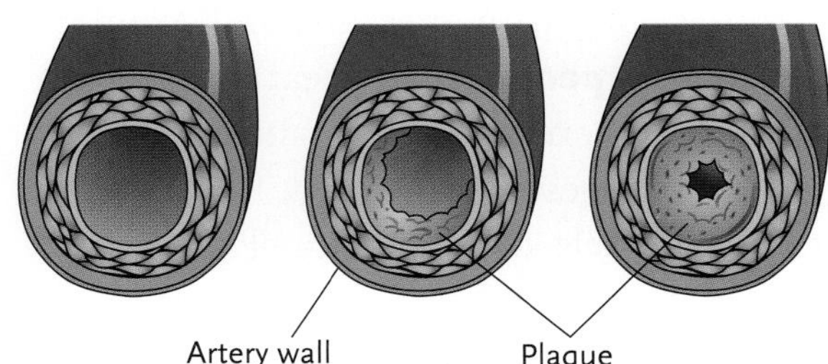

Fig. 4-13. Arteries may harden or narrow because of a buildup of plaque. Hardened arteries are one cause of high blood pressure.

Hypertension can develop in people of any age. Signs and symptoms of hypertension are not always obvious, especially in the early stages. Often it is only discovered when blood pressure is measured by a healthcare provider. A person may complain of headaches, blurred vision, and dizziness.

Guidelines: Hypertension

- Hypertension can lead to serious problems such as CVA, heart attack, kidney disease, or blindness. Treatment to control it is vital. Residents may take medication that lowers blood pressure. They may take diuretics. **Diuretics** are medications that reduce fluid in the body. Offer trips to the bathroom regularly. Answer call lights promptly.
- Residents may also have prescribed exercise programs or special diets, such as low-fat or low-sodium diets. Encourage residents to follow their diet and exercise programs. Measure blood pressure as directed.

Coronary Artery Disease (CAD)

Coronary artery disease occurs when the blood vessels in the coronary arteries narrow. This reduces the supply of blood to the heart muscle and deprives it of oxygen and nutrients. Over time, as fatty deposits block the artery, the muscle that was supplied by the blood vessel dies. CAD can lead to heart attack or stroke.

The heart muscle that is not getting enough oxygen causes chest pain, pressure, or discomfort, called **angina pectoris**. The heart needs more oxygen during exercise, stress, and excitement, as well as to digest a heavy meal. In CAD, narrow blood vessels keep the extra blood with oxygen from getting to the heart (Fig. 4-14).

The pain of angina pectoris is usually described as pressure or tightness. It occurs in the left side or the center of the chest, behind the sternum or breastbone. Some people have pain moving down the inside of the left arm or to the neck and left side of the jaw. A person suffering from angina pectoris may sweat or look pale. The person may feel dizzy and have trouble breathing.

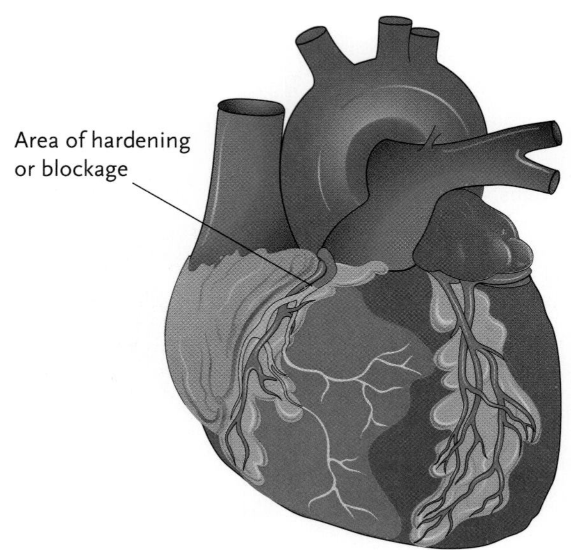

Fig. 4-14. *Angina pectoris is pain or pressure that results from the heart not getting enough oxygen.*

Guidelines: Angina Pectoris

- Encourage residents to rest. Rest is extremely important. Rest reduces the heart's need for extra oxygen. It helps blood flow return to normal, often within three to 15 minutes.
- Medication is also needed to relax the walls of the coronary arteries. This allows them to open and get more blood to the heart. This medication, nitroglycerin, is a small tablet that the resident places under the tongue. There it dissolves and is rapidly absorbed. Residents who have angina pectoris may keep nitroglycerin on hand to use as symptoms arise. To maintain potency, the nitroglycerin bottle should be kept tightly closed. Nursing assistants are not allowed to give any medication unless they have had special training. Tell the nurse if a resident needs help taking the medication.

  Nitroglycerin is also available as a patch. Do not remove the patch. Tell the nurse immediately if the patch comes off. Nitroglycerin may also come in the form of a spray that the resident sprays onto or under the tongue.

G Residents may also need to avoid heavy meals, overeating, intense exercise, and cold or hot and humid weather.

Myocardial Infarction (MI) or Heart Attack

When blood flow to the heart muscle is blocked, oxygen and nutrients fail to reach the cells in that area (Fig. 4-15). Waste products are not removed. The muscle cells die. This is called a myocardial infarction (MI) or heart attack. A myocardial infarction is a medical emergency that can result in serious heart damage or death. Chapter 2 has a list of warning signs of an MI.

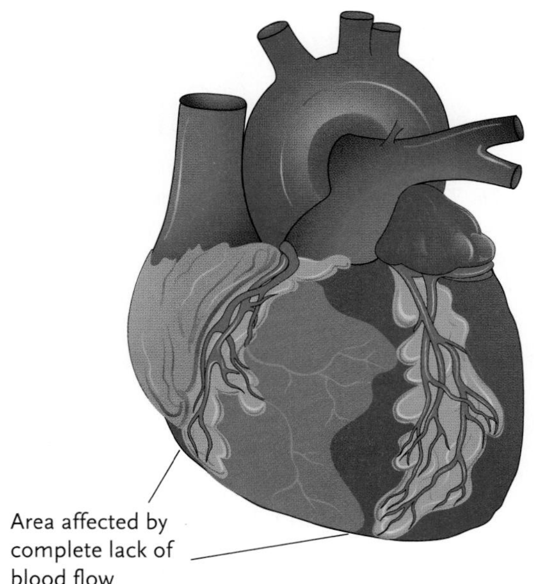

Fig. 4-15. *A heart attack occurs when all or part of the blood flow to the heart is blocked.*

Guidelines: Myocardial Infarction

G After a myocardial infarction, cardiac rehabilitation is usually ordered. This ongoing program consists of the following:

- Low-cholesterol, low saturated fat, and low-sodium diet
- Regular exercise program
- Medications to regulate heart rate and blood pressure, to lower cholesterol, and to lower triglycerides
- Regular blood testing
- Stopping smoking
- Avoiding cold temperatures
- Stress management program

G Encourage residents to follow their special diets and to follow their exercise programs.

G Be encouraging if residents have quit or are trying to quit smoking.

G Reduce stress as much as possible. Listen when residents want to talk. Report signs of and complaints of stress to the nurse.

Congestive Heart Failure (CHF)

Coronary artery disease, myocardial infarction, hypertension, and other disorders may all damage the heart. When the heart muscle has been severely damaged, it fails to pump effectively. When the left side of the heart is affected, blood backs up into the lungs. When the right side of the heart is affected, blood backs up into the legs, feet, or abdomen. When one or both sides of the heart stop pumping blood properly, it is called congestive heart failure (CHF).

Guidelines: Congestive Heart Failure

G Although CHF is a serious illness, it can be treated and controlled. Medications can strengthen the heart muscle and improve its pumping.

G Assist the resident as needed with getting to the toilet or commode. Medications help remove excess fluids. This means more trips to the bathroom. Answer call lights promptly.

G Encourage residents to follow diet orders or restrictions. A low-sodium diet or fluid restrictions may be ordered.

G A weakened heart may make it hard for residents to walk, carry items, or climb stairs.

Limited activity or bedrest may be prescribed. Allow for a period of rest after an activity.

- Measure intake and output of fluids as ordered.
- Weigh residents as instructed. Residents may be weighed daily at the same time to watch for weight gain from fluid retention.
- Apply elastic leg stockings as ordered to reduce swelling in feet and ankles.
- Assist with range of motion (ROM) exercises as ordered. These exercises improve muscle tone when activity and exercise are limited.
- Extra pillows may help residents who have trouble breathing. Keeping the head of the bed elevated may also help with breathing.
- Help with personal care and ADLs as needed.
- A common side effect of medications for congestive heart failure is dizziness. This may result from a lack of potassium, although not all medications for CHF deplete potassium. Report dizziness to the nurse.

Peripheral Vascular Disease (PVD)

Peripheral vascular disease (PVD) is a disease in which the legs, feet, arms, or hands do not have enough blood circulation. This is due to fatty deposits in the blood vessels that harden over time. The legs, feet, arms, and hands feel cool or cold. Nail beds and/or feet become ashen or blue. Swelling occurs in the hands and feet. Ulcers of the legs and feet may develop and can become infected. Pain may be very severe when walking, but it is usually relieved with rest. Risk factors for PVD include smoking, diabetes, high cholesterol, hypertension, inactivity, and obesity. Treatment includes quitting smoking, medications, exercise, and surgery.

5. Describe the respiratory system and related conditions

Respiration, the body taking in oxygen and removing carbon dioxide, involves breathing in, **inspiration**, and breathing out, **expiration**. The lungs accomplish this process (Fig. 4-16). The functions of the respiratory system are to bring oxygen into the body and to eliminate carbon dioxide produced as the body uses oxygen.

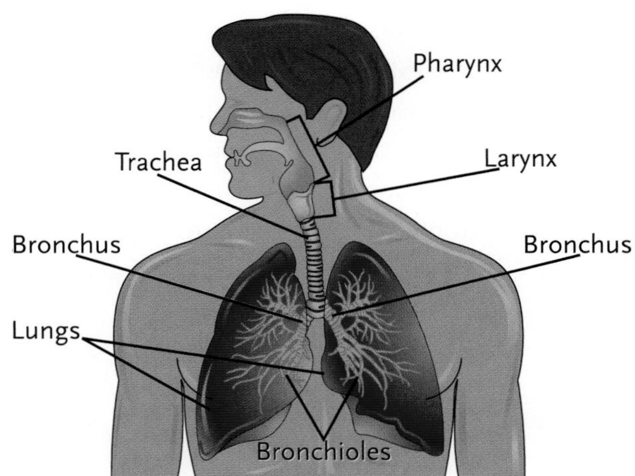

Fig. 4-16. *The respiratory process begins with inspiration through the nose or mouth. The air travels through the trachea and into the lungs via the bronchi, which then branch into bronchioles.*

Normal changes of aging include the following:

- Lung strength decreases.
- Lung capacity decreases.
- Oxygen in the blood decreases.
- Voice weakens.

How the NA Can Help

Residents with acute or chronic upper respiratory conditions should not be exposed to cigarette smoke or polluted air. The NA should provide rest periods as needed and encourage exercise and regular movement. The NA should assist with deep breathing exercises as ordered. Residents who have difficulty breathing will usually be more comfortable sitting up rather than lying down.

Observing and Reporting: Respiratory System

Observe and report these signs and symptoms:

- Change in respiratory rate

- O/R Shallow breathing or breathing through pursed lips
- O/R Coughing or wheezing
- O/R Nasal congestion or discharge
- O/R Sore throat, difficulty swallowing, or swollen tonsils
- O/R The need to sit after mild exertion
- O/R Pale, bluish, or gray color of the lips, arms, and/or legs
- O/R Pain in the chest area
- O/R Discolored sputum, mucus a person coughs up from the lungs (green, yellow, blood-tinged, or gray)

Chronic Obstructive Pulmonary Disease (COPD)

Chronic obstructive pulmonary disease (COPD) is a chronic disease. This means a person may live for years with it but never be cured. COPD causes trouble with breathing, especially in getting air out of the lungs. There are two chronic lung diseases that are grouped under COPD: chronic bronchitis and emphysema.

Bronchitis is an irritation and inflammation of the lining of the bronchi. Chronic bronchitis is a form of bronchitis that is usually caused by cigarette smoking. Symptoms include coughing that brings up sputum (phlegm) and mucus. Breathlessness and wheezing may be present. Treatment includes stopping smoking and possibly medications.

Emphysema is a chronic disease of the lungs that usually results from chronic bronchitis and cigarette smoking. People with emphysema have trouble breathing. Other symptoms are coughing, breathlessness, and a fast heartbeat. There is no cure for emphysema. Treatment includes managing symptoms and pain. Oxygen therapy, as well as medications, may be ordered. Quitting smoking is very important.

Over time, a person with either of these lung disorders becomes chronically ill and weakened. There is a high risk for acute lung infections, such as pneumonia. Pneumonia is an illness that can be caused by a bacterial, viral, or fungal infection. Acute inflammation occurs in lung tissue. The affected person develops a high fever, chills, cough, greenish or yellow sputum, chest pains, and rapid pulse. Treatment includes antibiotics, along with plenty of fluids. Recovery from pneumonia may take longer for older adults and persons with chronic illnesses.

When the lungs and brain do not get enough oxygen, all body systems are affected. Residents may have a constant fear of not being able to breathe. This can cause them to sit upright to try to improve their ability to expand the lungs. These residents can have poor appetites. They usually do not get enough sleep. All of this can add to feelings of weakness and poor health. They may feel they have lost control of their bodies, particularly their breathing. They may fear suffocation.

Residents with COPD may have these symptoms:

- Chronic cough or wheeze
- Trouble breathing, especially with inhaling and exhaling deeply
- Shortness of breath, especially during physical effort
- Pale, blue, or reddish-purple skin
- Confusion
- General state of weakness
- Trouble completing meals due to shortness of breath
- Fear and anxiety

Guidelines: COPD

- G Colds or viruses can make COPD worse. Always observe and report signs and symptoms of colds or illness.

- G Help residents sit upright or lean forward. Offer pillows for support (Fig. 4-17).

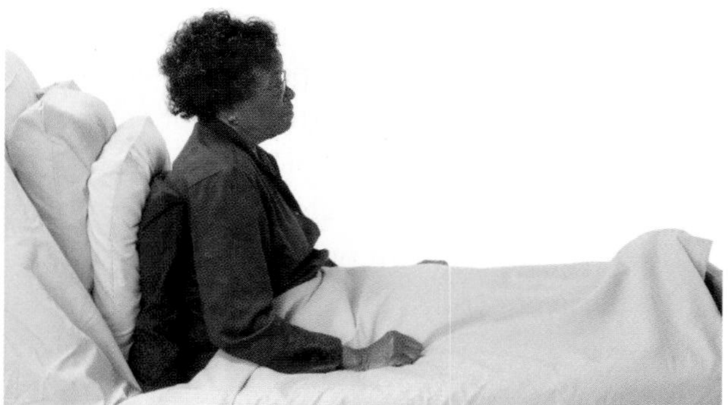

***Fig. 4-17.** It helps residents with COPD to sit upright and lean forward slightly.*

- G Offer plenty of fluids and small, frequent meals.
- G Encourage a well-balanced diet.
- G Keep an oxygen supply available as ordered.
- G Being unable to breathe or fearing suffocation can be very frightening. Be calm and supportive.
- G Use infection prevention practices. Wash your hands often and encourage the resident to do the same. Dispose of used tissues promptly.
- G Encourage as much independence with ADLs as possible.
- G Remind residents to avoid exposure to infections, especially colds and the flu.
- G Encourage pursed-lip breathing. Pursed-lip breathing involves inhaling slowly through the nose and exhaling slowly through pursed lips (as if about to whistle). A nurse should teach residents how to do this.
- G Encourage residents to save energy for important tasks. Encourage residents to rest.
- G Report any of these to the nurse:
  - Temperature over 101°F
  - Changes in breathing patterns, including shortness of breath
  - Changes in color or consistency of lung secretions
  - Changes in mental state or personality
  - Refusal to take medications as ordered
  - Excessive weight loss
  - Increasing dependence upon caregivers and family

6. Describe the urinary system and related conditions

The urinary system is composed of two kidneys, two ureters, one urinary bladder, a single urethra, and a meatus (Fig. 4-18 and Fig. 4-19). The urinary system has two important functions. Through urine, the urinary system eliminates waste products created by the cells. The urinary system also maintains the water balance in the body.

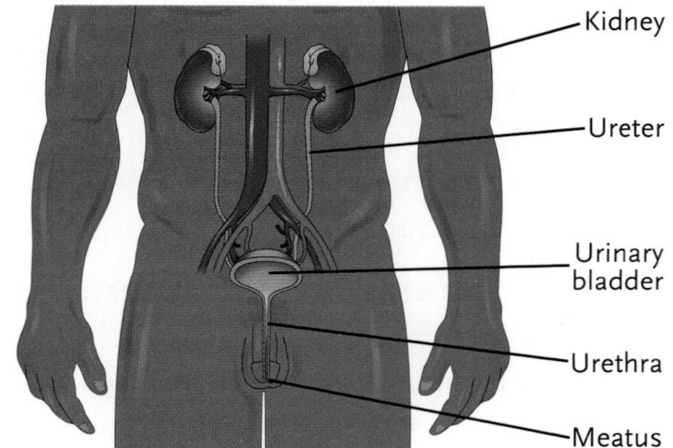

***Fig. 4-18.** This is an illustration of the male urinary system.*

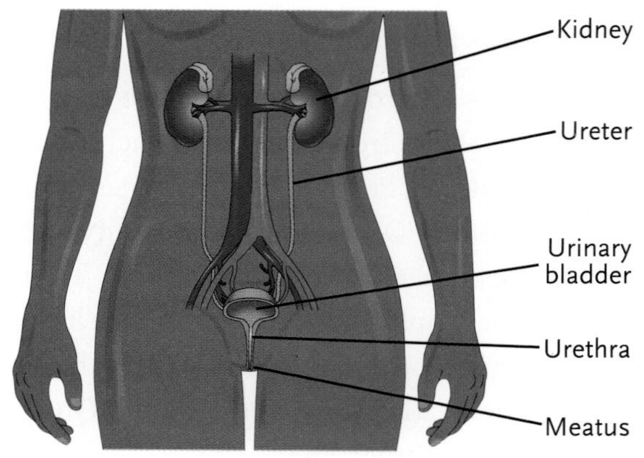

***Fig. 4-19.** The female urethra is shorter than the male urethra. This is one reason why the female bladder is more likely to become infected by bacteria.*

Normal changes of aging include the following:

- The ability of kidneys to filter blood decreases.
- Bladder muscle tone weakens.
- The bladder holds less urine, which causes more frequent urination.
- The bladder may not empty completely, causing a greater risk of infection.

How the NA Can Help

The NA should encourage fluids and offer frequent trips to the bathroom. Residents should wipe from front to back after elimination. If residents are incontinent, the NA should not show frustration or anger. **Urinary incontinence** is the inability to control the bladder, which leads to an involuntary loss of urine. Residents should be kept clean and dry.

Observing and Reporting: Urinary System

Observe and report these signs and symptoms:

O/R Weight loss or gain

O/R Swelling in upper or lower extremities

O/R Pain or burning during urination

O/R Changes in urine, such as cloudiness, odor, or color

O/R Changes in frequency and amount of urination

O/R Swelling in the abdominal/bladder area

O/R Complaints that bladder feels full or painful

O/R Urinary incontinence/dribbling

O/R Pain in the kidney or back/flank region

O/R Inadequate fluid intake

O/R Confusion

Urinary Incontinence

Urinary incontinence can occur in residents who are confined to bed, ill, elderly, paralyzed, or who have circulatory or nervous system diseases or injuries. Incontinence is not a normal part of aging. Nursing assistants should always report incontinence.

Guidelines: Urinary Incontinence

G Offer a bedpan, urinal, commode, or trip to the bathroom often. Follow toileting schedules in the care plan.

G Answer call lights and requests for help immediately.

G Urinary incontinence is a major risk factor for pressure injuries. Document all episodes of incontinence carefully and accurately.

G Cleanliness and careful skin care are important. Urine is very irritating to the skin. It should be washed off immediately and completely. Keep residents clean, dry, and free from odor. Observe the skin carefully when bathing and giving perineal care.

G Change wet or soiled clothing immediately. Change bed linen any time it is wet or soiled. Use absorbent pads under bed linen for residents who are incontinent.

G Some residents will wear disposable incontinence pads or briefs for adults. They keep body wastes away from the skin. Change wet briefs immediately. Do not refer to an incontinence brief as a diaper. Residents are not children. Using that term is disrespectful.

G Encourage residents to drink plenty of fluids.

G Residents who are incontinent need reassurance and understanding. Be professional and kind when dealing with incontinence.

Urinary Tract Infection (UTI)

A urinary tract infection (UTI) is a bacterial infection of the urethra, bladder, ureter, or kidney.

This results in painful burning during urination. It also causes a frequent feeling of needing to urinate. UTIs are more common in women. This is due, in part, to the female urethra being shorter (one to one and one-half inches) than the male urethra (seven to eight inches). In addition, the female urethra is located directly in front of the vagina and anus. This means it is closer to potential sources of bacteria. Bacteria can reach a woman's bladder more easily.

Guidelines: Preventing UTIs

- **G** Encourage residents to wipe from front to back after elimination (Fig. 4-20). When you give perineal care, make sure you do this too.

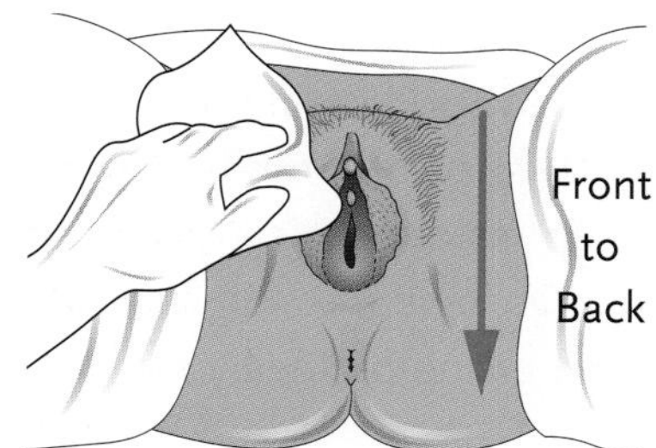

Fig. 4-20. *After elimination, wipe from front to back to prevent infection.*

- **G** Give careful perineal care when changing incontinence briefs.
- **G** Encourage plenty of fluids. Drinking water and other fluids helps prevent UTIs. Cranberry, orange, and blueberry juices, which are rich in vitamin C, help to acidify urine. This can prevent infection.
- **G** Offer a bedpan or a trip to the toilet at least every two hours. Answer call lights promptly.
- **G** Taking showers, rather than baths, helps prevent UTIs.
- **G** Report cloudy, dark, or foul-smelling urine, or if a resident urinates often and in small amounts.
- **G** Report if the resident has a fever. Report new or worsening confusion.

7. Describe the gastrointestinal system and related conditions

The gastrointestinal (GI) system, also called the digestive system, is made up of the gastrointestinal tract and the accessory digestive organs (Fig. 4-21). The gastrointestinal system has these functions: digestion, absorption, and elimination. **Digestion** is the process of preparing food physically and chemically so that it can be absorbed into the cells. **Absorption** is the transfer of nutrients from the intestines to the cells. **Elimination** is the process of expelling wastes (made up of the waste products of food and fluids) that are not absorbed into the cells.

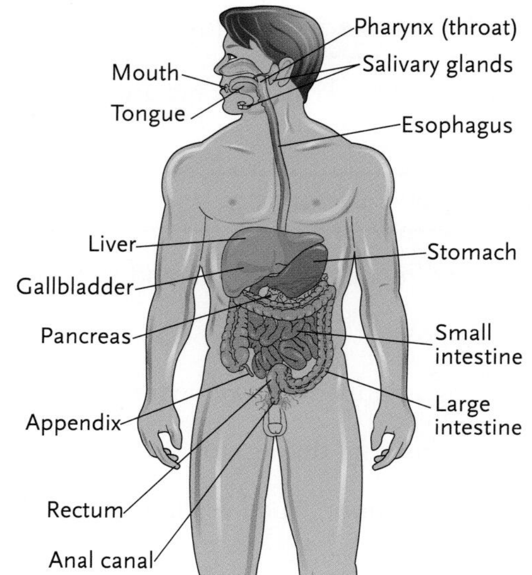

Fig. 4-21. *The GI system consists of all the organs needed to digest food and process waste.*

Normal changes of aging include the following:

- Decreased saliva production affects the ability to chew and swallow.
- Dulled sense of taste may result in poor appetite.
- Absorption of vitamins and minerals decreases.
- The process of digestion takes longer and is less efficient.
- Body waste moves more slowly through the intestines, causing more frequent constipation.

How the NA Can Help

Fluids and nutritious, appealing meals should be encouraged. The NA should allow time to eat and make mealtime enjoyable. Regular oral care should be provided. Dentures must fit properly and should be cleaned regularly. Residents who have trouble chewing and swallowing are at risk of choking. The NA should offer fluids during mealtime. Residents should eat a diet that contains fiber and drink plenty of fluids to help prevent constipation. Residents should be given the opportunity to have a bowel movement around the same time each day.

Observing and Reporting: Gastrointestinal System

Observe and report these signs and symptoms:

- O/R Difficulty swallowing or chewing, including denture problems, tooth pain, or mouth sores
- O/R **Fecal incontinence** (inability to control the bowels, leading to an involuntary passage of stool)
- O/R Weight gain or weight loss
- O/R Loss of appetite
- O/R Abdominal pain and cramping
- O/R Diarrhea
- O/R Nausea and vomiting (especially vomitus that looks like coffee grounds)
- O/R Constipation
- O/R Flatulence
- O/R Hiccups or belching
- O/R Bloody, black, or hard stools
- O/R Heartburn
- O/R Poor nutritional intake

Constipation

Constipation is the inability to eliminate stool (have a bowel movement) or the infrequent, difficult, and often painful elimination of a hard, dry stool. Constipation occurs when the feces move too slowly through the intestine. This can result from decreased fluid intake, poor diet, inactivity, medications, aging, disease, or ignoring the urge to eliminate. Signs of constipation include abdominal swelling, gas, irritability, and a record of no recent bowel movement.

Treatment often includes increasing fiber and fluid intake, increasing activity level, and possibly medication. Accurate documentation of bowel movements is important. An enema or rectal suppository may be ordered to help. An **enema** is a specific amount of water, with or without an additive, that is introduced into the colon to eliminate stool. A rectal suppository is a medication given rectally to cause a bowel movement.

Fecal Impaction

A fecal impaction is a hard stool that is stuck in the rectum and cannot be expelled. It results from unrelieved constipation. Symptoms include no stool for several days, oozing of liquid stool, cramping, abdominal swelling, and rectal pain. When an impaction occurs, a nurse or doctor will insert one or two gloved fingers into the rectum and break the mass into fragments so that it can be passed. Prevention of fecal impactions includes a high-fiber diet, plenty of fluids, an increase in activity level, and possibly medication. Early assessments of constipation may also help prevent impactions.

Hemorrhoids

Hemorrhoids are enlarged veins in the rectum. They may also be visible outside the anus. Chronic constipation, obesity, pregnancy, chronic diarrhea, overuse of laxatives and enemas, and straining during bowel movements are common causes. Rectal itching, burning, pain, and bleeding during bowel elimination are signs and symptoms of hemorrhoids. Treatment includes increasing fiber and fluid intake. Medications, compresses, and sitz baths are also used for treatment. Surgery may be necessary. When cleaning the anal area, the NA should be careful to avoid causing pain and bleeding.

Diarrhea

Diarrhea is the frequent elimination of liquid or semi-liquid feces. Abdominal cramps, urgency, nausea, and vomiting can accompany diarrhea, depending on the cause. Infections, microorganisms in food and water, irritating foods, and medications can cause diarrhea. Treatment usually involves medication, an increase in certain fluids, and a change of diet.

Gastroesophageal Reflux Disease (GERD)

Gastroesophageal reflux disease, commonly referred to as *GERD*, is a chronic condition in which the liquid contents of the stomach back up into the esophagus. The liquid can inflame and damage the lining of the esophagus. It can cause bleeding or ulcers. In addition, scars from tissue damage can narrow the esophagus and make swallowing difficult.

Heartburn is the most common symptom of GERD. Heartburn must be reported to the nurse. Heartburn and GERD are usually treated with medications. Serving the evening meal three to four hours before bedtime may help. The resident should not lie down until at least two to three hours after eating. Extra pillows should be used to keep the body more upright during sleep. Serving the largest meal of the day at lunchtime, serving several small meals throughout the day, and reducing fast foods, fatty foods, and spicy foods may also help. Stopping smoking, not drinking alcohol, and wearing loose-fitting clothes are helpful as well.

Ostomies

An **ostomy** is the surgical creation of an opening from an area inside the body to the outside. The terms *colostomy* and *ileostomy* refer to the surgical removal of a portion of the intestines. In a resident with one of these ostomies, the end of the intestine is brought out of the body through an artificial opening in the abdomen. This opening is called a **stoma**. Stool, or feces, are eliminated through the ostomy rather than through the anus. An ostomy may be necessary due to bowel disease, cancer, or trauma. It may be temporary or permanent.

The terms *colostomy* and *ileostomy* tell what part of the intestine was removed and the type of stool that will be eliminated. A colostomy is a surgically created opening into the large intestine to allow stool to be expelled. With a colostomy, stool will generally be semi-solid. An ileostomy is a surgically created opening into the end of the small intestine to allow stool to be expelled. Stool will be liquid and may be irritating to the resident's skin. Residents who have had an ostomy wear a disposable pouching system that fits over the stoma to collect the feces (Fig. 4-22). The pouching system is attached to the skin by adhesive. A belt may also be used to secure it.

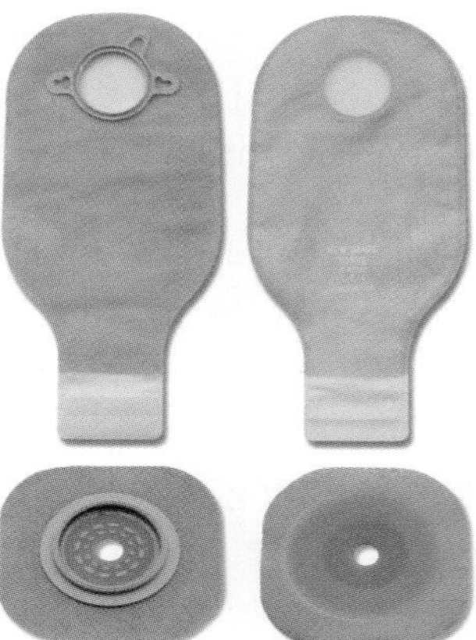

Fig. 4-22. *This photo shows the front and back of a two-piece system. The top is an ostomy drainage pouch, and the bottom is a skin barrier.* (PHOTOS COURTESY OF HOLLISTER INCORPORATED, LIBERTYVILLE, ILLINOIS, HOLLISTER.COM)

Many people manage the ostomy appliance by themselves. Nursing assistants should receive training before providing ostomy care. NAs should give careful skin care. They should empty and clean or replace the ostomy pouch whenever stool is eliminated. NAs should always wear gloves and wash hands carefully when providing ostomy care. They can help by teaching proper handwashing to residents with ostomies.

Residents' Rights

Ostomies

Many residents with ostomies feel they have lost control of a basic bodily function. They may be embarrassed or angry about the ostomy. NAs should be sensitive and supportive and should always provide privacy for ostomy care.

Caring for an ostomy

Equipment: disposable bed protector, bath blanket, clean ostomy pouching system, belt (if needed), disposable wipes (made for ostomy care), basin of warm water, washcloth, 2 towels, plastic disposable bag, gloves

1. Identify yourself by name. Identify the resident by name.
   Resident has right to know identity of his or her caregiver. Identifying resident by name shows respect and establishes correct identification.
2. Wash your hands.
   Provides for infection prevention.
3. Explain procedure to the resident. Speak clearly, slowly, and directly. Maintain face-to-face contact whenever possible.
   Promotes understanding and independence.
4. Provide for resident's privacy with curtain, screen, or door.
   Maintains resident's right to privacy and dignity.
5. Adjust bed to a safe level, usually waist high. Lock bed wheels.
   Prevents injury to you and to resident.
6. Put on gloves.
   Provides for infection prevention.
7. Place bed protector under resident. Cover resident with a bath blanket. Pull down the top sheet and blankets. Expose only the ostomy site. Offer resident a towel to keep clothing dry.
   Maintains resident's right to privacy and dignity.
8. Undo the ostomy belt if used. Remove the ostomy pouch carefully. Place it in the plastic bag. Note the color, odor, consistency, and amount of stool in the pouch.
   Changes in stool can indicate a problem.
9. Wipe the area around the stoma with disposable wipes for ostomy care. Discard the wipes in the plastic bag.
10. Using a washcloth and warm water, wash the area in one direction, away from the stoma (Fig. 4-23). Rinse. Pat dry with another towel.
    Keeping skin clean and dry prevents skin breakdown.

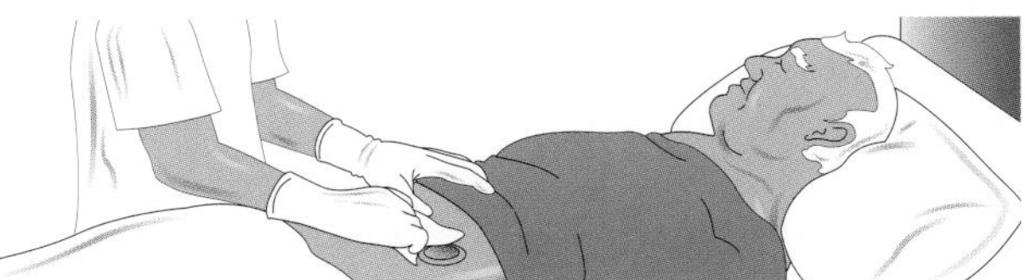

Fig. 4-23. *Wash the area gently, moving away from the stoma.*

11. Place the clean ostomy drainage pouch on the resident. Hold in place and seal securely. Make sure the bottom of the pouch is clamped.
12. Remove the bed protector and discard. Place soiled linens in the proper container. Discard the plastic bag properly.
13. Remove and discard gloves.
14. Wash your hands.
    Provides for infection prevention.
15. Return bed to lowest position. Remove privacy measures.
    Lowering the bed provides for safety.
16. Place call light within resident's reach.
    A call light allows resident to communicate with staff as necessary.
17. Report any changes in resident to the nurse. Note any changes in stoma and surrounding area. A normal stoma is red and moist and looks like the lining of the mouth. Call the nurse if the stoma is very red or blue or if swelling or bleeding is present. Report any signs of skin breakdown around the stoma.
18. Document procedure using facility guidelines.
    If you do not document the care you gave, legally it did not happen.

8. Describe the endocrine system and related conditions

The endocrine system is made up of glands in different areas of the body (Fig. 4-24). **Glands** are organs that produce and secrete chemicals called hormones. **Hormones** are chemical substances created by the body that control numerous body functions. Hormones are carried in the blood to various organs. The functions of the endocrine system are to:

- Maintain homeostasis through hormone secretion
- Influence growth and development
- Maintain blood sugar levels
- Regulate levels of calcium and phosphate in the body
- Regulate the body's ability to reproduce
- Determine how fast cells burn food for energy

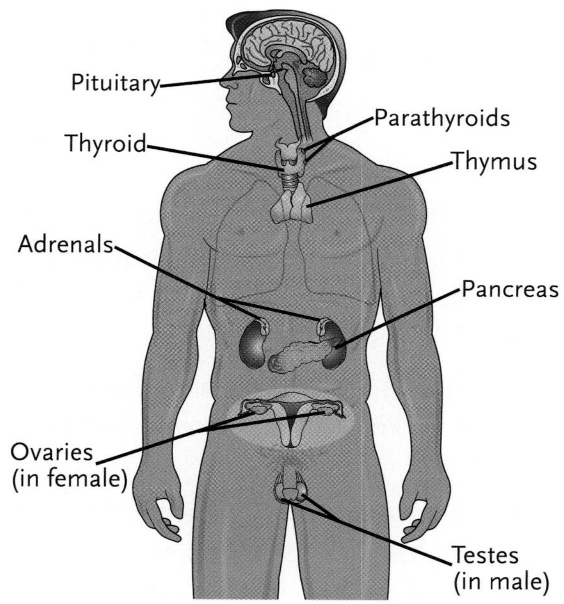

Fig. 4-24. *The endocrine system includes organs that produce hormones that regulate body processes.*

Normal changes of aging include the following:

- Levels of hormones, such as estrogen and progesterone, decrease.
- Insulin production lessens.
- The body is less able to handle stress.

How the NA Can Help

The NA should encourage proper nutrition and try to eliminate or reduce stressors. Stressors are anything that causes stress. Exercise can help reduce stress and should be encouraged. The NA can also help by listening to residents.

Observing and Reporting: Endocrine System

Observe and report these signs and symptoms:

- O/R Headache
- O/R Weakness
- O/R Blurred vision
- O/R Dizziness
- O/R Irritability
- O/R Sweating/excessive perspiration
- O/R Change in "normal" behavior
- O/R Confusion
- O/R Change in mobility
- O/R Change in sensation
- O/R Numbness or tingling in arms or legs
- O/R Weight gain or weight loss
- O/R Loss of appetite or increased appetite
- O/R Increased thirst
- O/R Frequent urination or any change in urine output
- O/R Hunger
- O/R Dry skin
- O/R Skin breakdown
- O/R Sweet or fruity breath
- O/R Sluggishness or fatigue
- O/R Hyperactivity

Diabetes

Diabetes mellitus, commonly called **diabetes**, occurs when the pancreas produces too little insulin or does not properly use insulin. **Insulin** is a hormone that works to move **glucose**, or natural sugar, from the blood and into the cells for energy for the body. Without insulin to process glucose, these sugars collect in the blood and cannot get to cells. This causes problems with circulation and can damage vital organs.

Diabetes is common in people with a family history of the illness, in the elderly, and in people who are obese. Diabetes is a chronic disease that has two major types: type 1 and type 2.

Type 1 diabetes is usually diagnosed in children and young adults. In type 1 diabetes, the pancreas does not produce any insulin. The condition will continue throughout a person's life. Type 1 diabetes is managed with daily injections of insulin or an insulin pump and a special diet. Regular blood glucose testing must be done.

Type 2 diabetes is the most common form of diabetes. In type 2 diabetes, either the body does not produce enough insulin or the body fails to properly use insulin. This is known as *insulin resistance*. Type 2 diabetes usually develops slowly. It is the milder form of diabetes. It typically develops after age 35. The risk of getting this type increases with age. However, the number of children with type 2 diabetes is growing rapidly.

Type 2 diabetes often occurs in obese people or those with a family history of the disease. It can usually be controlled with diet and/or oral medications. Blood glucose levels should be tested regularly.

Pre-diabetes occurs when a person's blood glucose levels are above normal but not high enough for a diagnosis of type 2 diabetes. Research indicates that some damage to the body, especially the heart and circulatory system, may already be occurring during pre-diabetes.

Pregnant women who have never had diabetes before but who have high blood sugar (glucose) levels during pregnancy are said to have **gestational diabetes**.

People with diabetes may have these signs and symptoms:

- Excessive thirst
- Extreme hunger
- Frequent urination
- Weight loss
- High blood sugar levels
- Glucose (sugar) in the urine
- Sudden vision changes
- Tingling or numbness in hands or feet
- Feeling very tired much of the time
- Very dry skin
- Sores that are slow to heal
- More infections than usual

Diabetes can lead to further complications:

- Changes in the circulatory system can cause heart attack and stroke, reduced circulation, poor wound healing, and kidney and nerve damage.
- Damage to the eyes can cause vision loss and blindness.
- Poor circulation and impaired wound healing may cause leg and foot ulcers, infected wounds, and gangrene. Gangrene can lead to amputation.
- Insulin reaction and diabetic ketoacidosis can be serious complications of diabetes. Chapter 2 has more information.

Diabetes must be carefully controlled to prevent complications and severe illness. When working with people with diabetes, NAs must follow care plan instructions carefully.

Guidelines: Diabetes

G Follow diet instructions exactly. The intake of carbohydrates, including breads, potatoes, grains, pastas, and sugars, must be regulated. Meals must be eaten at the same time each day. The resident must eat all that is served. If a resident will not eat what is served, or if you suspect that he is not following the diet, tell the nurse.

G Encourage the resident to follow his exercise program. Regular exercise is important. Exercise affects how quickly bodies use food. Exercise also improves circulation. Exercise may include walking or other activities. It may also include passive range of motion exercises. Help with exercise as necessary. Be positive. Try to make it fun. A walk can be a chore or it can be the highlight of the day.

G Observe the resident's management of insulin. Doses are calculated exactly. They are given at the same time each day. NAs are not allowed to inject insulin, but they need to know when residents take insulin and when their meals should be served. There must be a balance between the insulin level and food intake.

G Perform blood tests as directed. A fingerstick blood glucose test is one type of blood test that may be used to check blood sugar. This is a simple test that is performed by quickly piercing the fingertip, then placing the blood on a chemically active disposable strip. The strip is inserted into a blood glucose meter, a special glucose monitoring machine (Fig. 4-25). The strip will indicate the result. Sometimes the care plan will specify a daily blood test for insulin levels. Not all states allow NAs to do this. Know your state's rules. Your facility will provide training if you are allowed to do this test. Wear gloves when helping with glucose monitoring. Perform tests only as directed and allowed.

G Proper foot care is vitally important for people with diabetes. Give foot care as directed. People with diabetes have poor circulation. Even a small sore on the leg or foot can grow into a large wound that may not heal. This can result in amputation. Careful foot care, including regular, daily inspection, is very important. The goals of diabetic foot care are to check for irritation or sores, to promote blood circulation, and to prevent infection.

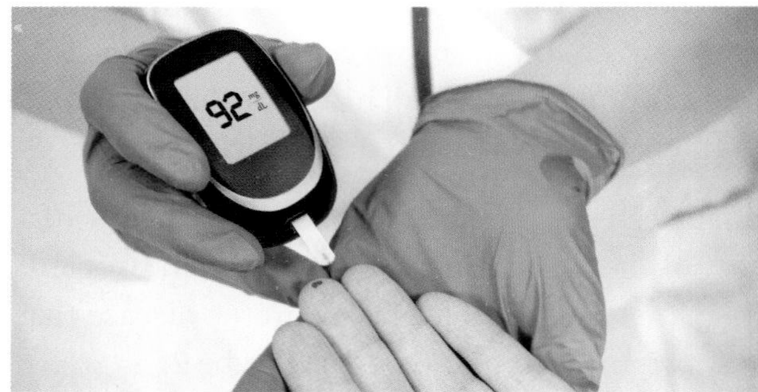

***Fig. 4-25.** There are different types of equipment to measure glucose levels in the blood.*

G Encourage residents to wear comfortable, supportive well-fitting shoes that do not hurt their feet. Shoes made of material that breathes, such as leather, cotton, or canvas, help prevent buildup of moisture. To avoid injuries to the feet, residents should not go barefoot. Socks made of natural fibers such as cotton or wool are best because they absorb sweat. Socks should not be too tight. NAs should not trim or clip toenails. Only a nurse or doctor should do this.

9. Describe the reproductive system and related conditions

The reproductive system is made up of the reproductive organs. They are different in men and women (Fig. 4-26 and Fig. 4-27). The reproductive system allows human beings to **reproduce**, or create new human life. Reproduction begins when a male's and female's sex cells (sperm and ovum) join. These sex cells are formed in the male and female sex glands. These sex glands are called the **gonads**.

For males, the function of the reproductive system is to manufacture sperm and the male hormone testosterone. For females, the reproductive system manufactures ova (eggs) and the female hormones estrogen and progesterone. It also provides an environment for the development of a fetus and produces milk for the nourishment of a baby after birth.

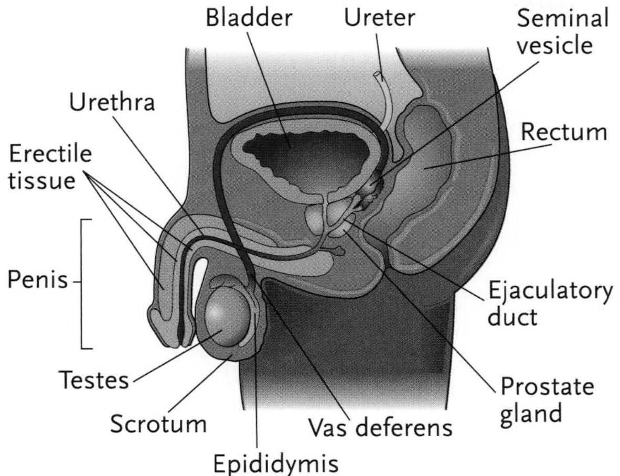

Fig. 4-26. *The male reproductive system.*

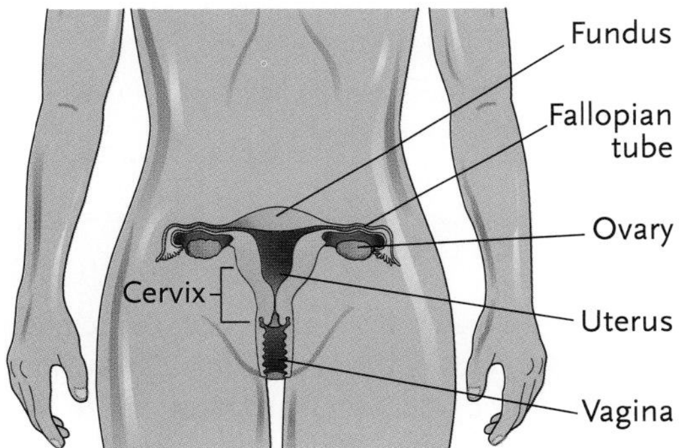

Fig. 4-27. *The female reproductive system.*

Normal changes of aging for males include the following:

- Sperm production decreases.
- The prostate gland enlarges, which can interfere with urination.

Normal changes of aging for females include the following:

- Menstruation ends. Menopause is the end of menstruation. It occurs when a woman has not had a menstrual period for 12 months.
- A decrease in estrogen may lead to a loss of calcium. This can cause brittle bones and, potentially, osteoporosis.
- Vaginal walls become drier and thinner.

How the NA Can Help

Sexual needs and desires continue as people age. The NA should provide privacy when necessary for sexual activity. The NA must respect residents' sexual needs and never judge any sexual behavior. However, any behavior that makes the NA uncomfortable or seems inappropriate should be reported. Inappropriate behavior is not a normal sign of aging and could be a sign of illness.

Observing and Reporting: Reproductive System

Observe and report these signs and symptoms:

- O/R Discomfort or difficulty with urination
- O/R Discharge from the penis or vagina
- O/R Swelling of the genitals
- O/R Blood in urine or stool
- O/R Breast changes, including size, shape, lumps, or discharge from the nipple
- O/R Sores on the genitals
- O/R Redness or rash on the genitals
- O/R Genital itching
- O/R Resident reports of erectile dysfunction (ED) (trouble getting or keeping an erection)
- O/R Resident reports painful intercourse

Vaginitis

Vaginitis is an inflammation of the vagina. It may be caused by a bacteria, protozoa (one-celled animals), or fungus (yeast). It may also be caused by hormonal changes after menopause. Women who have vaginitis have a white vaginal discharge. This is accompanied by itching and burning. These symptoms should be reported to the nurse. Treatment of vaginitis includes oral medications, as well as vaginal creams or suppositories.

Benign Prostatic Hypertrophy (BPH)

Benign prostatic hypertrophy is a disorder that is common in men over the age of 60. The prostate becomes enlarged and causes pressure on the urethra. This pressure leads to frequent urination, dribbling of urine, and difficulty in starting the flow of urine. Urinary retention (urine remaining in the bladder) may also occur, causing urinary tract infection. Urine can also back up into the ureters and kidneys, causing damage to these organs. Medications or surgery are used to treat this disorder. A test is also available to screen for cancer of the prostate. As men age, they are at increased risk for prostate cancer. Prostate cancer is usually slow-growing and responsive to treatment if detected early.

Residents' Rights

Sexual Expression and Privacy

Residents have the right to sexual freedom and expression. Residents have the right to privacy and to meet their sexual needs.

10. Describe the immune and lymphatic systems and related conditions

The immune system protects the body from disease-causing bacteria, viruses, and microorganisms in two ways. Nonspecific immunity protects the body from disease in general. Specific immunity protects against a particular disease that is invading the body at a given time.

The lymphatic system removes excess fluids and waste products from the body's tissues. It also helps the immune system fight infection. It is closely related to both the immune and the circulatory systems. The lymphatic system consists of lymph vessels and lymph capillaries in which a fluid called lymph circulates (Fig. 4-28). Lymph is a clear, yellowish fluid that carries disease-fighting cells called lymphocytes.

Normal changes of aging include the following:

- The immune system weakens, increasing the risk of all types of infections.
- It may take longer for a person to recover from an illness.
- The number and size of lymph nodes decrease, which results in the body being less able to contract a fever to fight infection.
- Response to vaccines decreases.

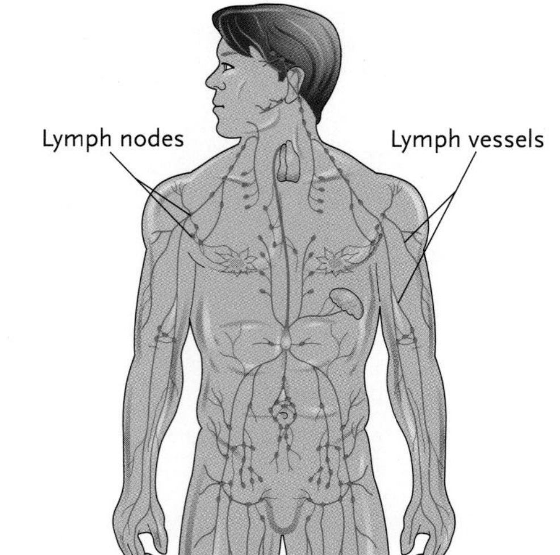

Fig. 4-28. *Lymph nodes work to fight infection and are located throughout the body.*

How the NA Can Help

Factors that weaken the immune system include not enough sleep, poor nutrition, chronic illness, and stress. Preventing infection is important. The NA should wash her hands often and keep the resident's environment clean. She can help with personal hygiene as needed. Proper nutrition and fluid intake should be encouraged. A slight temperature increase may indicate that a resident is fighting an infection. The NA should measure vital signs accurately.

Observing and Reporting: Immune and Lymphatic Systems

Observe and report these signs and symptoms:

- O/R Recurring infections (such as pneumonia, fevers, and diarrhea)
- O/R Swelling of the lymph nodes
- O/R Increased fatigue

HIV and AIDS

Acquired immunodeficiency syndrome (AIDS) is a disease caused by the human immunodeficiency virus (HIV). HIV attacks the body's immune system. It gradually weakens and disables it. AIDS is caused by acquiring the HIV virus through blood or body fluids from an infected person. AIDS is the final stage of HIV infection in which infections, tumors, and symptoms appear due to a weakened immune system that is unable to fight infection. It can take years for HIV to develop into AIDS.

HIV is a sexually transmitted disease. It is also spread through the blood and from infected needles.

In general, HIV affects the body in stages. The first stage shows symptoms like the flu, with fever, muscle aches, cough, fatigue, and swollen lymph glands. These are signs of the immune system fighting the infection. As the infection worsens, the immune system overreacts. It attacks not only the virus, but also normal tissue.

When the virus weakens the immune system in later stages, a group of problems may appear. These include infections, tumors, and central nervous system symptoms. These would not occur if the immune system were healthy. This stage of the disease is known as AIDS. The diagnosis of AIDS is made when a person's CD4+ lymphocyte (a type of white blood cell) count falls to 200 or below. In the late stages of AIDS, damage to the central nervous system may cause memory loss, poor coordination, paralysis, and confusion. These symptoms together are known as AIDS dementia complex.

These are signs and symptoms of HIV infection and AIDS:

- Flu-like symptoms, including fever, cough, weakness, and severe or constant fatigue
- Appetite loss
- Weight loss
- Night sweats
- Swollen lymph nodes in the neck, underarms, or groin
- Severe diarrhea
- Dry cough
- Skin rashes
- Painful white spots in the mouth or on the tongue
- Cold sores or fever blisters on the lips and flat, white ulcers in the mouth
- Cauliflower-like warts on the skin and in the mouth
- Inflamed and bleeding gums
- Bruising that does not go away
- Low resistance to infection, particularly to pneumonia, but also to tuberculosis, herpes, bacterial infections, and hepatitis
- Kaposi's sarcoma, a form of skin cancer that appears as purple, red, or brown skin lesions
- *Pneumocystis jiroveci* pneumonia, a lung infection
- AIDS dementia complex

Infections, such as pneumonia, tuberculosis, or hepatitis, invade the body when the immune system is weak and cannot defend itself. These illnesses worsen AIDS. They further weaken the immune system. It is hard to treat these infections. Over time, a person with AIDS may develop a resistance to some antibiotics. These infections can cause death in people with AIDS.

There is no cure for this disease, and there is no vaccine to prevent the disease. People who are infected with HIV are treated with drugs that slow the progress of the disease. Without medication, however, a weakened resistance to infections may lead to AIDS and eventually to death.

A combination of medications can help people with HIV live longer. The medicines must be taken at precise times. They have many unpleasant side effects. For some people, the medications work less well than for others. Other aspects of HIV treatment include relief of symptoms and prevention of infection.

Guidelines: HIV and AIDS

- **G** Follow Standard Precautions. In addition, follow Transmission-Based Precautions if they are ordered.
- **G** People with poor immune system function are more sensitive to infections. Wash your hands often. Keep everything clean.
- **G** Involuntary weight loss occurs in almost all people who develop AIDS. High-protein, high-calorie, and high-nutrient meals can help maintain a healthy weight.
- **G** Some people with HIV/AIDS lose their appetites and have trouble eating. Encourage these residents to relax before meals and to eat in a pleasant setting. Familiar and favorite foods should be served. Report appetite loss or trouble eating to the nurse. If appetite loss continues, the doctor may prescribe an appetite stimulant.
- **G** Residents with infections of the mouth may need food that is low in acid and neither cold nor hot. Spicy seasonings should be removed. Soft or pureed foods may be easier to swallow. Drinking liquid meals and fortified drinks may help ease the pain of chewing. Warm rinses may help painful mouth sores. Careful mouth care is vital.
- **G** A person who has nausea or vomiting should eat small, frequent meals and should eat slowly. The person should avoid high-fat and spicy foods and eat a soft, bland diet. Residents should drink fluids in between meals. Proper intake of fluids to balance lost fluids is important.
- **G** Residents with mild diarrhea may have small, frequent meals that are low in fat, fiber, and milk products. The doctor may order a BRAT (bananas, rice, applesauce, and toast) diet. This diet is helpful for short-term use. Diarrhea rapidly depletes the body of fluids. Fluid replacement is necessary. Good rehydration fluids include water, juice, caffeine-free soda, and broth. Caffeinated drinks should be avoided.
- **G** Numbness, tingling, and pain in the feet and legs is usually treated with medications. Wearing loose, soft slippers may be helpful. If blankets cause pain, a bed cradle can keep sheets and blankets from resting on legs and feet (Fig. 4-29).

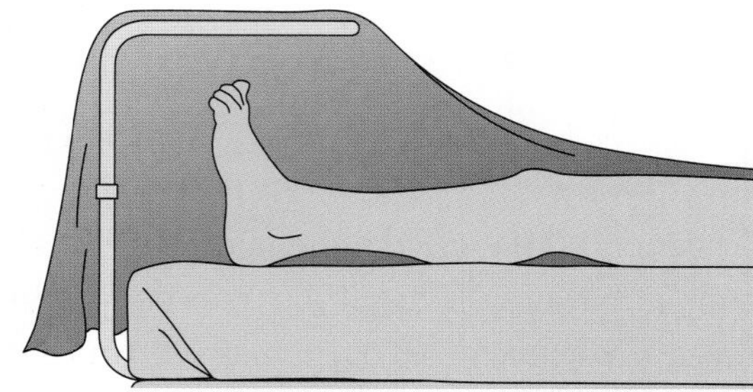

Fig. 4-29. *A bed cradle helps keep covers from resting on the feet.*

- **G** Give emotional support, as well as physical care. Residents with HIV/AIDS may have anxiety and depression. In addition, they are often judged by family, friends, and society. Some people blame them for their illness. People with HIV/AIDS may feel tremendous stress. They may be uncertain about their illness, health care, and finances. They may also have lost friends who have died from AIDS. Listen closely to residents to understand their needs. This is part of providing person-centered care. Treat residents with respect. Help give needed emotional support. Residents with this disease need support from others. This may come from family; friends; religious, community, and support groups; and from the care team.
- **G** Withdrawal, avoidance of tasks, and mental slowness are early symptoms of HIV infection. Medications may also cause side effects of this type. AIDS dementia complex may cause further mental problems. There may also be muscle weakness and loss of muscle control, making falls a risk. Residents will need a safe environment and close supervision in their ADLs.

Residents' Rights

The Facts about HIV and AIDS

A handshake or a hug cannot spread HIV. The disease cannot be transmitted by telephones, doorknobs, tables, chairs, toilets, mosquitoes, or by breathing the same air as an infected person. NAs should spend time with residents who have HIV or AIDS. These residents need the same thoughtful, personal attention that NAs give to all residents.

Cancer

Cancer is a general term used to describe a disease in which abnormal cells grow in an uncontrolled way. Cancer usually occurs in the form of a tumor or tumors growing on or within the body. A **tumor** is a group of abnormally growing cells. Benign tumors are considered noncancerous. They usually grow slowly in local areas. Malignant tumors are cancerous. They can grow rapidly and invade surrounding tissues.

Cancer invades local tissue and can spread to other parts of the body. When it spreads from the site where it first appeared, it can affect other body systems. In general, treatment is more difficult and cancer is more deadly after this has occurred. Cancer often appears first in the breast, colon, rectum, uterus, prostate, lungs, or skin. There is no known cure for cancer, but some treatments are effective.

Known causes of cancer include the following:

- Genetic factors
- Tobacco use
- Alcohol use
- Poor diet/obesity
- Lack of physical activity
- Certain infections
- Environmental exposure, such as radiation
- Sun exposure

When diagnosed and treated early, cancer can often be controlled. The American Cancer Society has identified some warning signs of cancer:

- Unexplained weight loss
- Fever
- Fatigue
- Pain
- Skin changes, such as a change in skin color
- Change in bowel or bladder function
- Sores that do not heal
- Unusual bleeding or discharge
- Thickening or lump in the breast, testicle, or other parts of the body
- Indigestion or difficulty swallowing
- New mole or recent change in appearance of a mole, wart, or spot
- Nagging cough or hoarseness

People with cancer can live longer and sometimes recover if they are treated early. Often these treatments are combined:

- Surgery
- Chemotherapy
- Radiation therapy (radiotherapy)
- Targeted therapy
- Immunotherapy

Guidelines: Cancer

G Each case is different. Cancer is a general term. It refers to many individual situations. Residents may live many years or only several months. Treatment affects each person differently. Do not make assumptions about a resident's condition.

G Residents may want to talk or may avoid talking. Respect each resident's needs. Be honest. Never say "Everything will be okay." Be sensitive. Remember that cancer is a disease. Its cause is unknown. Have a positive attitude (Fig. 4-30).

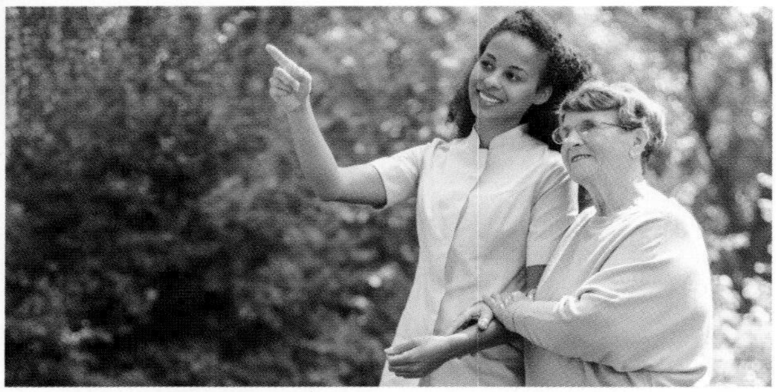

Fig. 4-30. *Have a positive attitude and focus on concrete details. For example, comment if a resident seems stronger, or mention that the sun is shining outside.*

- **G** Proper nutrition is important for residents with cancer. Follow the care plan carefully. Residents frequently have poor appetites. Encourage a variety of food and small portions. Liquid nutrition supplements may be used in addition to, not in place of, meals. If nausea or swallowing is a problem, foods such as soups, gelatin, or starches may appeal to the resident. Use plastic utensils for a resident receiving chemotherapy. It makes food taste better. Metal utensils cause a bitter taste.
- **G** Cancer can cause great pain, especially in the late stages. Watch for signs of pain (Chapter 7). Report them to the nurse. Help with comfort measures, such as repositioning and providing conversation, music, or reading materials. Report if pain seems to be uncontrolled.
- **G** Give back rubs for comfort and to increase circulation. For residents who spend many hours in bed, moving to a chair for a period of time may improve comfort as well. Residents who are weak or immobile need to be repositioned at least every two hours.
- **G** Check the skin often to help prevent pressure injuries. Keep the skin clean and dry. Use lotion on dry or delicate skin. Do not apply lotion to areas receiving radiation therapy. Do not remove markings that are used in radiation therapy. Follow any skin care orders (for example, no hot or cold packs, no soap or cosmetics, or no tight stockings).
- **G** Help residents brush teeth regularly. Medications, nausea, vomiting, or mouth infections may cause pain and a bad taste in the mouth. You can help by using a soft-bristled toothbrush, rinsing with baking soda and water, or using a prescribed rinse. Do not use a commercial mouthwash. For residents with mouth sores, use oral swabs rather than toothbrushes. Be gentle when giving care.
- **G** People with cancer may have a poor self-image because they are weak and their appearance has changed. For example, hair loss is a common side effect of chemotherapy. Help with grooming if desired.
- **G** If visitors help cheer your resident, encourage them. Do not intrude. If some times of day are better than others, suggest this. It may help a person with cancer to think of something else for a while. Pursue other topics. Get to know your residents' interests. Report any signs of depression.
- **G** Having a family member with cancer can be very difficult. Be alert to needs that are not being met or stresses created by the illness.
- **G** Report any of these to the nurse:
  - Increased weakness or fatigue
  - Weight loss
  - Nausea, vomiting, or diarrhea
  - Changes in appetite
  - Fainting
  - Signs of depression
  - Confusion
  - Blood in stool or urine
  - Change in mental status
  - Changes in skin
  - New lumps, sores, or rashes
  - Increase in pain, or unrelieved pain
  - Blood in the mouth

Community resources for residents who are ill are located at the end of Chapter 3.

5 Confusion, Dementia, and Alzheimer's Disease

1. Discuss confusion and delirium

Confusion is the inability to think clearly. A confused person has trouble focusing his attention and may feel disoriented. Confusion interferes with the ability to make decisions. The person's personality may change. He may not know his name, the date, other people, or where he is. A confused person may be angry, depressed, or irritable.

Confusion may come on suddenly or gradually. It can be temporary or permanent. Confusion is more common in the elderly. It may occur when a person is in the hospital. Some causes of confusion include the following:

- Urinary tract infection (UTI)
- Low blood sugar
- Head trauma or head injury
- Dehydration
- Nutritional problems
- Fever
- Sudden drop in body temperature
- Lack of oxygen
- Medications
- Infections
- Brain tumor
- Diseases or illnesses
- Loss of sleep
- Seizures

Guidelines: Confusion

- **G** Do not leave a confused resident alone.
- **G** Stay calm. Provide a quiet environment.
- **G** Speak in a lower tone of voice. Speak clearly and slowly.
- **G** Introduce yourself each time you see the resident.
- **G** Remind the resident of his location, name, and the date. A calendar can help.
- **G** Explain what you are going to do, using simple instructions.
- **G** Be patient. Do not rush the resident.
- **G** Talk to the resident about plans for the day. Keeping a routine may help.
- **G** Encourage the use of eyeglasses and hearing aids. Make sure they are clean and are not damaged.
- **G** Promote self-care and independence.
- **G** Do not leave cleaning agents or personal care products where the resident can access them. A person who is confused may try to eat or drink these products.
- **G** Report observations to the nurse.

Delirium is a state of severe confusion that occurs suddenly; it is usually temporary. Possible causes include infections, disease, fluid imbalances, and poor nutrition. Drugs and alcohol may also cause delirium. Signs and symptoms include the following:

- Agitation
- Anger
- Depression
- Irritability
- Disorientation
- Trouble focusing
- Problems with speech
- Changes in sensation and perception
- Changes in consciousness
- Decrease in short-term memory

NAs should report these signs and symptoms to the nurse. The goal of treatment is to control or reverse the cause. Emergency care may be needed, as well as a stay in a hospital.

Confusion and Delirium

When communicating with a person who is confused or disoriented, the NA should

- Not raise her voice or shout
- Use the person's name, and speak clearly in simple sentences
- Use facial expressions and body language to aid in understanding
- Reduce distractions by taking action, such as turning down the TV
- Be gentle and try to decrease fears

2. Describe dementia and discuss Alzheimer's disease

As a person ages, some of the ability to think logically and clearly may be lost. This ability is called **cognition**. When some of this ability is lost, a person is said to have **cognitive impairment**. How much ability is lost depends on the individual. Cognitive impairment affects concentration and memory. Elderly residents may lose their memories of recent events. This can be frustrating for them. NAs can help by encouraging them to make lists of things to remember. Writing down names and phone numbers may also help. Other normal changes of aging in the brain are slower reaction time, trouble finding or using the right words, and sleeping less.

Dementia is a general term that refers to a serious loss of mental abilities such as thinking, remembering, reasoning, and communicating. As dementia advances, these losses make it hard to perform activities of daily living such as eating, bathing, dressing, and eliminating. Dementia is not a normal part of aging (Fig. 5-1).

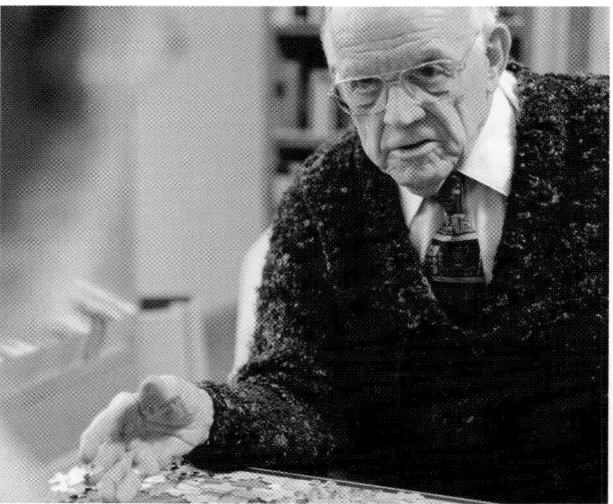

Fig. 5-1. *Some loss of cognitive ability is normal; however, dementia is not a normal part of aging.*

These are some common causes of dementia:

- Alzheimer's disease
- Multi-infarct or vascular dementia (a series of strokes causing damage to the brain)
- Lewy body dementia
- Parkinson's disease
- Huntington's disease

Alzheimer's disease (AD) is the most common cause of dementia in the elderly. The Alzheimer's Association (alz.org/facts) estimates that 5.5 million Americans are living with Alzheimer's disease. One in 10 people aged 65 and older has Alzheimer's disease. Women are more likely than men to have Alzheimer's disease and dementia. African-Americans are about two times as likely to get Alzheimer's disease as older whites, while Hispanics are about 1.5 times as likely. The risk of getting AD increases with age, but it is not a normal part of aging.

Alzheimer's disease causes tangled nerve fibers and protein deposits to form in the brain. They eventually cause dementia. There is no known cause of AD, and there is no cure. Diagnosis is difficult, involving many physical and mental tests to rule out other causes. The only sure way to determine AD at this time is by autopsy (examination of the body after death). The length of time it takes AD to progress from onset to death varies greatly. It may take anywhere from four to 20 years.

Symptoms of AD appear gradually. It begins with memory loss. As the disease progresses, it causes greater and greater loss of health and abilities. People with AD may get disoriented. They may be confused about time and place. Communication problems are common. They may lose their ability to read, write, speak, or understand. Mood and behavior changes. Aggressiveness, wandering, and withdrawal are all part of AD. Alzheimer's disease generally progresses in stages. In each stage, the symptoms become worse. The majority of victims are eventually completely dependent on others for care.

Each person with AD will show different symptoms at different times. For example, one resident may continue to read, but not be able to recognize a family member. Another may be able to play a musical instrument, but may not know how to use the phone. Skills a person has used over a lifetime are usually kept longer (Fig. 5-2). It is important for NAs to encourage independence, regardless of what signs a resident shows. The resident should be encouraged to do whatever he is able to do. This helps keep the resident's mind and body as active as possible (Fig. 5-3). Working, socializing, reading, problem solving, and exercising should be encouraged. Tasks should be challenging but not frustrating. NAs can help residents succeed in doing these tasks.

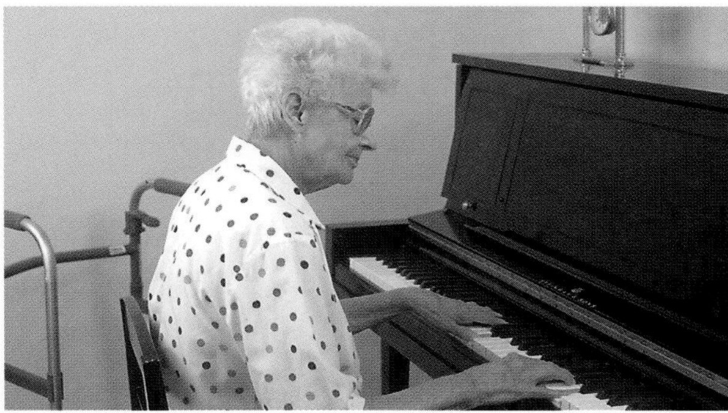

Fig. 5-2. *A person with AD may continue to have skills she has used her whole life.*

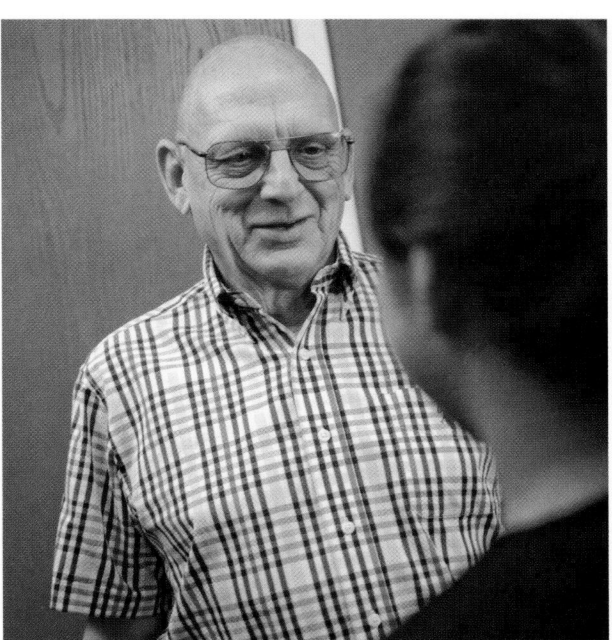

Fig. 5-3. *Nursing assistants should encourage residents to do whatever they are able to do.*

These attitudes help nursing assistants give the best possible care to residents with AD:

- Do not take things personally.
- Be empathetic.
- Work with the symptoms and behaviors noted.
- Work as a team.
- Be aware of difficulties associated with caregiving.

- Work with family members.
- Remember the goals of the care plan.

3. List strategies for better communication with residents with Alzheimer's disease

Many things can be done to improve communication with residents who have Alzheimer's disease. Providing person-centered care means responding to each resident as an individual.

Guidelines: Communicating with Residents Who Have Alzheimer's Disease

- G Always approach from the front, and do not startle the resident.
- G Smile and look happy to see the resident. Be friendly.
- G Determine how close the resident wants you to be.
- G Communicate in a calm area with little background noise and distraction.
- G Always identify yourself and use the resident's name. Continue to use the resident's name during the conversation.
- G Speak slowly, using a lower tone of voice. This is calming and easier to understand.
- G Repeat yourself. Use the same words and phrases as often as needed.
- G Use signs, pictures, gestures, or written words to help communicate.
- G Break complex tasks into smaller, simpler ones. Give simple, step-by-step instructions as necessary.

In addition, residents with AD can be helped by using these techniques for specific situations:

If the resident is frightened or anxious:

- G Speak slowly in a low, calm voice. Speak in a quiet area with few distractions.
- G Try to see and hear yourself as the resident might. Always describe what you are going to do.
- G Use simple words and short sentences. If helping with care, list steps one at a time.
- G Check your body language; make sure you are not tense or hurried.

If the resident forgets or shows memory loss:

- G Repeat yourself. Use the same words if you need to repeat an instruction or question. However, you may be using a word the resident does not understand, such as *tired*. Try other words like *nap*, *lie down*, or *rest*. Repetition can also be soothing. Many people with AD will repeat words, phrases, questions, or actions. This is called **perseveration**. Do not try to stop a resident who is perseverating. Answer the questions, using the same words each time, until he stops. Even though responding over and over may frustrate you, it communicates comfort and security.
- G Keep messages simple. Break complex tasks into smaller, simpler ones.

If the resident has trouble finding words or names:

- G Suggest a word that sounds correct. If this upsets the resident, learn from it. Try not to correct a resident who uses an incorrect word. As words become more difficult, smiling, touching, and hugging can help show care and concern. Remember, however, that some people find touch unwelcome.

If the resident seems not to understand basic instructions or questions:

- G Ask the resident to repeat your words. Use short words and sentences, and allow time to answer.
- G Note the communication methods that are effective and use them.

- Watch for nonverbal cues as the ability to talk lessens. Observe body language—eyes, hands, and face.
- Use signs, pictures, gestures, or written words. For example, a picture of a toilet on the bathroom door can help remind a resident where the bathroom is. Combining verbal and nonverbal communication is helpful. For example, you can say, "Let's get dressed now," while holding up clothes.

If the resident wants to say something but cannot:

- Ask the resident to point, gesture, or act it out.
- If the resident is upset but cannot explain why, offer comfort with a smile, or try to distract him. Verbal communication may be frustrating.

If the resident does not remember how to perform basic tasks:

- Break each activity into simple steps. For instance, "Let's go for a walk. Stand up. Put on your sweater. First the right arm..." Always encourage residents to do what they can.

If the resident insists on doing something that is unsafe or not allowed:

- Redirect activities toward something else. Try to limit the times you say "don't."

If the resident hallucinates (sees or hears things that are not really happening) or is paranoid or accusing:

- Try not to take it personally.
- Try to redirect behavior or ignore it. People with AD often have a limited attention span. This behavior usually passes quickly.

If the resident is depressed or lonely:

- Take time, one-on-one, to ask how he is feeling and really listen to the answer.
- Try to involve the resident in activities. Always report signs of depression to the nurse (Chapter 3).

If the resident repeatedly asks to go home:

- Ask the resident to tell you what his home was like and how he felt being there.
- Redirect or guide the conversation and/or the resident's activities to something he enjoys.
- Expect that the resident may continue to ask to go home and be patient and gentle in your response.

If the resident is verbally abusive or uses bad language:

- Remember it is the dementia speaking, not the person. Try to ignore the language, and redirect attention to something else.

If the resident has lost most verbal skills:

- Use nonverbal skills. As speaking abilities decline, people with AD will still understand touch, smiles, and laughter for much longer. However, some people do not like to be touched. Approach touching slowly and be gentle. Softly touch the hand or place your arm around the resident. A smile can show affection and say you want to help (Fig. 5-4).

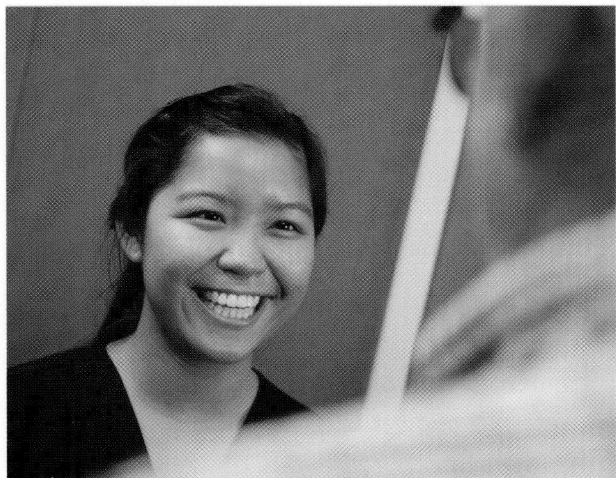

Fig. 5-4. *Smiling can communicate positivity and a willingness to help.*

- **G** Even after verbal skills are lost, signs, labels, and gestures can reach people with dementia.
- **G** Assume people with AD can understand more than they can express. Do not talk about them as though they were not there or treat them like children.

4. List and describe interventions for problems with common activities of daily living (ADLs)

Nursing assistants should use the same procedures for personal care and ADLs for residents with Alzheimer's disease as they would with other residents. However, these general principles will help them give the best care:

1. **Develop a routine and stick to it.** Being consistent is important for residents who are confused and easily upset.
2. **Promote self-care.** Helping residents care for themselves as much as possible will help them cope with this difficult disease.
3. **Take good care of themselves, both mentally and physically.** This will help give the best care.

As Alzheimer's disease worsens, residents will have trouble with their ADLs. Below are techniques that can help with these problems.

Guidelines: Assisting with ADLs for Residents Who Have Alzheimer's Disease

If the resident has problems with bathing:

- **G** Schedule bathing when the resident is least agitated. Be organized so the bath can be quick. Give sponge baths if the resident resists a shower or tub bath.
- **G** Prepare the resident before bathing. Hand him the supplies (washcloth, soap, shampoo, and towels). This serves as a visual aid.
- **G** Take a walk with the resident down the hall. Stop at the tub or shower room, rather than talking directly about the bath.
- **G** Make sure the bathroom is well lit and is at a comfortable temperature.
- **G** Provide privacy during the bath.
- **G** Be calm and quiet when bathing a resident. Keep the process simple.
- **G** Be sensitive when talking to a resident about bathing.
- **G** Give the resident a washcloth to hold. This can distract him while you finish the bath.
- **G** Always follow safety precautions. Ensure safety by using nonslip mats, tub seats, and handholds.
- **G** Be flexible about when to bathe a resident. A resident may not always be in the mood. Also, not everyone bathes with the same frequency. Understand if a resident does not want to bathe.
- **G** Be relaxed and allow the resident to enjoy the bath. Offer praise.
- **G** Let the resident do as much as possible during the bath.
- **G** Check the skin regularly for signs of irritation or breakdown during the bath.

If the resident has problems with grooming and dressing:

- **G** Help with grooming to help the resident feel attractive.
- **G** Avoid delays or interruptions while dressing.
- **G** Provide privacy by closing doors and curtains. Dress the resident in her room.
- **G** Show the resident some of her clothing. This brings up the idea of dressing.
- **G** Encourage the resident to pick clothes to wear. Simplify this by giving just a few choices. Make sure the clothing is clean and

appropriate. Lay out clothes in the order in which they are to be put on (Fig. 5-5). Choose clothes that are simple to put on. Some people with AD layer clothing regardless of the weather.

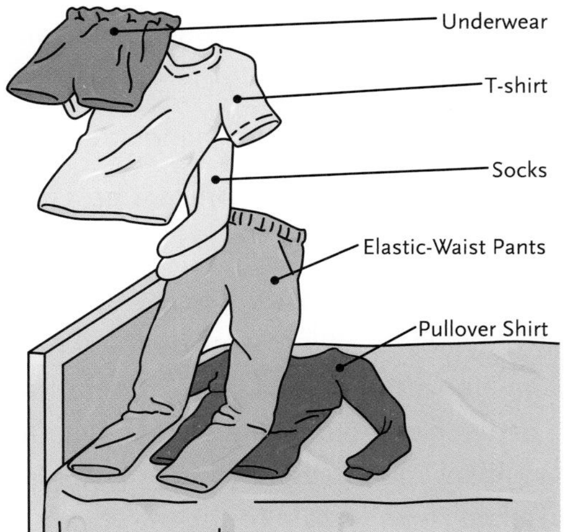

Fig. 5-5. *Clothes should be laid out in the order in which they should be put on.*

- **G** Break the task down into simple steps. Introduce one step at a time. Do not rush the resident.
- **G** Use a friendly, calm voice when speaking. Praise and encourage the resident at each step.

If the resident has problems with elimination:

- **G** Encourage fluids. Never withhold or discourage fluids because a resident has problems with urinary incontinence. Report to the nurse if the resident is not drinking fluids. Follow the schedule in the care plan for drinking fluids.
- **G** Mark the bathroom with a sign or a picture. This is a reminder of both where it is and to use the toilet.
- **G** Make sure there is enough light in the bathroom and on the way there.
- **G** Note when the resident is incontinent over two to three days. Check her every 30 minutes. This can help determine "bathroom times." Take the resident to the bathroom just before her bathroom time.
- **G** Observe toilet patterns for two to three nights to try to determine nighttime bathroom times.
- **G** Take the resident to the bathroom after drinking fluids. Take the resident to the bathroom before and after meals and before bedtime. Make sure the resident actually urinates before getting off the toilet.
- **G** Put lids on trash cans, wastebaskets, or other containers if the resident urinates or defecates in them.
- **G** Family or friends may be upset by their loved one's incontinence. Be professional when cleaning after episodes of incontinence. Do not show disgust or irritation.

If the resident has problems with nutrition:

- **G** Encourage nutritious food. Food may not interest a resident with AD, or he may forget to eat. It may be of great interest, but he may only want to eat a few types of food. A resident with AD is at risk for malnutrition.
- **G** Have meals at regular times each day. You may need to remind the resident that it is mealtime. Familiar, appetizing foods should be served.
- **G** Make sure there is proper lighting.
- **G** Keep noise and distractions low during meals.
- **G** Keep the task of eating simple. If the resident is restless, try smaller, more frequent meals. Finger foods (foods that are easy to pick up with the fingers) work best. They allow residents to choose the food they want to eat. Examples of finger foods that may be good to serve are sandwiches cut into fourths, chicken nuggets or small pieces of cooked boneless chicken, fish sticks, cheese cubes, halved hard-boiled eggs, and cut fresh fruit and soft vegetables.
- **G** Do not serve steaming or very hot foods or drinks.

- Use a simple place setting with a single eating utensil. Remove other items from the table (Fig. 5-6). Plain plates without patterns or colors work best.

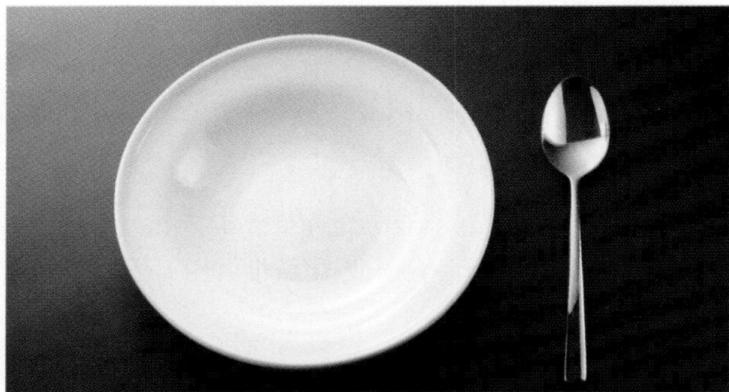

Fig. 5-6. *Plain white plates on a contrasting-colored surface may help avoid confusion and distraction.*

- Put only one item of food on the plate at a time. Multiple kinds of food on a plate or a tray may be overwhelming.
- Give simple, clear instructions. Residents with AD may not understand how to eat or use utensils. Help the resident taste a sample of the meal first. Place a spoon to the lips. This will encourage the resident to open her mouth. Ask the resident to open her mouth.
- Guide the resident through the meal. Provide simple instructions. Offer regular drinks of water, juice, and other fluids to prevent dehydration.
- Use adaptive equipment for eating, such as special spoons and bowls, as needed.
- If the resident needs to be fed, do so slowly. Offer small pieces of food.
- Make mealtimes simple and relaxed, not rushed. Give the resident time to swallow before the next bite or drink.
- Seat the resident with others at small tables. This encourages socializing.
- Observe and report eating or swallowing problems. Report changes in eating habits. Monitor weight accurately and frequently.

To promote the resident's physical health:

- Prevent infections and follow Standard Precautions.
- Observe the resident's physical health and report any potential problems. People with dementia may not notice their own health problems.
- Help residents wash their hands frequently.
- Give careful skin care to prevent pressure injuries.
- Watch for signs of pain. A person who has AD may not be able to express that he is in pain. Nonverbal signs that a resident may be in pain include grimacing or clenching fists. A resident may be agitated or angry. Report possible signs of pain to the nurse.
- Maintain a daily exercise routine.

To promote the resident's mental and emotional health:

- Maintain self-esteem by encouraging independence in activities of daily living.
- Share in enjoyable activities, such as looking at pictures and talking.
- Reward positive and independent behavior with smiles and warm touches.

5. List and describe interventions for common difficult behaviors related to Alzheimer's disease

Below are some common difficult behaviors that NAs may face with residents who have AD. Each resident is different, and NAs should work with each person as an individual.

Agitation: A resident who is excited, restless, or troubled is said to be agitated. Feeling insecure or frustrated, encountering new people or places, and changing a routine can all trigger this behavior. A trigger is a situation that leads to agitation. Even watching television can cause agitation, as a person with AD may lose his ability to tell fiction from reality. If a resident is agitated, the NA should

- Try to remove triggers, keep a routine, and avoid frustration. Redirect attention.
- Reduce noise and distractions. Focus on a familiar activity, such as sorting things or looking at pictures.
- Stay calm and use a low, soothing voice. This may reassure the resident.

Sundowning: When a person with AD gets restless and agitated in the late afternoon, evening, or night, it is called **sundowning**. Sundowning may be caused by hunger or fatigue, a change in routine or caregiver, or any new or frustrating situation. If a resident experiences this, the NA should

- Avoid stressful situations during this time. Activities, appointments, and visits should be limited.
- Play soft music.
- Set a bedtime routine and keep it.
- Recognize when sundowning occurs. A calming activity can be done just before.
- Remove caffeine from the diet.
- Provide snacks.
- Give a soothing back massage.
- Distract the resident with a simple, calm activity like looking at a magazine.
- Maintain a daily exercise routine.

Catastrophic Reactions: When a person with AD overreacts to something, it is called a **catastrophic reaction**. It may be triggered by any of the following:

- Fatigue
- Change of routine, environment, or caregiver
- Overstimulation (too much noise or activity)
- Difficult choices or tasks
- Physical pain or discomfort, including hunger or a need to use the toilet

An NA can respond to catastrophic reactions as she would to agitation or sundowning. For example, she can remove triggers. She can help the resident focus on a soothing activity.

Violent Behavior: A resident who attacks, hits, or threatens someone is using violence. Frustration or overstimulation may trigger violence. It can also be triggered by a change in routine, environment, or caregiver. If a resident is violent, the NA should

- Call for help if needed.
- Block blows but never hit back.
- Step out of reach and stay calm.
- Avoid leaving the resident alone.
- Try to remove triggers.
- Use the same techniques to calm residents as for agitation.

Pacing and Wandering: A resident who walks back and forth in the same area is **pacing**. A resident who walks aimlessly around the facility is **wandering** (Fig. 5-7). These are some causes of pacing and wandering:

- Restlessness
- Hunger
- Disorientation
- Incontinence or the need to use the bathroom
- Constipation
- Pain
- Forgetting how or where to sit down
- Too much daytime napping
- Need for exercise

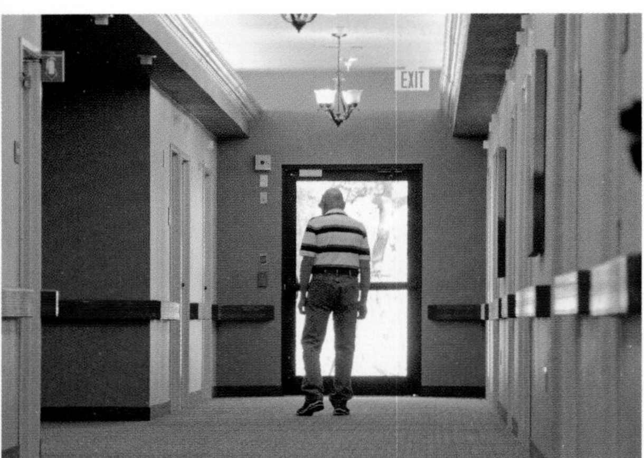

Fig. 5-7. *A resident with AD who is walking aimlessly around the facility or facility grounds is wandering.*

If a resident paces or wanders, the NA should

- Remove causes when she can. For example, give nutritious snacks, encourage an exercise routine, and maintain a toileting schedule.
- Let residents pace and wander in a safe and secure (locked) area. Staff should keep an eye on them.
- Redirect attention to something the resident enjoys, such as suggesting going on a walk together.
- Mark rooms with signs or pictures, such as stop signs or "closed" signs. This may prevent residents from wandering into areas where they should not go.

Elopement

Residents with AD may try to **elope**, or leave a facility unsupervised and unnoticed. It is very important that residents who elope are located and returned to the facility as soon as possible. The longer a resident is gone, the greater the danger he might encounter. If an NA believes a resident might have eloped, she must tell her supervisor immediately. Residents who elope are often found near where they were last seen. The earlier a search is begun, the more likely the resident is to be found nearby and safe.

Hallucinations or Delusions: A resident who sees, hears, smells, tastes, or feels things that are not there is having **hallucinations**. A resident who believes things that are not true is having **delusions**. If a resident is experiencing hallucinations and/or delusions, the NA should

- Ignore harmless hallucinations and delusions.
- Reassure a resident who seems agitated or worried.
- Not argue with a resident who is imagining things. Challenging the resident serves no purpose and can make matters worse. The feelings are real to him. The NA should not tell the resident that she sees or hears his hallucinations. She should redirect the resident to other activities or thoughts.
- Be calm and reassure the resident that she is there to help.

Depression: People who become withdrawn, lack energy, and stop eating or doing things they used to enjoy may be depressed. Depression may have many causes, including the following:

- Loss of independence
- Inability to cope
- Feelings of failure or fear
- Reality of facing a progressive, incurable illness
- Chemical imbalance

If a resident is depressed, the NA should

- Report signs of depression to the nurse immediately. It is an illness that can be treated with medication and/or therapy. Any threats of suicide should be reported immediately.
- Observe for triggers that cause changes in mood.
- Encourage independence, self-care, and activity.
- Listen to the resident if she wants to share her feelings or talk about her mood.
- Encourage social interaction.

Perseveration or Repetitive Phrasing: A resident who has dementia may repeat words, phrases, questions, or activities over and over again. This is called perseverating or repetitive phrasing. This may be caused by disorientation or confusion. The NA should be patient and not try to silence or stop the resident. She should answer questions each time they are asked. She should use the same words each time.

Disruptiveness: Disruptive behavior is anything that disturbs others, such as yelling, banging on furniture, and slamming doors. Often this behavior is triggered by pain, constipation, frustration, or a wish for attention. To prevent or respond to disruptive behavior, the NA should

- Be calm and friendly, and try to find out why the behavior is occurring. There may be a physical reason, such as pain or discomfort.
- Gently direct the resident to a private area.
- Notice and praise improvements in the resident's behavior. Be careful to avoid treating the resident like a child.
- Tell the resident about any changes in schedules, routines, or the environment in advance. Involving the resident in developing routine activities and schedules may help.
- Encourage the resident to join in independent activities that are safe (for example, folding towels). This helps the resident feel in charge. It can prevent feelings of powerlessness. Independence is power.
- Help the resident find ways to cope. Focusing on activities the resident may still be able to do, such as knitting or crafts, can provide a diversion.

Inappropriate Social Behavior: Inappropriate social behavior may be cursing, name calling, or yelling. As with violent or disruptive behavior, there may be many reasons why a resident is behaving this way. The NA should try not to take it personally. The resident may only be reacting to frustration or other stress. The NA should stay calm and be reassuring. She can try to find out what caused the behavior. Possible causes include too much noise, too many people, and too much stress, pain, or discomfort. If the resident is disturbing others, the NA should gently direct him to a private area. Any physical abuse or serious verbal abuse should be reported to the nurse.

Inappropriate Sexual Behavior: Inappropriate sexual behavior, such as removing clothes, touching one's own genitals in public, or trying to touch others can disturb or embarrass those who see it. It is helpful to stay calm when this behavior occurs. The NA should not overreact, as this may reinforce the behavior. Trying to determine the cause may help. Is the behavior actually intentional? Is it consistent? If distracting the resident does not work, the NA can gently direct him to a private area. She should tell the nurse. A resident may be reacting to a need for physical stimulation or affection. Ways to provide physical stimulation include back rubs, a soft stuffed animal to cuddle, comforting blankets, or physical touch that is appropriate.

Hoarding and Rummaging: **Rummaging** is going through drawers, closets, or personal items that belong to oneself or others. **Hoarding** is collecting and putting things away in a guarded way. These behaviors are not within the control of a person with Alzheimer's disease. They should not be considered stealing. Stealing is planned. It requires a conscious effort. In most cases, the person with AD is only collecting something that catches his attention. It is common for those with AD to wander and collect things. They may carry these objects around for a while and then leave them in other places. This is not intentional. Residents with AD will often take their own things and leave them in another room, not knowing what they are doing. If a resident hoards or rummages, the NA should

- Label all personal belongings with the resident's name and room number. This way there is no confusion about what belongs to whom.

- Place a label, symbol, or object on the resident's door. This helps the resident find his own room.
- Not tell the family that their loved one is "stealing" from others.
- Prepare the family so they are not upset when they find items that do not belong to their family member.
- Ask the family to tell staff if they notice unfamiliar items in the room.
- Regularly check areas where residents store items. They may store uneaten food in these places. Providing a rummage drawer—a drawer with items that are safe for the resident to take with him—can help.

Sleep Disturbances: Residents with AD may experience a number of sleep disturbances. If a resident experiences sleep problems, the NA should

- Make sure that the resident gets moderate exercise/activity throughout the day. The NA can encourage him to participate in activities he enjoys.
- Allow the resident to spend some time each day in natural sunlight if possible. Exposure to light and dark can help establish restful sleep patterns.
- Reduce light and noise as much as possible during nighttime hours.
- Discourage sleeping during the day.

Suspicion: A person with AD often becomes suspicious as the disease progresses. Residents may accuse staff or family members of lying to them or stealing from them. Suspicion may escalate to paranoia (having intense feelings of distrust and believing others are "out to get them"). When a resident is acting suspicious, the NA should not argue with him. Arguing just increases defensiveness. Instead, the NA should offer reassurance and be understanding and supportive.

Residents' Rights

Abuse and Alzheimer's Disease

People with Alzheimer's disease may be at a higher risk for abuse. One reason for this is that caring for someone with Alzheimer's disease is very difficult. There are many psychological and physical demands placed on caregivers.

To help manage the stress of caring for people with AD, NAs should take care of themselves, both mentally and physically. This will help them give the best care. If needed, a supervisor can provide more resources to help an NA cope.

NAs must never abuse residents in any way. If an NA notices someone else abusing a resident, he is legally required to report it. All NAs are responsible for residents' safety and should take this responsibility seriously.

6. Describe creative therapies for residents with Alzheimer's disease

Although Alzheimer's disease cannot be cured, there are ways to improve life for residents with AD.

Validation therapy is letting residents believe they live in the past or in imaginary circumstances. **Validating** means giving value to or approving. When using validation therapy, the NA should make no attempt to reorient the resident to actual circumstances (Fig. 5-8). She can explore the resident's beliefs. She should not argue with or correct him. Validating can give comfort and reduce agitation. Validation therapy is useful in cases of severe dementia.

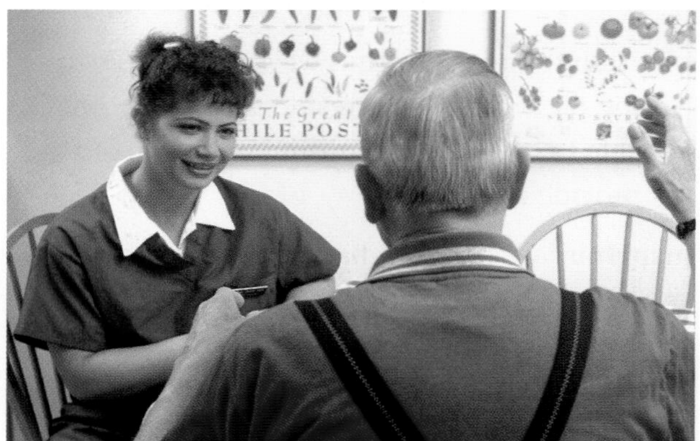

Fig. 5-8. *Validation therapy accepts a resident's fantasies without attempting to reorient him to reality.*

Example: Mr. Baldwin tells the NA that he does not want to eat lunch today because he is going out to a restaurant with his wife. The NA knows his wife has been dead for many years and that Mr. Baldwin can no longer eat out. Instead of telling him that he is not going out to eat, the NA asks what restaurant he is going to and what he will have. She suggests that he eat a good lunch now because sometimes the service is slow in restaurants.

Reminiscence therapy is encouraging residents to remember and talk about the past. The NA can explore memories by asking about details. Reminiscence therapy can help elderly people remember pleasant times in their past. It also allows caregivers to increase their understanding of residents. It is useful in many stages of AD, but especially with moderate to severe dementia.

Example: Mr. Benton, an 83-year-old man with Alzheimer's disease, fought in the Korean War. In his room are many mementos of the war. He has pictures of his war buddies, a medal he was given, and more. The NA asks him to tell him where he was sent in the war. The NA asks him more detailed questions. Eventually the resident shares a lot: the friends he made in the service, why he was given the medal, times he was scared, and how much he missed his family (Fig. 5-9).

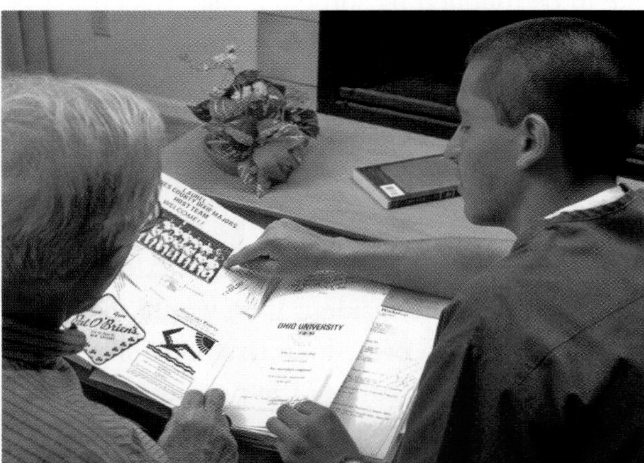

Fig. 5-9. *Reminiscence therapy encourages a resident to remember and talk about his past.*

Activity therapy uses activities that the resident enjoys to prevent boredom and frustration. These activities also promote self-esteem. The NA can help the resident take walks, do puzzles, listen to music, read, or do other things she enjoys (Fig. 5-10). Activities may be done in groups or one-on-one. Activity therapy is useful in most stages of AD.

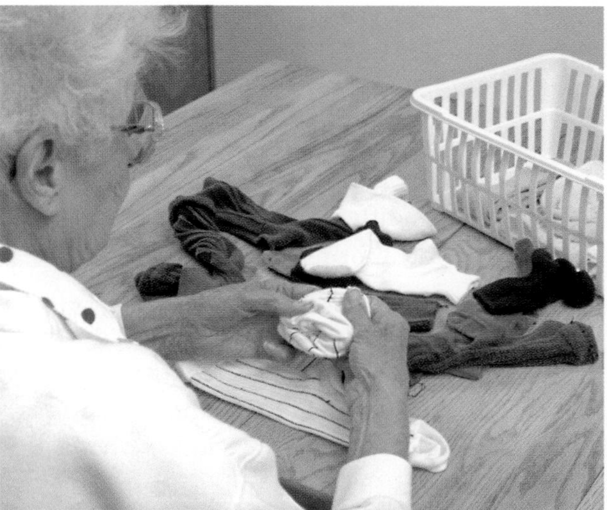

Fig. 5-10. *Activities that are not frustrating can be helpful for residents with AD. They promote mental exercise.*

Example: Mrs. Hoebel, a 70-year-old woman with AD, was a librarian for almost 45 years. She loves books and reading, but she cannot read much anymore. The NA obtains books from the facility that are filled with pictures. Mrs. Hoebel sits with the books, sorting them, turning pages, and looking at pictures.

Music Therapy

Music therapy involves using music to accomplish specific goals, such as managing stress and improving mood and cognition. This type of therapy has been used successfully with people who have Alzheimer's disease. Music is a form of sensory stimulation. Hearing familiar songs can cause a response in people with dementia who do not respond well or at all to other treatments. Music & Memory is a nonprofit organization that brings personalized music into the lives of the elderly. Their website, musicandmemory.org, provides more information.

6 Personal Care Skills

1. Explain personal care of residents

Personal care is different from other tasks that NAs may perform for residents, such as measuring vital signs or tidying a unit. The term *personal* refers to tasks that are concerned with the person's body, appearance, and hygiene. It suggests privacy may be important. **Hygiene** is the term used to describe ways to keep bodies clean and healthy. Bathing and brushing teeth are two examples. **Grooming** refers to practices like caring for fingernails and hair. Hygiene and grooming activities, as well as dressing, eating, transferring, and eliminating, are called *activities of daily living* (*ADLs*). NAs will help residents with these tasks every day. These activities are often called *a.m. care* or *p.m. care*. This refers to the time of day that they are done.

Assisting with a.m. care includes

- Offering a bedpan or urinal or helping the resident to the bathroom and helping with perineal care as needed
- Helping the resident wash face and hands
- Assisting with hair care, dressing, and shaving
- Assisting with mouth care before or after breakfast

Assisting with p.m. care includes

- Offering a bedpan or urinal or helping the resident to the bathroom
- Helping the resident wash face and hands
- Giving a snack
- Assisting with mouth care
- Assisting with changing into nightclothes
- Giving a back rub

The way NAs help residents with personal care plays a large part in promoting residents' independence and dignity. The help NAs give will be different for each resident. It will depend on each resident's abilities. For example, a resident who has recently had a stroke may need more help than one who has a broken foot that is almost healed. Promoting independence is an important part of care.

Many people have been doing personal care tasks for themselves their entire lives. They may feel uncomfortable about having anyone help them with these tasks. Some residents may not like to be touched by someone else. NAs must be sensitive to these issues. They should be professional when helping with these tasks.

Before beginning any task, the NA should explain to the resident exactly what she will be doing. Having care explained is a resident's legal right. It may also help lessen anxiety. The NA should ask the resident if he would like to use the bathroom or bedpan first. She should provide privacy by pulling the privacy curtain around the bed and closing the door. The resident should be allowed to make as many decisions as possible about when, where, and how a procedure is done (Fig. 6-1). This promotes independence and is part of providing person-centered care. Other ways for NAs to promote respect, dignity, and privacy include the following:

- Encouraging residents to do as much as they are able to do and be patient
- Knocking and waiting for permission to enter the resident's room if the resident is able to give permission
- Not interrupting residents while they are in the bathroom
- Leaving the room when residents receive or make phone calls
- Respecting residents' private time and personal things
- Not interrupting residents while they are dressing
- Keeping residents covered whenever possible when helping with dressing

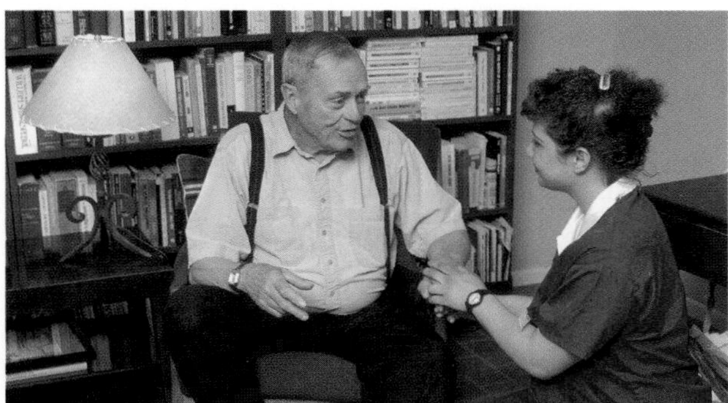

Fig. 6-1. *Nursing assistants should let the resident make as many decisions as possible about personal care.*

During personal care, the NA should look for any problems or changes that have occurred. Communication is very important during personal care. Some residents will share symptoms, feelings, and concerns with the NA. The NA should keep a small notepad in a pocket to note exactly how the resident describes these symptoms. These comments should be reported to the nurse and documented. NAs must also look for physical or mental changes. The resident's environment should be checked for anything unsafe. These issues should also be reported.

During the procedure, if the resident appears tired, the NA should stop and take a short break. The resident should not be rushed. After care, the NA should always ask if the resident would like anything else. She should leave the resident's area clean and tidy. Before leaving, the NA must make sure the call light is left within the resident's reach. The room should be at a comfortable temperature. The walkways must be clear. The bed should be left in its lowest position unless the care plan instructs otherwise.

Observing and Reporting: Personal Care

O/R Skin color, temperature, redness

O/R Mobility

O/R Flexibility

O/R Comfort level or pain or discomfort

O/R Strength and the ability to perform ADLs

O/R Mental and emotional state

O/R Resident's complaints

2. Identify guidelines for providing skin care and preventing pressure injuries

Immobility reduces the amount of blood that circulates to the skin. Residents who have restricted mobility are at greater risk of skin deterioration at pressure points. **Pressure points** are areas of the body that bear much of its weight. Pressure points are mainly located at bony prominences. **Bony prominences** are areas of the body where the bone lies close to the skin. The skin here is at a much higher risk for skin breakdown. These areas include elbows, shoulder blades, the tailbone, hips and knees (inner and outer parts), ankles, heels, toes, and the back of the head. Other areas at risk are the ears, the area under the breasts or scrotum, the area between the folds of the buttocks or abdomen, and the skin between the legs (Fig. 6-2).

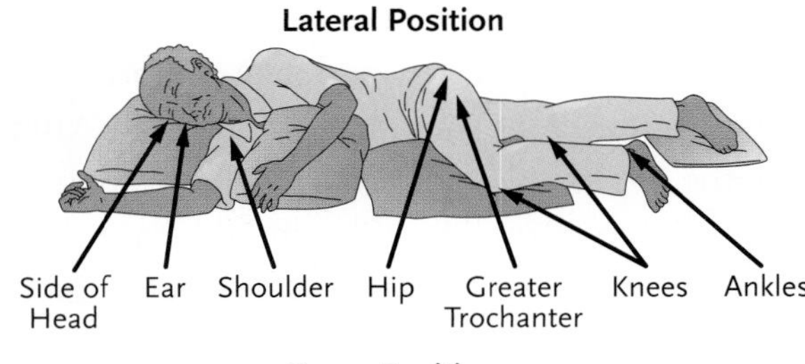

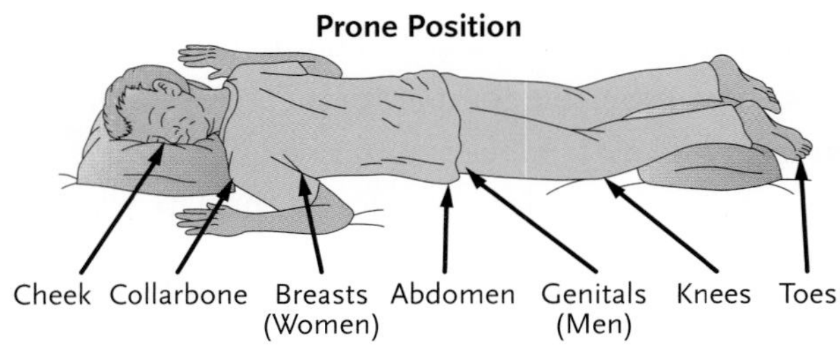

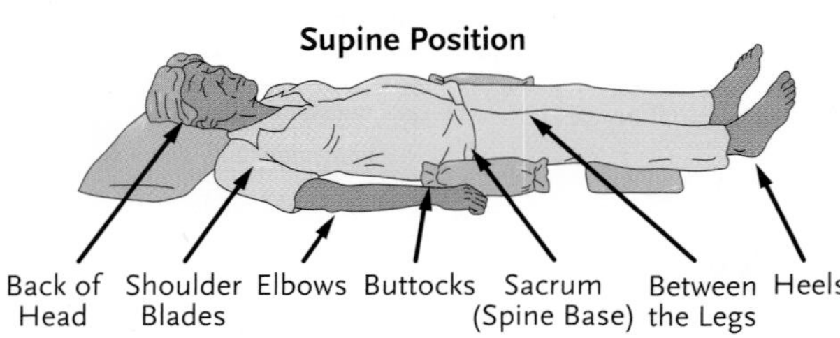

Fig. 6-2. *Pressure injury danger zones.*

Pressure on these areas reduces circulation, decreasing the amount of oxygen the cells receive. Warmth and moisture also add to skin breakdown. Once the surface of the skin is weakened, injuries can occur and may become infected. This can cause damage to the underlying tissue. When infection occurs, the healing process slows. The injuries that result from skin deterioration and shearing are called **pressure injuries** (also called *pressure ulcers, pressure sores, decubitus ulcers*, or *bed sores*). **Shearing** is rubbing or friction that results from the skin moving one way and the bone underneath it remaining fixed or moving in the opposite direction.

If caught early, a break in the skin can heal fairly quickly without other problems. However, if not caught early, a pressure injury can get bigger, deeper, and infected. Pressure injuries are painful and are difficult to heal. They can lead to life-threatening infections. Prevention is important. It is the key to skin health. Stages of pressure injuries are:

- **Stage 1**: Skin is intact, but it may look red, and the redness is not relieved after removing pressure. Darker skin may not look red but may appear to be a different color than the surrounding area. The area may be swollen, painful, firm, soft, or warmer or cooler when compared to the area around it.
- **Stage 2**: There is partial-thickness skin loss involving the outer and/or inner layers of skin. The injury is pink or red and moist, and may also look like a blister.
- **Stage 3**: There is full-thickness skin loss in which fat is visible in the injury. Slough and/or eschar may be present. *Slough* is yellow, tan, gray, green, or brown tissue that is usually moist. *Eschar* is dead tissue that is hard or soft in texture and black, brown, or tan, and may be similar to a scab. The damage may extend down to, but not through, the tissue that covers muscle.
- **Stage 4**: There is full-thickness skin loss extending through all layers of the skin, tissue, muscle, bone, and other structures, such as tendons. The injury will look like a deep crater and slough and/or eschar may be visible (Fig. 6-3).
- **Unstageable Pressure Injury**: There is full-thickness skin and tissue loss, but the extent of the damage cannot be determined because it is covered with slough or eschar. Once the slough and/or eschar is removed, the injury can then be staged (either Stage 3 or Stage 4).
- **Deep Tissue Pressure Injury**: The skin area is intact or nonintact and is deep red, purple, or maroon. The wound may appear as a blood-filled blister. The area may be painful and may be warmer or cooler than the surrounding tissue. Discoloration may be different in darker skin.

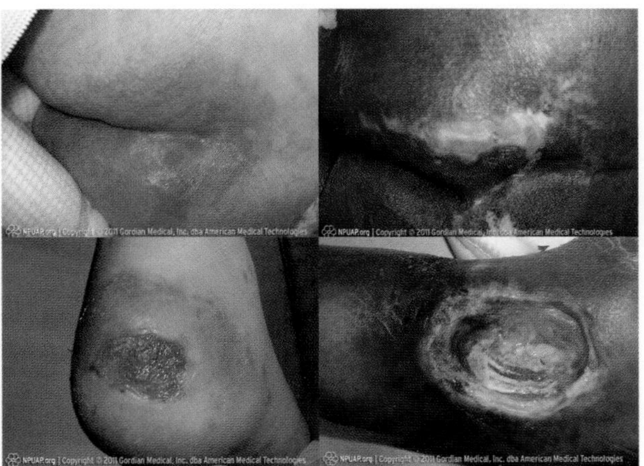

Fig. 6-3. Pressure injury stages as described by the National Pressure Ulcer Advisory Panel (NPUAP). (a) Photo of a Stage 1 pressure injury on the buttocks. (b) Photo of a Stage 2 pressure injury on the buttocks. (c) Photo of a Stage 3 pressure injury on the heel. (d) Photo of a Stage 4 pressure injury on the foot. (PHOTOS COPYRIGHT © NATIONAL PRESSURE ULCER ADVISORY PANEL, NPUAP.ORG, USED WITH PERMISSION)

Observing and Reporting: Resident's Skin

Report any of these to the nurse:

- O/R Pale, white, reddened, gray, or purple skin
- O/R Blisters, bruises, or wounds on the skin
- O/R Differences in temperature of the skin when compared to the area around it
- O/R Complaints of tingling, warmth, or burning of the skin
- O/R Dry, cracked, or flaking skin
- O/R Itching or scratching
- O/R Rash or any skin discoloration
- O/R Swelling
- O/R Fluid or blood draining from the skin
- O/R Broken skin anywhere on the body, including between the toes or around the toenails
- O/R Changes in existing injury (size, depth, drainage, color, or odor)

Breaks in the skin can cause serious, even life-threatening, problems. It is better to prevent skin problems and keep the skin healthy than it is to treat problems after they happen.

Guidelines: Basic Skin Care

- G Report any changes in a resident's skin.
- G Provide regular, daily care for skin to keep it clean and dry. Check the skin daily, even when complete baths are not given or taken every day.
- G Reposition immobile residents often (at least every two hours).
- G Give frequent, thorough skin care as often as needed for residents who are incontinent. Change clothing and linens often as well. Check on residents at least every two hours.
- G Do not scratch or irritate the skin in any way. Keep rough, scratchy fabrics away from the resident's skin. Report to the nurse if a resident wears shoes that cause blisters.
- G Massage the skin often. Use light, circular strokes to increase circulation. Do not massage bony areas. Do not massage a white, red, or purple area or put any pressure on it. Massage the healthy skin and tissue around the area.
- G Be gentle during transfers. Avoid pulling or tearing fragile skin.
- G Residents who are overweight may have poor circulation and extra folds of skin. Pay careful attention to the skin under the folds. Keep it clean and dry. Report signs of skin irritation.
- G Encourage well-balanced meals and plenty of fluids. Proper nutrition is important for keeping skin healthy.
- G Keep plastic or rubber materials from coming into contact with the resident's skin. These materials prevent air from circulating, which causes the skin to sweat.
- G Follow the care plan. It may include instructions about special skin care, such as washing the skin with a special soap.

For residents who are not mobile or cannot change positions easily, do the following:

- Keep the bottom bedsheet tight and free of wrinkles. Keep the bed free from crumbs. Keep clothing or gowns free of wrinkles, too.
- Do not pull the resident across the sheets during transfers or repositioning. This causes shearing, which can lead to skin breakdown.
- Place an absorbent bed pad under the back and buttocks to absorb moisture that may build up. This also protects the skin from irritating bed linens. Absorbent pads are also available for wheelchairs.
- Relieve pressure under bony prominences. Use pillows and other devices to keep elbows and heels from resting on the surface of the bed (Fig. 6-4).

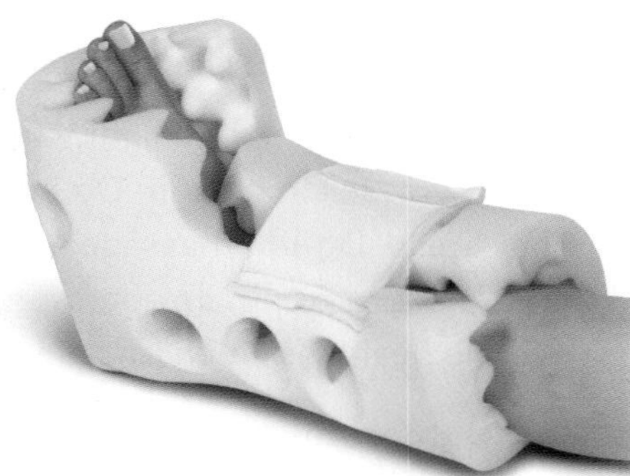

Fig. 6-4. *This foam boot suspends the heel to help reduce pressure.* (© MEDLINE INDUSTRIES INC.)

- A bed or chair can be made softer with flotation cushions or special foam overlays.
- Use a bed cradle to keep top sheets from rubbing the resident's skin.
- Residents in chairs or wheelchairs need to be repositioned often, too. Reposition residents at least every hour if they are in a wheelchair or chair and cannot change positions easily.

Many positioning devices are available to help make residents safer and more comfortable.

Guidelines: Positioning Devices

- Backrests provide support. They can be regular pillows or special wedge-shaped foam pillows.
- Bed cradles or foot cradles are used to keep the bed covers from resting on a resident's legs and feet.
- **Draw sheets** may be placed under residents who cannot help with turning, lifting, or moving up in bed. Draw sheets help prevent skin damage from shearing. A regular bed sheet folded in half can be used as a draw sheet.
- Footboards are padded boards placed against the resident's feet to keep them properly aligned. They help prevent foot drop. **Foot drop** is a weakness of muscles in the feet and ankles that causes problems with the ability to flex the ankles and walk normally. Foot splints may also be used to help prevent foot drop. Footboards are used to keep bed covers off the feet. Rolled blankets or pillows can also be used as footboards.
- Handrolls are cloth-covered or rubber items that keep the hand and/or fingers in a normal, natural position (Fig. 6-5). A rolled washcloth, gauze bandage, or rubber ball placed inside the palm may be used to keep the hand in a natural position. Handrolls can help prevent finger, hand, or wrist contractures.

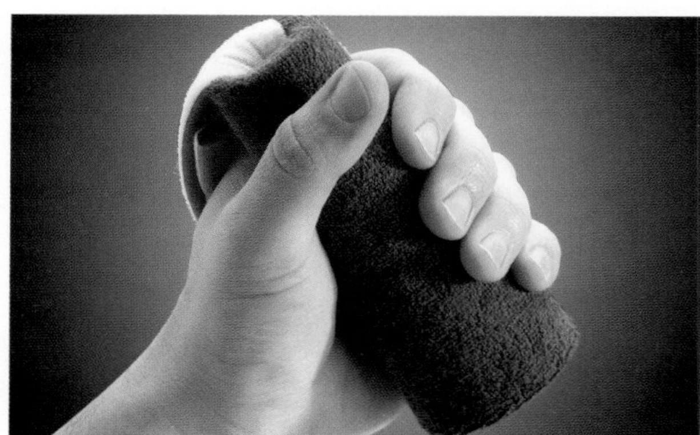

Fig. 6-5. *Handrolls keep the fingers and hand in a natural position, helping to prevent contractures.* (REPRINTED WITH PERMISSION OF TIDI PRODUCTS, LLC)

- An **orthotic device**, or **orthosis**, is a device that helps support and align a limb and improve its functioning (Fig. 6-6). It may be prescribed to keep a resident's joints in the correct position. Orthoses also help prevent or correct deformities. Splints are a type of orthotic device. Splints and the skin area around them should be cleaned at least once daily and as needed. Do not apply a splint unless you have been trained in its use.

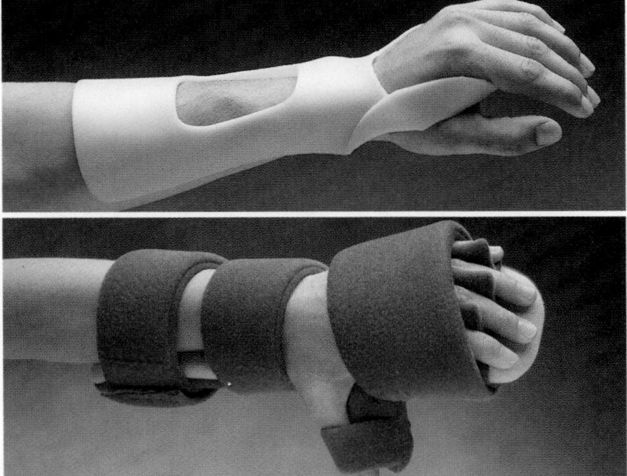

Fig. 6-6. Different types of orthotic splints. (PHOTOS COURTESY OF NORTH COAST MEDICAL, INC., WWW.NCMEDICAL.COM, 800-821-9319)

- **G** Trochanter rolls are rolled towels or blankets used to keep a resident's hips and legs from turning outward.
- **G** Abduction pillows/wedges/splints/pads or hip wedges keep hips in the proper position after hip surgery. Pillows between the legs from knees to ankles, while in the lateral position, can help keep the spine, hips, and knees in the proper position.

3. Describe guidelines for assisting with bathing

Bathing promotes health and well-being. It removes perspiration, dirt, oil, and dead skin cells from the skin. It helps to prevent skin irritation and body odor. Bathing can also be relaxing. The bed bath is an excellent time for moving arms and legs. It increases circulation. Bathing gives NAs an opportunity to observe residents' skin carefully.

Residents may have a bath in bed, or they may take a shower or have a tub bath. They may have a **partial bath**, which is a bath given on days when a complete bed bath, tub bath, or shower is not done. It includes washing the face, hands, axillae (underarms), and perineum. The **perineum** is the genital and anal area.

Guidelines: Bathing

- **G** The face, hands, underarms, and perineum should be washed every day. A complete bath can be taken every other day or less often.
- **G** Older skin produces less perspiration and oil. Elderly people with dry, fragile skin should bathe only once or twice a week. This prevents further dryness. Be gentle with the skin when bathing residents.
- **G** Use only products approved by the facility or that the resident prefers.
- **G** Before bathing a resident, make sure the room is warm enough.
- **G** Be familiar with available safety and assistive devices.
- **G** Gather supplies before giving a bath so the resident is not left alone.
- **G** Before bathing, make sure the water temperature is safe and comfortable. Test the water temperature with a thermometer or against the inside of your wrist to make sure it is not too hot. Then have the resident test the water temperature. The resident is best able to choose a comfortable water temperature.
- **G** Wear gloves while bathing a resident and change your gloves before performing perineal care.
- **G** Make sure all soap is removed from the skin before completing the bath.
- **G** Keep a record of the bathing schedule for each resident. Follow the care plan.

Giving a complete bed bath

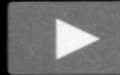

Equipment: bath blanket, bath basin, soap, bath thermometer (if available), 2–4 washcloths, 2–4 bath towels, disposable absorbent pads, clean

clothes, 2 pairs of gloves, orangewood stick, lotion, deodorant, brush or comb

When bathing, move the resident's body gently and naturally. Avoid force and overextension of limbs and joints.

1. Identify yourself by name. Identify the resident by name.
   Resident has right to know identity of his or her caregiver. Identifying resident by name shows respect and establishes correct identification.

2. Wash your hands.
   Provides for infection prevention.

3. Explain procedure to the resident. Speak clearly, slowly, and directly. Maintain face-to-face contact whenever possible.
   Promotes understanding and independence.

4. Provide for resident's privacy with curtain, screen, or door. Be sure the room is at a comfortable temperature and there are no drafts.
   Maintains resident's right to privacy and dignity.

5. Adjust bed to a safe level, usually waist high. Lock bed wheels.
   Prevents injury to you and to resident.

6. Place a bath blanket or towel over the resident (Fig. 6-7). Ask him to hold onto it as you remove or fold back the top bedding to the foot of the bed. Remove top clothing, while keeping resident covered with the bath blanket. Place clothing in proper container.

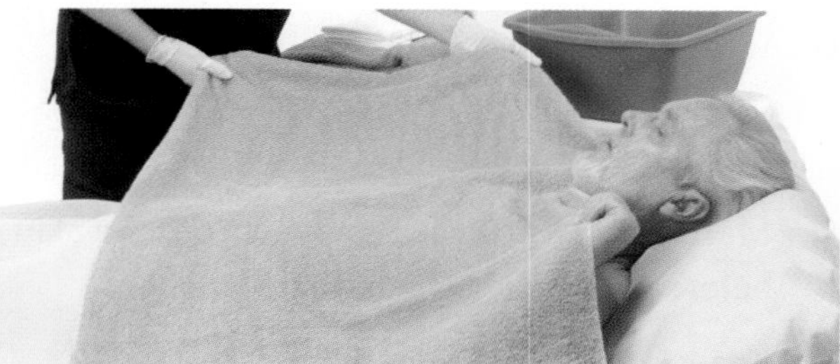

Fig. 6-7. *Cover the resident with a bath blanket or towel before removing the top bedding.*

7. Fill the basin with warm water. Test water temperature with a thermometer or against the inside of your wrist. Water temperature should be no higher than 105°F. Have resident check water temperature to see if it is comfortable. Adjust if necessary. The water will cool quickly. Change the water when it becomes too cool, soapy, or dirty.
   Resident's sense of touch may be different than yours; therefore, resident is best able to identify a comfortable water temperature.

8. Put on gloves.
   Protects you from contact with body fluids.

9. Ask the resident to participate in washing. Help him do this when needed.
   Promotes independence.

10. Uncover only one part of the body at a time. Place a towel or absorbent pad under the part being washed.
    Promotes resident's dignity and right to privacy. Also helps keep resident warm. A towel or pad under the body part helps keep the bed dry.

11. Wash, rinse, and dry one part of the body at a time. Start at the head. Work down, and complete the front first. When washing, use a clean area of the washcloth for each stroke.

    Eyes, Face, Ears, and Neck: With a wet washcloth (no soap), begin with the eye farther away from you. Wash inner to outer area (Fig. 6-8). Use a different area of the washcloth for each stroke. Repeat for the other eye. Wash the face from the middle outward. Use firm but gentle strokes. Wash the ears and behind the ears. Wash the neck. Rinse and pat dry.

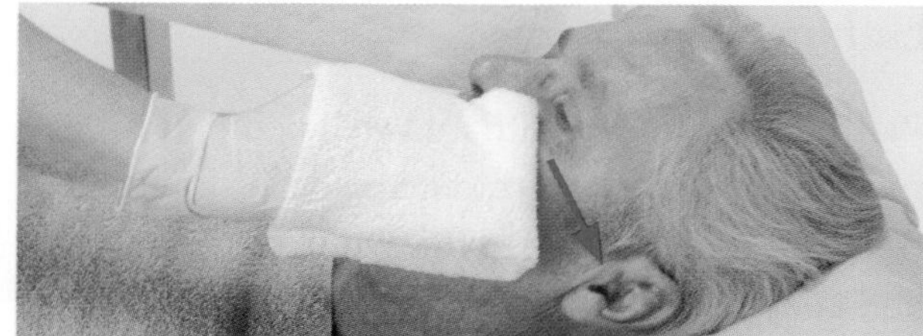

Fig. 6-8. *First wash the far eye from the inner to outer area, using a different area of the washcloth for each stroke.*

Arms and Axillae: Begin with the arm farther away from you. Remove the arm from under the towel. With a soapy washcloth, wash the upper arm and underarm. Use long strokes from the shoulder down to the wrist. Rinse and pat dry. Repeat for the other arm (Fig. 6-9).

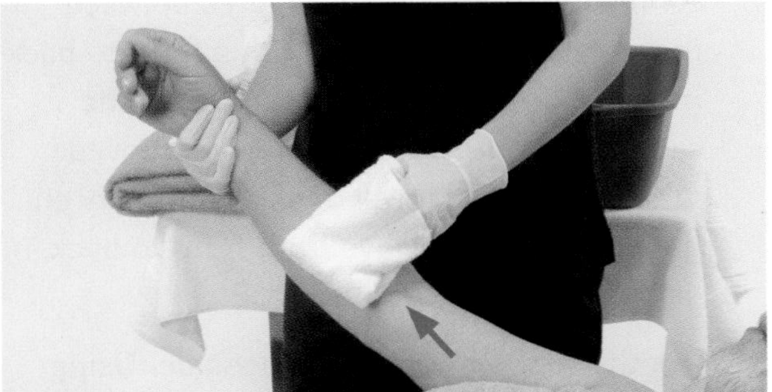

Fig. 6-9. *Support the wrist while washing the shoulder, arm, underarm, and elbow.*

Hands: Wash the far hand, including the fingers and fingernails. Clean under the nails with an orangewood stick. Rinse and pat dry. Make sure to dry between the fingers. Give nail care (see procedure later in this chapter). Repeat for the other hand. Put lotion on the resident's elbows and hands.

Chest: Place the towel across the resident's chest. Pull the blanket down to the waist. Lift the towel only enough to wash the chest. Rinse it and pat dry. For a female resident, wash, rinse, and dry breasts and under breasts. Check the skin in this area for signs of irritation.

Abdomen: Keep towel across chest. Fold the blanket down so that it still covers the pubic area. Wash the abdomen, rinse, and pat dry. If the resident has an ostomy, give skin care around the opening (Chapter 4). Cover with the towel. Pull the cotton blanket up to the resident's chin. Remove the towel.

Legs and Feet: Expose the far leg. Place a towel under it. Wash the thigh. Use long downward strokes. Rinse and pat dry. Do the same from the knee to the ankle (Fig. 6-10).

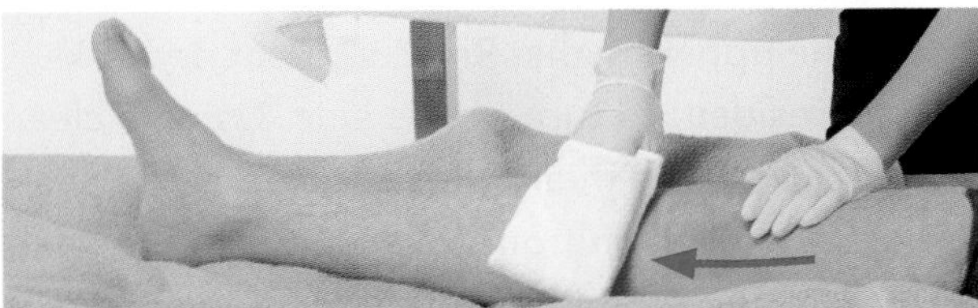

Fig. 6-10. *Use long, downward strokes when washing the legs.*

Place another towel under the far foot. Move the basin to the towel. Place the foot into the basin. Wash the foot and between the toes (Fig. 6-11). Rinse the foot and pat dry. Make sure the area between the toes is dry. Apply lotion to the foot if ordered, especially at the heels. Do not apply lotion between the toes. Repeat steps for the other leg and foot.

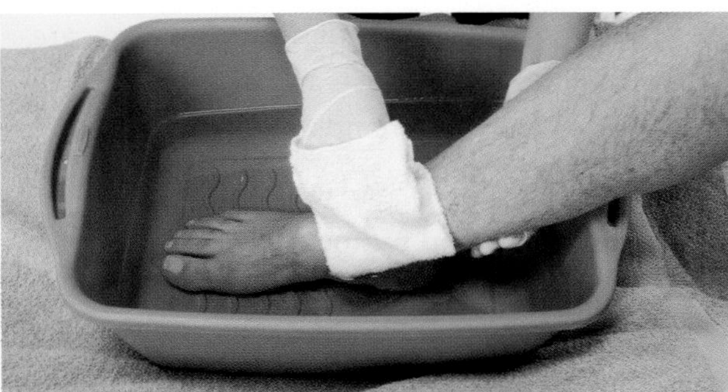

Fig. 6-11. *Washing the feet includes cleaning between the toes.*

Back: Help resident move to the center of the bed. Raise the far side rail (if used) for safety. Help the resident to turn onto his side, toward the raised side rail. Return to the working side of the bed. His back should be facing you. Fold the blanket away from the back. Place a towel lengthwise next to the back. Wash the back and neck with long, downward strokes (Fig. 6-12). Rinse and pat dry. Apply lotion if ordered.

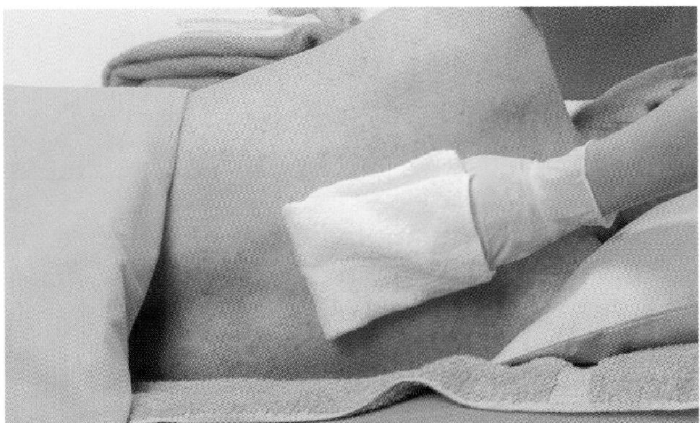

Fig. 6-12. *Wash the back with long downward strokes.*

12. Place the towel under the buttocks and upper thighs. Help the resident turn onto his back. If the resident is able to wash his perineal

area, place a basin of clean, warm water, a washcloth, and a towel within reach. Hand items to the resident as needed. If the resident wants you to leave the room, remove and discard gloves. Wash your hands. Leave side rails up (if used). Return bed to its lowest position. Leave supplies and the call light within reach.

13. If the resident cannot perform perineal care, you will do so. Remove and discard your gloves. Wash your hands and put on clean gloves. Provide privacy at all times.

14. **Perineal area and buttocks**: Change the bath water. Place a towel or pad under the perineal area, including the buttocks. Wash, rinse, and dry perineal area. Work from front to back (clean to dirty). Expose the perineal area only.

    For a female resident: Using water and a small amount of soap, wash the perineum from front to back. Use single strokes (Fig. 6-13). Use a clean area of washcloth or a clean washcloth for each stroke.

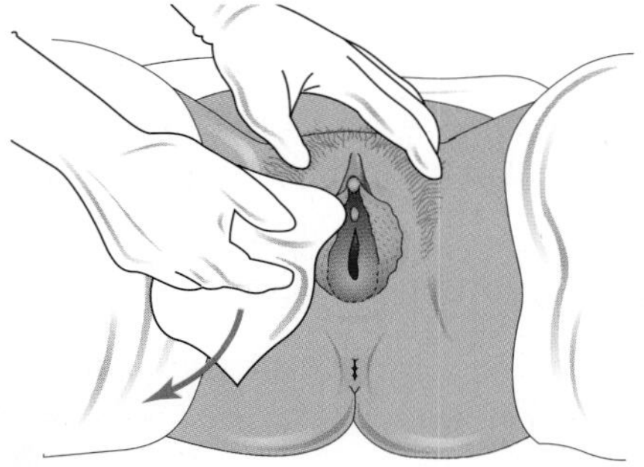

Fig. 6-13. Always work from front to back when performing perineal care. This helps prevent infection.

Working from front to back, wipe one side of the labia majora, the outside folds of perineal skin that protect the urinary meatus and the vaginal opening. Then wipe the other side, using a clean part of the washcloth. With your thumb and forefinger, gently separate the labia majora. Wipe from front to back on one side with a clean washcloth, using a single stroke. Using a clean area of the washcloth, wipe from front to back on the other side. Using another clean area of the washcloth, wipe from front to back down the center. Clean the perineum (area between the vagina and anus) last with a front-to-back motion. Rinse the area thoroughly in the same way. Make sure all soap is removed. With a clean, dry towel or washcloth, dry entire perineal area. Move from front to back, using a blotting motion.

Ask the resident to turn on her side. Using a clean washcloth, wash and rinse buttocks and anal area. Work from front to back. Clean the anal area without contaminating the perineal area. With a clean, dry towel or washcloth, dry buttocks and anal area.

For a male resident: If the resident is uncircumcised, pull back the foreskin first. Gently push the skin toward the base of penis. Hold the penis by the shaft. Wash in a circular motion from the tip down to the base (Fig. 6-14). Use a clean area of washcloth or clean washcloth for each stroke.

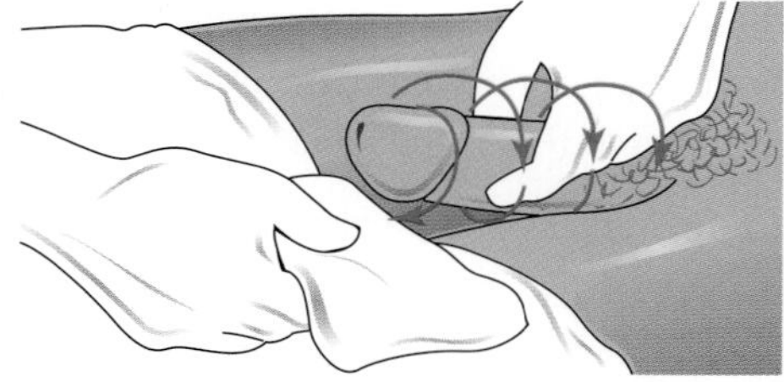

Fig. 6-14. Wash the penis in a circular motion from the tip down to the base.

Thoroughly rinse the penis and pat dry with a clean, dry towel or washcloth. If the resident is uncircumcised, gently return the foreskin to normal position. Then wash the scrotum and groin. The groin is the area from the pubis (area around the penis and scrotum) to the upper thighs. Rinse and pat dry. Ask the resident to turn on his side. Using a clean washcloth, wash and rinse buttocks and anal area. Work from front to back. Clean the anal area without contaminating the perineal area. With a clean, dry towel or washcloth, dry buttocks and anal area.

15. Cover the resident with the blanket.
16. Empty, rinse, and dry bath basin. Place basin in designated dirty supply area or return to storage, depending on facility policy.
17. Place soiled clothing and linens in proper containers.
18. Remove and discard gloves.
19. Wash your hands.
20. Provide deodorant. Place a towel over the pillow and brush or comb the resident's hair (see procedure later in this chapter). Help the resident put on clean clothing. Help the resident into a comfortable position with proper body alignment.
21. Return bed to lowest position. Leave side rails in the ordered position. Remove privacy measures.
    Lowering the bed provides for safety.
22. Place call light within resident's reach.
    Allows resident to communicate with staff as necessary.
23. Wash your hands.
    Provides for infection prevention.
24. Report any changes in resident to the nurse.
    Provides nurse with information to assess resident.
25. Document procedure using facility guidelines.
    If you do not document the care, legally it did not happen.

Back rubs help relax tired muscles, relieve pain, and increase circulation. Back rubs are often given after baths. After giving a back rub, any changes in a resident's skin should be noted.

Giving a back rub

Equipment: cotton blanket or towel, lotion

1. Identify yourself by name. Identify the resident by name.
   Resident has right to know identity of his or her caregiver. Addressing resident by name shows respect and establishes correct identification.
2. Wash your hands.
   Provides for infection prevention.
3. Explain procedure to resident. Speak clearly, slowly, and directly. Maintain face-to-face contact whenever possible.
   Promotes understanding and independence.
4. Provide for resident's privacy with curtain, screen, or door.
   Maintains resident's right to privacy and dignity.
5. Adjust bed to a safe level, usually waist high. Lower the head of the bed. Lock bed wheels.
   Prevents injury to you and to resident.
6. Position the resident lying on his side or his stomach. Cover resident with a blanket or towel. Fold back the bed covers. Expose the back to the top of the buttocks. Back rubs can also be given with the resident sitting up.
7. Warm lotion by putting the bottle in warm water for five minutes. Run your hands under warm water. Pour lotion on your hands. Rub them together. Always put lotion on your hands first, rather than on the resident's skin.
   Increases resident's comfort.
8. Place hands on each side of upper part of the buttocks. Use the full palm of each hand. Make long, smooth upward strokes with both hands. Move along each side of the spine, up to the shoulders (Figs. 6-15 and 6-16). Circle your hands outward. Move back along outer edges of the back. At the buttocks, make another circle. Move your hands back up to the shoulders. Without taking your hands off the resident's skin, repeat this motion for three to five minutes.
   Long upward strokes release muscle tension; circular strokes increase circulation in muscle areas.

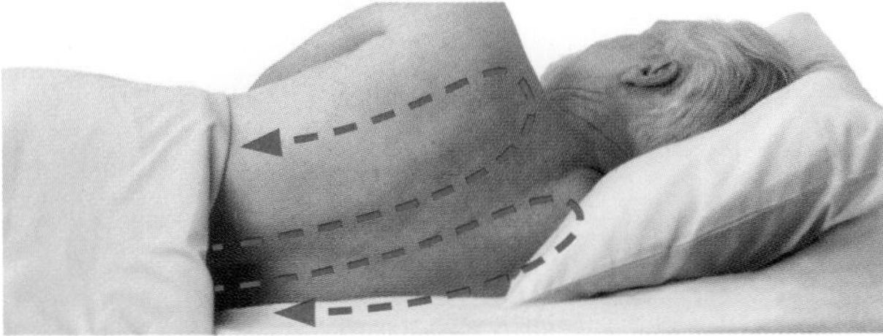

Fig. 6-15. *Move along each side of the spine, up to the shoulders.*

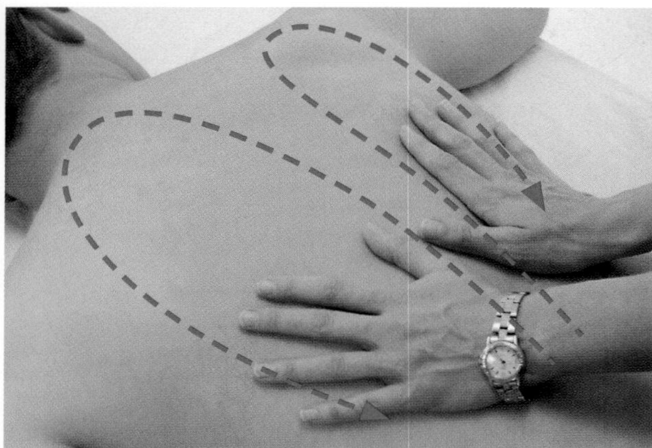

Fig. 6-16. Long, upward strokes help release muscle tension.

9. Knead with the first two fingers and thumb of each hand. Place them at the base of the spine. Move upward together along each side of the spine. Apply gentle downward pressure with fingers and thumbs. Follow the same direction as with the long smooth strokes, circling at the shoulders and buttocks.

10. Gently massage bony areas (spine, shoulder blades, hip bones). Use circular motions of your fingertips. Use little or no pressure. If any of these areas are white, red, or purple, do not massage them.
    Discoloration indicates that skin is already irritated and fragile. Include this information in your report to the nurse.

11. Let the resident know when you are almost through. Finish with some long, smooth strokes.

12. Dry the back if extra lotion remains on it.

13. Remove blanket or towel.

14. Help the resident get dressed. Help resident into comfortable position.

15. Store supplies. Place soiled clothing and linens in proper containers.

16. Return bed to lowest position. Remove privacy measures.
    Provides for resident's safety.

17. Place call light within resident's reach.
    Allows resident to communicate with staff as necessary.

18. Wash your hands.
    Provides for infection prevention.

19. Report any changes in resident to the nurse.
    Provides nurse with information to assess resident.

20. Document procedure using facility guidelines.
    If you do not document the care, legally it did not happen.

Hair care is an important part of cleanliness. Shampooing the hair removes dirt, bacteria, oils, and other materials from the hair. Residents who can get out of bed may have their hair shampooed in the sink, tub, or shower. For residents who cannot get out of bed, shampoo basins can be used. There are also special types of shampoo that do not require the use of water (Fig. 6-17). Gloves should be worn if a resident has open sores on his scalp.

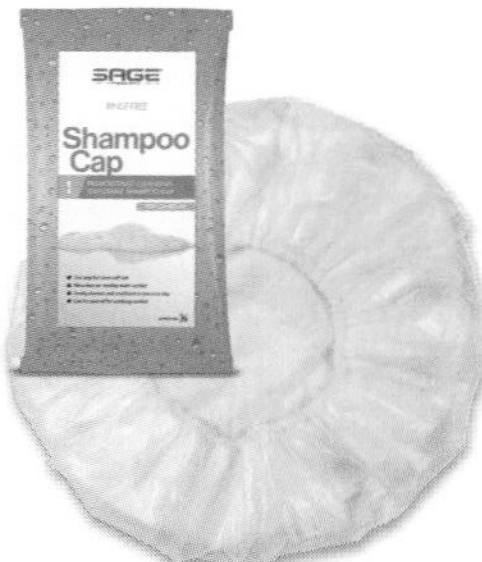

Fig. 6-17. This is a rinse-free shampoo cap that does not require the use of water. (PERMISSION GRANTED BY SAGE PRODUCTS LLC)

Shampooing hair in bed

Equipment: shampoo, hair conditioner (if requested), 2 bath towels, washcloth, bath thermometer, pitcher or handheld shower or sink attachment, waterproof pad, bath blanket, shampoo basin, comb and brush, hair dryer

1. Identify yourself by name. Identify the resident by name.
   Resident has right to know identity of his or her caregiver. Addressing resident by name shows respect and establishes correct identification.

2. Wash your hands.
   Provides for infection prevention.

3. Explain procedure to resident. Speak clearly, slowly, and directly. Maintain face-to-face contact whenever possible.
   Promotes understanding and independence.

4. Provide for resident's privacy with curtain, screen, or door. Be sure room is at a comfortable temperature and there are no drafts.
   Maintains resident's right to privacy and dignity.

5. Arrange the supplies within reach.

6. Test water temperature with thermometer or against the inside of your wrist. Water temperature should be no higher than 105°F. Have resident check water temperature. Adjust if necessary.
   Resident's sense of touch may be different than yours; therefore, resident is best able to identify a comfortable water temperature.

7. Remove all pillows and place the resident in a flat position. Adjust bed to a safe level, usually waist high. Lock bed wheels.
   Prevents injury to you and to resident.

8. Place the waterproof pad under the resident's head and shoulders. Cover the resident with the bath blanket. Fold back the top sheet and regular blankets.
   Protects bed linen.

9. Place the basin under the resident's head. Place one towel across the resident's shoulders.

10. Protect resident's eyes with a dry washcloth.

11. Use the pitcher or attachment to wet hair thoroughly. Apply a small amount of shampoo to your hands and rub them together.

12. Using both hands, massage the shampoo into a lather in the resident's hair. With your fingertips (not fingernails), massage the scalp in a circular motion, from front to back (Fig. 6-18). Do not scratch the scalp.

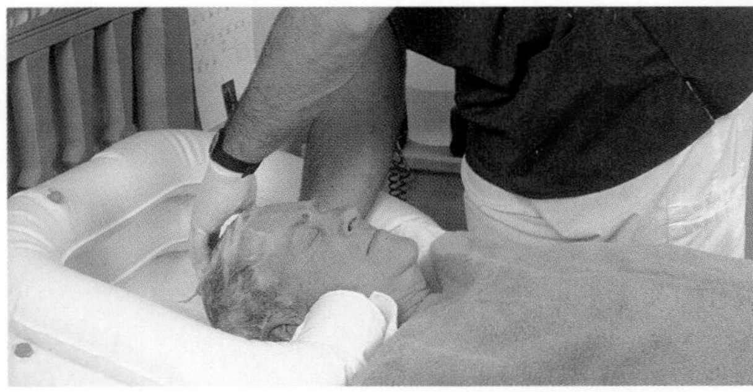

Fig. 6-18. *Use your fingertips, not your fingernails, to work shampoo into a lather. Be gentle so that you do not scratch the scalp.*

13. Rinse the hair until water runs clear. Use conditioner if resident wants it. Rinse as directed on container. Be sure to rinse the hair thoroughly to prevent the scalp from getting dry and itchy.

14. Wrap resident's hair in a clean towel. Remove the basin. Dry his face and neck with the washcloth or a towel.

15. Raise the head of the bed.

16. Gently rub the scalp and hair with the towel.

17. Comb or brush hair. Dry hair with a hair dryer on low setting if facility allows this. Style hair as resident prefers.

18. Return bed to lowest position. Remove privacy measures.
    Lowering the bed provides for safety.

19. Place call light within resident's reach.
    Allows resident to communicate with staff as necessary.

20. Empty, rinse, and wipe bath basin and pitcher. Take to proper area.

21. Clean comb or brush. Return hair dryer and comb or brush to proper storage.

22. Place soiled linen in proper container.

23. Wash your hands.
    Provides for infection prevention.

24. Report any changes in resident to nurse.
    Provides nurse with information to assess resident.

25. Document procedure using facility guidelines.
    If you do not document the care, legally it did not happen.

Many people prefer showers or tub baths to bed baths (Fig. 6-19). The NA must check with the nurse first to make sure a shower or tub bath is allowed.

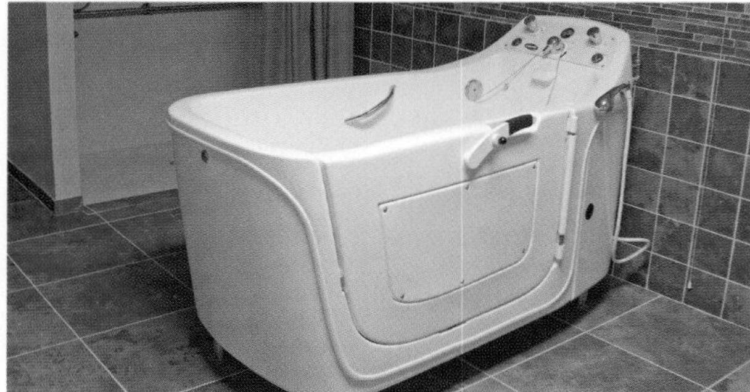

Fig. 6-19. *A common style of tub in long-term care facilities.*

Guidelines: Safety for Showers and Tub Baths

- **G** Clean tub or shower before and after use.
- **G** Make sure bathroom or shower room floor is dry.
- **G** Be familiar with available safety and assistive devices. Check that handrails, grab bars, and lifts are in working order.
- **G** Have resident use safety bars to get into or out of the tub or shower.
- **G** Place all needed items within reach.
- **G** Do not leave the resident alone.
- **G** Do not use bath oils, lotions, or powders in showers or tubs. They make surfaces slippery.
- **G** Test water temperature with thermometer or against the inside of your wrist before resident gets into the tub or shower. Water temperature should be no higher than 105°F. Make sure temperature is comfortable for resident.

Residents' Rights

Privacy when Bathing

Privacy is very important when residents are having a shower or tub bath. Doors should be kept closed. Residents should be covered when possible. Their bodies should not be unnecessarily exposed. For facilities that have communal shower areas, make sure females only shower with other females, and males with other males.

Giving a shower or a tub bath

Equipment: bath blanket, soap, shampoo, bath thermometer, 2–4 washcloths, 2–4 bath towels, clean clothes, nonskid footwear, 2 pairs of gloves, lotion, deodorant, hair dryer

1. Wash your hands.
   Provides for infection prevention.
2. Place equipment in shower or tub room. Put on gloves. Clean shower or tub area and shower chair. Place bucket under the shower chair (in case resident has a bowel movement). Turn on heat lamp to warm the room, if available.
   Cleaning reduces pathogens and prevents the spread of infection.
3. Remove and discard gloves. Wash your hands.
   Provides for infection prevention.
4. Go to resident's room. Identify yourself by name. Identify the resident by name.
   Resident has right to know identity of his or her caregiver. Addressing resident by name shows respect and establishes correct identification.
5. Wash your hands.
   Provides for infection prevention.
6. Explain procedure to resident. Speak clearly, slowly, and directly. Maintain face-to-face contact whenever possible.
   Promotes understanding and independence.
7. Provide for resident's privacy with curtain, screen, or door.
   Maintains resident's right to privacy and dignity.
8. Help the resident to put on nonskid footwear. Transport resident to shower or tub room.
   Nonskid footwear helps lessen the risk of falls.
9. Wash your hands. Put on clean gloves.
10. Help resident remove clothing and shoes.

For a shower:

11. If using a shower chair, place it close to resident. Lock its wheels (Fig. 6-20). Safely transfer the resident into the shower chair.
    Chair may slide if resident attempts to get up.

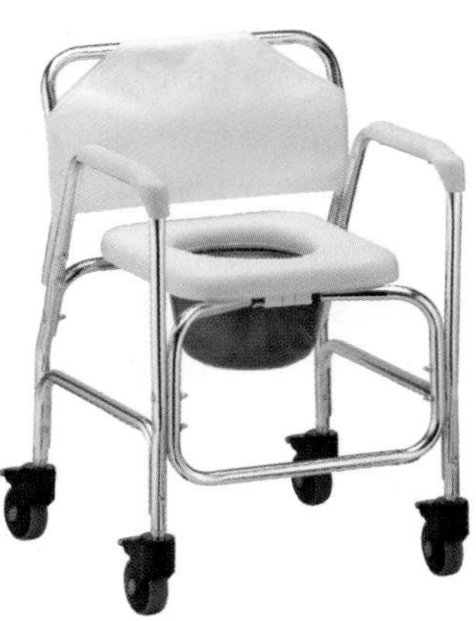

***Fig. 6-20.** A shower chair is a sturdy chair designed to be placed in a bathtub or shower. It is water- and slip-resistant. The chair allows a person who is unable to get into a tub or is too weak to stand in a shower to bathe in the tub or shower, rather than in bed. A shower chair must be locked before transferring a resident into it.* (PHOTO COURTESY OF NOVA MEDICAL PRODUCTS, WWW.NOVAMEDICALPRODUCTS.COM)

12. Turn on water. Test water temperature with thermometer or against the inside of your wrist. Water temperature should be no higher than 105°F. Have resident check water temperature. Adjust if necessary. Check temperature throughout the shower.
    Resident's sense of touch may be different than yours; therefore, resident is best able to identify a comfortable water temperature.
13. Unlock the shower chair and move it into the shower stall. Lock its wheels.
14. Stay with the resident during the procedure.
    Provides for resident's safety.
15. Let resident wash as much as possible. Help her to wash her face.
    Encourages resident to be independent.
16. Help the resident shampoo and rinse hair.
17. Using soap, help to wash and rinse the entire body. Move from head to toe (clean to dirty).
18. Turn off water. Unlock shower chair wheels. Roll the resident out of the shower.

For a tub bath:

11. Residents may need help to get into the bath, depending on their level of mobility. Safely transfer the resident onto a chair or tub lift, or help the resident into the bath.
12. Fill the tub halfway with warm water. Test water temperature with thermometer or against the inside of your wrist. Water temperature should be no higher than 105°F. Have resident check water temperature. Adjust if necessary.
13. Stay with the resident during the procedure.
    Provides for resident's safety.
14. Let resident wash as much as possible. Help her to wash her face.
    Encourages resident to be independent.
15. Help the resident shampoo and rinse hair.
16. Using soap, help to wash and rinse the entire body. Move from head to toe (clean to dirty).
17. Drain the tub. Cover resident with the bath blanket while the tub drains.
    Maintains resident's dignity and right to privacy by not exposing body. Keeps resident warm.
18. Help resident out of the tub and onto a chair.

Remaining steps for either procedure:

19. Give the resident a towel and help her to pat dry. Pat dry under the breasts, between skin folds, in the perineal area, and between toes.
    Patting dry prevents skin tears and reduces chafing.
20. Apply lotion and deodorant as needed.
21. Place soiled clothing and linens in proper containers.
22. Remove and discard gloves.
23. Wash your hands.
    Provides for infection prevention.
24. Help resident dress and comb hair before leaving shower or tub room. Offer a hair dryer if needed. Put on nonskid footwear. Return resident to her room.
    Combing hair in shower room allows resident to maintain dignity when returning to room.
25. Make sure resident is comfortable.

26. Place call light within resident's reach.
    Allows resident to communicate with staff as necessary.

27. Report any changes in resident to nurse.
    Provides nurse with information to assess resident.

28. Document procedure using facility guidelines.
    If you do not document the care, legally it did not happen.

4. Describe guidelines for assisting with grooming

Grooming affects the way people feel about themselves and how they look to others (Fig. 6-21). When helping with grooming, NAs should always let residents do all they can for themselves. Residents should make as many choices as possible. Residents may have particular ways of grooming themselves. They may have routines. These routines remain important even when people are elderly, sick, or disabled. Some residents may be embarrassed, depressed, or anxious because they need help with grooming tasks. NAs should be sensitive to this. Being respectful promotes person-centered care.

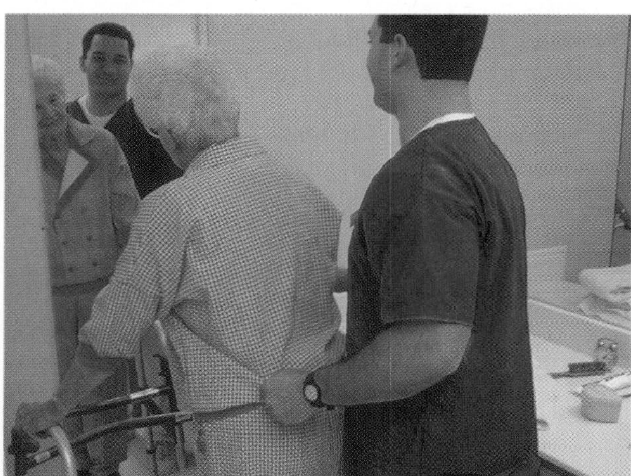

Fig. 6-21. *A well-groomed appearance helps a person feel good about herself.*

Fingernails can harbor bacteria. It is important to keep hands and nails clean to help prevent infection. Nail care should be given when nails are dirty or have jagged edges and whenever it has been assigned. Some facilities do not allow NAs to cut a resident's fingernails or toenails. Poor circulation can lead to infection if skin is accidentally cut while caring for nails. For a resident who has diabetes, such an infection can lead to a severe wound or even amputation. NAs should follow their facility's policies. The same nail equipment should not be used on more than one resident.

Providing fingernail care 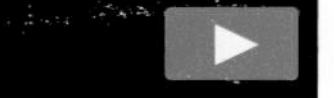

Equipment: orangewood stick, emery board, lotion, basin, soap, 2 washcloths, 2 towels, bath thermometer, gloves

1. Identify yourself by name. Identify the resident by name.
   Resident has right to know identity of his or her caregiver. Addressing resident by name shows respect and establishes correct identification.

2. Wash your hands.
   Provides for infection prevention.

3. Explain procedure to resident. Speak clearly, slowly, and directly. Maintain face-to-face contact whenever possible.
   Promotes understanding and independence.

4. Provide for resident's privacy with curtain, screen, or door.
   Maintains resident's right to privacy and dignity.

5. If resident is in bed, adjust bed to a safe level, usually waist high. Lock bed wheels.
   Prevents injury to you and to resident.

6. Fill the basin halfway with warm water. Test water temperature with thermometer or against the inside of your wrist. Water temperature should be no higher than 105°F. Have resident check water temperature. Adjust if necessary. Place basin at a comfortable level for the resident.
   Resident's sense of touch may be different than yours; therefore, resident is best able to identify a comfortable water temperature.

7. Put on gloves.

8. Soak the resident's hands and nails in the basin of water. Soak all 10 fingertips for at least five minutes.
   Nail care is easier if nails are first softened.

9. Remove hands from the water. Wash hands with a soapy washcloth. Rinse. Pat hands dry with a towel, including between the fingers. Remove the hand basin.

10. Place resident's hands on the towel. Gently clean under each fingernail with the orangewood stick (Fig. 6-22).
    Most pathogens on hands come from beneath the nails.

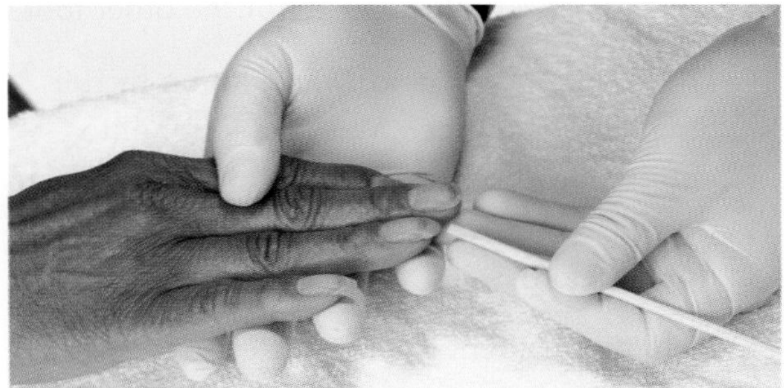

Fig. 6-22. *Be gentle when removing dirt from under the nails with an orangewood stick.*

11. Wipe the orangewood stick on the towel after cleaning under each nail. Wash the resident's hands again. With a clean, dry towel or washcloth, dry them thoroughly, especially between the fingers.

12. Shape nails with an emery board or file. Move in only one direction (not back and forth). File in a curve. Finish with nails smooth and free of rough edges.
    Filing in a curve smoothes nails and eliminates edges, which may catch on clothes or tear skin.

13. Apply lotion from fingertips to wrists. Remove excess, if any, with a towel or washcloth.

14. Empty, rinse, and dry basin. Place basin in designated dirty supply area or return to storage, depending on facility policy.

15. Place soiled clothing and linens in proper containers.

16. Remove and discard gloves. Wash your hands.
    Provides for infection prevention.

17. Return bed to lowest position. Remove privacy measures.
    Lowering the bed provides for safety.

18. Place call light within resident's reach.
    Allows resident to communicate with staff as necessary.

19. Report any changes in resident to the nurse.
    Provides nurse with information to assess resident.

20. Document procedure using facility guidelines.
    If you do not document the care, legally it did not happen.

Careful foot care is extremely important; it should be a part of daily care of residents.

Observing and Reporting: Foot Care

Report any of these to the nurse:

- O/R Dry, flaking skin
- O/R Nonintact or broken skin
- O/R Discoloration of the feet, such as reddened, gray, white, or black areas
- O/R Blisters
- O/R Bruises
- O/R Blood or drainage
- O/R Long, ragged toenails
- O/R Ingrown toenails
- O/R Swelling
- O/R Soft, fragile, or reddened heels
- O/R Differences in temperature of the feet

Providing foot care 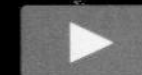

Equipment: basin, bath mat, soap, lotion, 2 washcloths, 2 towels, bath thermometer, clean socks, gloves

1. Identify yourself by name. Identify the resident by name.
   Resident has right to know identity of his or her caregiver. Addressing resident by name shows respect and establishes correct identification.

2. Wash your hands.
   Provides for infection prevention.

3. Explain procedure to resident. Speak clearly, slowly, and directly. Maintain face-to-face contact whenever possible.
   Promotes understanding and independence.

4. Provide for resident's privacy with curtain, screen, or door.
   Maintains resident's right to privacy and dignity.

5. If the resident is in bed, adjust bed to a safe level, usually waist high. Lock bed wheels.
   Prevents injury to you and to resident.

6. Fill the basin halfway with warm water. Test water temperature with thermometer or against the inside of your wrist. Water temperature should be no higher than 105°F. Have resident check water temperature. Adjust if necessary.
   Resident's sense of touch may be different than yours; therefore, resident is best able to identify a comfortable water temperature.

7. Place basin on the bath mat or bath towel on the floor (if the resident is in a chair) or on a towel at the foot of the bed (if the resident is in bed). Make sure basin is in a comfortable position for resident. Support the foot and ankle throughout the procedure.

8. Put on gloves.

9. Remove resident's socks. Completely submerge resident's feet in the water. Soak the feet for 10 to 20 minutes. Add warm water to basin as necessary.

10. Put soap on a wet washcloth. Remove one foot from the water. Wash entire foot, including between the toes and around the nail beds (Fig. 6-23).

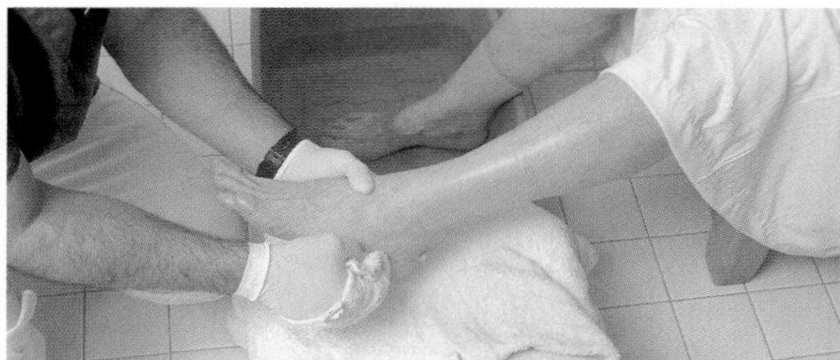

Fig. 6-23. *While supporting the foot and ankle, wash the entire foot with a soapy washcloth.*

11. Rinse entire foot, including between the toes.

12. With a clean, dry towel or washcloth, dry entire foot, including between the toes.

13. Repeat steps 10 through 12 for the other foot.

14. Put lotion in one hand. Warm lotion by rubbing hands together. Massage lotion into entire foot (top and bottom), **except between the toes**. Remove excess, if any, with a towel or washcloth.

15. Help the resident to put on clean socks.

16. Empty, rinse, and dry basin. Place basin in designated dirty supply area or return to storage, depending on facility policy.

17. Place soiled clothing and linens in proper containers.

18. Remove and discard gloves. Wash your hands.
    Provides for infection prevention.

19. Return bed to lowest position. Remove privacy measures.
    Lowering the bed provides for safety.

20. Place call light within resident's reach.
    Allows resident to communicate with staff as necessary.

21. Report any changes in resident to the nurse.
    Provides nurse with information to assess resident.

22. Document procedure using facility guidelines.
    If you do not document the care, legally it did not happen.

Because hair thins as people age, pieces of hair can be pulled out of the head while combing or brushing it. NAs must handle residents' hair very gently.

Pediculosis is the medical term for an infestation of lice. Lice are tiny bugs that bite into the skin and suck blood to live and grow. Three types of lice are head lice, body lice, and crab or pubic lice. Head lice are usually found on the scalp. Lice are hard to see. Symptoms include itching, bite marks on the scalp, skin sores, and matted, bad-smelling hair and scalp. Lice eggs may be visible on the hair, behind the ears, and on the neck. They are small and round and may be brown or white. Lice droppings look like a fine black powder. They may be on sheets or pillows. If NAs notice any of these symptoms, they should tell the nurse immediately. Lice can spread very quickly. Special creams, shampoos, lotions, sprays, or special combs may be used to treat the lice. People who have lice spread it to others. To help prevent the spread of lice, a resident's combs, brushes, clothes, wigs, and hats should not be shared with others.

Combing or brushing hair

Equipment: comb, brush, towel, mirror, hair care items requested by resident

Use hair care products that the resident prefers for his or her type of hair.

1. Identify yourself by name. Identify the resident by name.
   Resident has right to know identity of his or her caregiver. Addressing resident by name shows respect and establishes correct identification.
2. Wash your hands.
   Provides for infection prevention.
3. Explain procedure to resident. Speak clearly, slowly, and directly. Maintain face-to-face contact whenever possible.
   Promotes understanding and independence.
4. Provide for resident's privacy with curtain, screen, or door.
   Maintains resident's right to privacy and dignity.
5. If resident is in bed, adjust bed to a safe level, usually waist high. Raise the head of the bed so the resident is sitting up. Lock bed wheels. If resident is ambulatory, provide a chair.
   Prevents injury to you and to resident. Sitting upright puts resident in more natural position.
6. Place a towel under the resident's head or around the shoulders.
7. Remove any hair pins, hair ties, or clips.
8. Remove tangles first by dividing hair into small sections. Hold lock of hair just above the tangle so you do not pull at the scalp. Gently comb or brush through the tangle. If the resident agrees, use a small amount of detangler or leave-in conditioner.
   Reduces hair breakage, scalp pain, and irritation.
9. After tangles are removed, brush two-inch sections of hair at a time (Fig. 6-24).

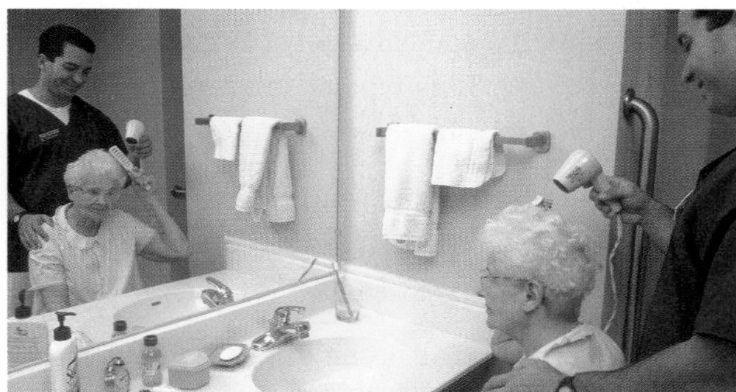

***Fig. 6-24.** Gently brush hair after tangles are removed.*

10. Neatly style hair as the resident prefers. Avoid childish hairstyles. Each resident may prefer different styles and hair products. Offer the mirror to the resident.
    Each resident has the right to choose. Promotes resident's independence.
11. Return supplies to proper storage. Clean hair from comb or brush. Clean comb or brush.
12. Dispose of soiled linen in the proper container.
13. Return bed to lowest position. Remove privacy measures.
    Lowering the bed provides for safety.

14. Place call light within resident's reach.
    Allows resident to communicate with staff as necessary.

15. Wash your hands.
    Provides for infection prevention.

16. Report any changes in resident to nurse.
    Provides nurse with information to assess resident.

17. Document procedure using facility guidelines.
    If you do not document the care, legally it did not happen.

Personal preferences for shaving must be respected. The NA should make sure the resident wants her to shave him or help him shave. NAs must wear gloves when shaving residents due to risk of exposure to blood. Razors should not be shared between residents. Different types of razors include the following:

- A **safety razor** has a sharp blade, which comes with a special safety casing to help prevent cuts. This type of razor requires shaving cream or soap.
- A **disposable razor** requires shaving cream or soap. It is discarded in a biohazard container for sharps after use.
- An **electric razor** is the safest and easiest type of razor to use. It does not require soap or shaving cream.

Shaving a resident

Equipment: razor, basin filled halfway with warm water (if using a safety or disposable razor), 2 towels, washcloth, mirror, shaving cream or soap (if using a safety or disposable razor), aftershave lotion, gloves

1. Identify yourself by name. Identify the resident by name.
   Resident has right to know identity of his or her caregiver. Addressing resident by name shows respect and establishes correct identification.

2. Wash your hands.
   Provides for infection prevention.

3. Explain procedure to resident. Speak clearly, slowly, and directly. Maintain face-to-face contact whenever possible.
   Promotes understanding and independence.

4. Provide for resident's privacy with curtain, screen, or door.
   Maintains resident's right to privacy and dignity.

5. If resident is in bed, adjust bed to a safe level, usually waist high. Lock bed wheels.
   Prevents injury to you and to resident.

6. Raise head of bed so that the resident is sitting up. Place a towel across the resident's chest, under his chin.
   Sitting upright puts resident in a more natural position. Towel protects resident's clothing and bed linen.

7. Put on gloves.
   Shaving may cause bleeding. Wearing gloves promotes infection prevention and follows Standard Precautions.

Shaving using a safety or disposable razor:

8. Soften the beard with a warm, wet washcloth on the face for a few minutes before shaving. Lather the face with shaving cream or soap and warm water.
   Warm water and lather soften skin and hair and make shaving more comfortable.

9. Hold skin taut. Shave in the direction of hair growth. Shave beard in short, downward, and even strokes on face and upward strokes on neck (Fig. 6-25). Rinse the blade often in the basin to keep it clean and wet.
   Shaving in the direction of hair growth maximizes hair removal.

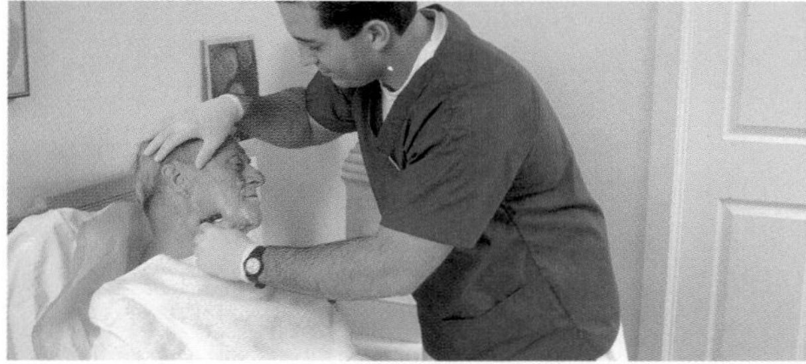

Fig. 6-25. *Holding the skin taut, shave in downward strokes on face and upward strokes on neck.*

10. When you have finished, wash and rinse the resident's face with a warm, wet washcloth. If he is able, let him use the washcloth himself. Use the towel to dry his face. Offer a mirror to the resident.
    Removes soap, which may cause irritation. Promotes independence.

Shaving using an electric razor:

8. Use a small brush to clean the razor. Do not use an electric razor near any water source or when oxygen is in use.
   Electricity near water may cause electrocution. Electricity near oxygen may cause an explosion.

9. Turn on the razor and hold skin taut. Shave with smooth, even movements (Fig. 6-26). If using a foil shaver, shave the beard with a back-and-forth motion in the direction of the beard growth. If using a three-head shaver, shave the beard in a circular motion. Shave the chin and under the chin.

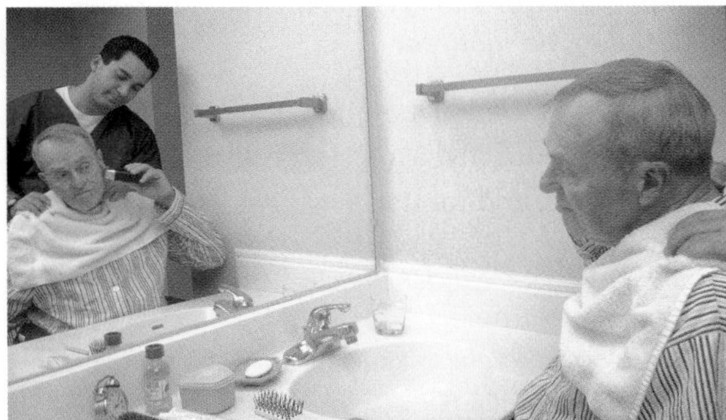

Fig. 6-26. *Shave, or have the resident shave, with smooth, even movements.*

10. Offer a mirror to the resident.
    Promotes independence.

Final steps:

11. Apply aftershave lotion if the resident wants it.
    Improves resident's self-esteem.

12. Remove the towel. Place the towel and washcloth in the proper container.

13. Clean the equipment and store it. Follow facility policy for a safety razor. For a disposable razor, dispose of it in a biohazard container for sharps. For an electric razor, clean the head of the razor. Remove whiskers, recap shaving head, and return razor to case.

14. Remove and discard gloves. Wash your hands.
    Provides for infection prevention.

15. Make sure that resident and environment are free of loose hairs.

16. Return bed to lowest position. Remove privacy measures.
    Lowering the bed provides for safety.

17. Place call light within resident's reach.
    Allows resident to communicate with staff as necessary.

18. Report any changes in resident to the nurse.
    Provides nurse with information to assess resident.

19. Document procedure using facility guidelines.
    If you do not document the care, legally it did not happen.

5. List guidelines for assisting with dressing

Dressing and undressing residents is an important part of daily care. When helping with dressing, the NA should know what limitations the resident has. Residents may have one side of the body that is weaker due to stroke or injury. That side is called the weaker, **affected**, or **involved side**. The NA should not refer to the weaker side as the "bad side," or talk about the "bad" leg or arm. When dressing, the NA should begin with the weaker side of the body. This helps reduce the risk of injury. The weaker arm is placed through a sleeve first. When one leg is weak, it is easier if the resident sits down to pull the pants over both legs.

Guidelines: Dressing and Undressing

G Ask about and follow the resident's preferences. This is part of promoting person-centered care. Let the resident choose clothing for the day. Check to see if it is clean, appropriate for the weather, and in good condition.

- **G** Encourage the resident to dress in regular clothes rather than nightclothes. Clothing with elastic waistbands and clothing that is a size larger than normal are easier to put on.
- **G** Let the resident do as much to dress or undress himself as possible. It may take longer, but it helps maintain independence. Ask where your help is needed. Assistive devices for dressing are available (Fig. 6-27). Use them as directed.

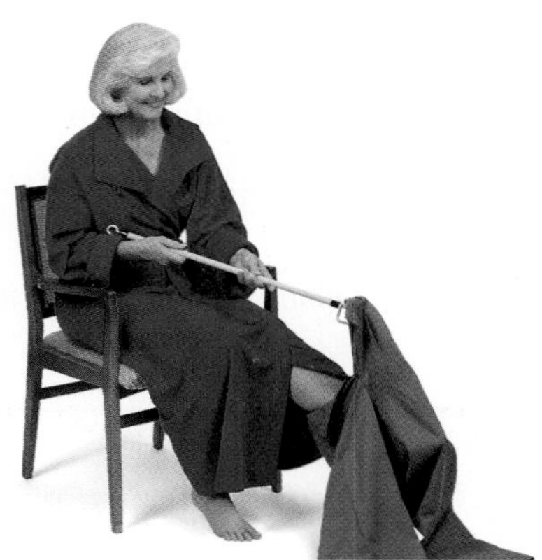

Fig. 6-27. *Special dressing aids promote independence by helping residents dress themselves.* (PHOTO COURTESY OF NORTH COAST MEDICAL, INC., WWW.NCMEDICAL.COM, 800-821-9319)

- **G** Provide privacy and never expose more than what is necessary.
- **G** Roll or fold socks or stockings down when putting them on. Slip over the toes and foot, then unroll them into place.
- **G** For a female resident, make sure bra cups fit over the breasts. A front-fastening bra is easier for residents to work by themselves. A bra that fastens in back can be put around the waist and fastened first. After fastening, rotate the bra around and move it up. Arms can be put through the straps last. This can be done in reverse for undressing.
- **G** Place the weaker arm or leg through the garment first. Then help with the stronger arm or leg. When undressing, start with the stronger, or unaffected, side (Fig. 6-28).

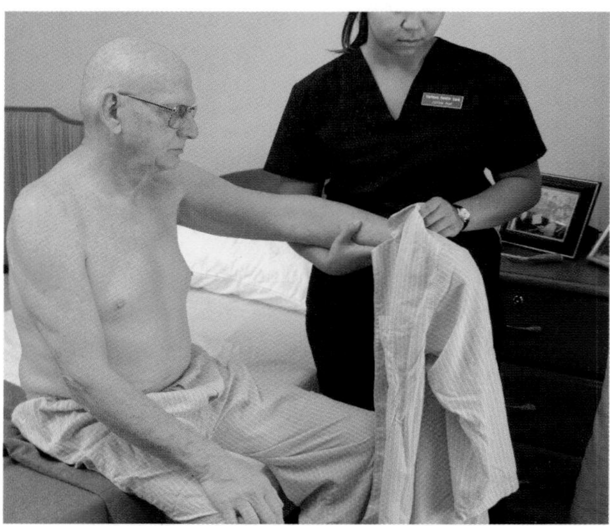

Fig. 6-28. *When dressing, the NA should start with the affected (weaker) side first.*

Dressing a resident 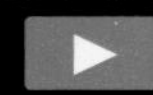

Equipment: bath blanket, clean clothes of resident's choice, nonskid footwear

When putting on items, move the resident's body gently and naturally. Avoid force and overextension of limbs and joints.

1. Identify yourself by name. Identify the resident by name.
   Resident has right to know identity of his or her caregiver. Addressing resident by name shows respect and establishes correct identification.
2. Wash your hands.
   Provides for infection prevention.
3. Explain procedure to resident. Speak clearly, slowly, and directly. Maintain face-to-face contact whenever possible.
   Promotes understanding and independence.
4. Provide for resident's privacy with curtain, screen, or door.
   Maintains resident's right to privacy and dignity.
5. If resident is in bed, adjust bed to a safe level, usually waist high. Lock bed wheels.
   Prevents injury to you and to resident.

6. Raise head of bed so that the resident is sitting up.
7. Ask resident what she would like to wear. Dress her in the outfit she chooses.
   Promotes resident's right to choose.
8. Place a bath blanket over the resident. Ask her to hold onto it as you remove or fold back the top bedding to the foot of the bed. Remove the gown or top. Keep the resident covered with the bath blanket. Take clothes off the stronger side first when undressing. Then remove from the weaker side. Place top clothing in the proper container. Move the bath blanket down to cover the lower body.
   Maintains resident's dignity and right to privacy.
9. Help the resident put on the top. If the top goes over the head, slide the top over the head first. Then place the weaker arm through the sleeve before placing the garment on the stronger arm. Help the resident lean forward and smooth the top down. If the top fastens in the front, slide your hand through one sleeve and grasp the resident's hand on the weaker side, pulling it through. Help the resident lean forward and arrange the top across the back. Pull the second sleeve onto the stronger side as you did with the first one. Fasten the top.
10. Remove the bath blanket and place it in the proper container. Help the resident put on a skirt or pants. Put the weaker leg through the skirt or pants first. Then place the stronger leg through the skirt or pants. Have the resident raise her buttocks or turn the resident from side to side to pull the pants over the buttocks up to the waist. Fasten the pants or skirt if needed and make sure the clothing is comfortable.
11. Roll one sock over the weaker foot. Make sure the heel of the sock is over the heel of the foot. Make sure there are no twists or wrinkles in the sock after it is on. Repeat for the other foot.
    Promotes resident's safety.
12. Starting with the weaker foot, slip on nonskid footwear. Use an assistive device if needed. Fasten one shoe securely and then put on the other shoe.
13. Finish with resident dressed appropriately. Make sure clothing is right-side-out and zippers and buttons are fastened.
14. Return bed to lowest position. Remove privacy measures.
    Lowering the bed provides for safety.
15. Place call light within resident's reach.
    Allows resident to communicate with staff as necessary.
16. Wash your hands.
    Provides for infection prevention.
17. Report any changes in resident to the nurse.
    Provides nurse with information to assess resident.
18. Document procedure using facility guidelines.
    If you do not document the care, legally it did not happen.

Intravenous therapy, often called IV therapy, is the delivery of medication, nutrition, or fluids through a vein. Medication, nutrition, or fluids either drip from a bag suspended on a pole or are pumped by a portable pump through a tube and into the vein. Chapter 7 has more information about IV therapy.

Guidelines: Dressing a Resident with an IV

G Never disconnect IV lines or turn off the pump. The nurse will be responsible for unhooking IV tubing from the pump.

G Always keep the IV bag higher than the IV site on the body.

G First remove clothing from the side without the IV. Then gather the clothing on the side with the IV. Lift clothing over the IV site. Move it up the tubing toward the IV bag.

Lift the IV bag off its pole. Carefully slide the clothing over the bag. Place the bag back on the pole.

G Lift the IV bag off its pole. Apply clean clothing to the side with the IV. Slide the clothing over the bag. Place the IV bag back on the pole. Move the clothing down the IV tubing, over the IV site, and onto the resident's arm. Put the other arm into the clothing.

G Check that the IV is dripping properly. Make sure none of the tubing is dislodged. Check to see that the IV site dressing is in place. Make sure tubing is not kinked after you are finished.

For cases of poor circulation to the legs and feet, elastic stockings are ordered. These stockings help prevent swelling and blood clots and aid circulation. They promote blood circulation by gently squeezing the legs to increase blood flow. Elastic stockings are also known as *anti-embolic stockings* or *TED hose*. They are referred to as anti-embolic because they help prevent embolisms. An **embolism** is an obstruction of a blood vessel, usually by a blood clot. The embolism can travel from where it was formed to another part of the body, blocking blood flow. It can cause serious damage and even death.

Elastic stockings may either be knee-high or thigh-high. They need to be put on in the morning, before the resident gets out of bed. Legs are at their smallest size then. The stockings are usually removed in the evening.

Applying knee-high elastic stockings 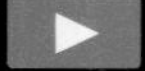

Equipment: elastic stockings

1. Identify yourself by name. Identify resident by name.
   Resident has right to know identity of his or her caregiver. Addressing resident by name shows respect and establishes correct identification.

2. Wash your hands.
   Provides for infection prevention.

3. Explain procedure to resident. Speak clearly, slowly, and directly. Maintain face-to-face contact whenever possible.
   Promotes understanding and independence.

4. Provide for resident's privacy with curtain, screen, or door.
   Maintains resident's right to privacy and dignity.

5. The resident should be in the supine position (on her back) in bed. With resident lying down, remove her socks, shoes, or slippers, and expose one leg. Expose no more than one leg at a time.

6. Take one stocking and turn it inside out at least to heel area (Fig. 6-29).

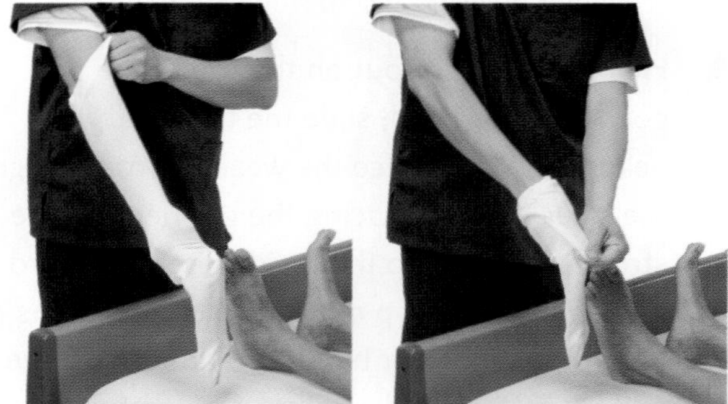

Fig. 6-29. *Turning the stocking inside out allows the stocking to roll on gently.*

7. Gently place the foot of the stocking over the toes, foot, and heel (Fig. 6-30). Make sure the heel is in the right place. The heel of the foot should be in the heel of the stocking.

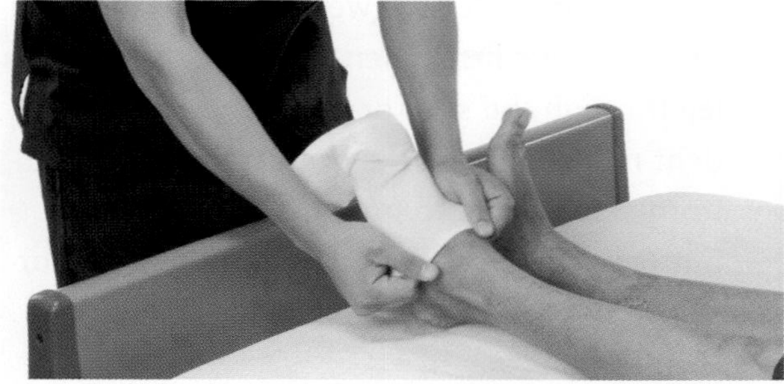

Fig. 6-30. *Place the foot of the stocking over the toes, foot, and heel. Promote the resident's comfort and safety. Avoid force and overextension of joints.*

8. Gently pull the top of the stocking over the foot, heel, and leg.

9. Make sure there are no twists or wrinkles in the stocking after it is on. It must fit smoothly (Fig. 6-31). Make sure the heel of the stocking is over the heel of the foot. If the stocking has an opening in the toe area, make sure the opening is either over or under the toe area. This depends on the manufacturer's instructions. Adjust if needed.

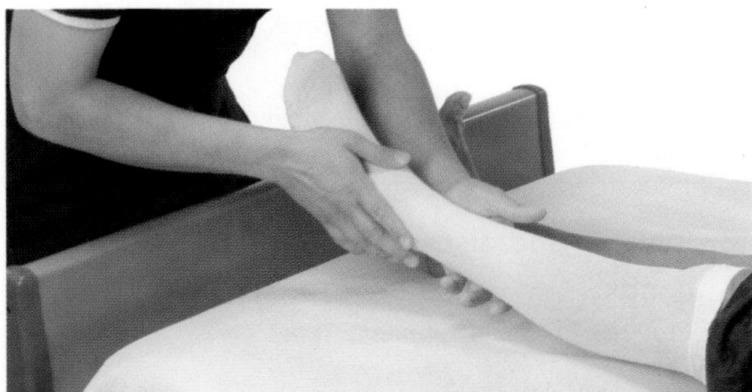

Fig. 6-31. *Make stocking smooth. Twists or wrinkles cause the stocking to be too tight, which reduces circulation.*

10. Repeat steps 6 through 9 for the other leg.
11. Place call light within resident's reach.
    Allows resident to communicate with staff as necessary.
12. Wash your hands.
    Provides for infection prevention.
13. Report any changes in resident to nurse.
    Provides nurse with information to assess resident.
14. Document procedure using facility guidelines.
    If you do not document the care, legally it did not happen.

6. Identify guidelines for proper oral hygiene

Oral care, or care of the mouth, teeth, and gums, is done at least twice each day to clean the mouth. Oral care should be done after breakfast and after the last meal or snack of the day. It may also be done before a resident eats. Oral care includes brushing the teeth, tongue, and gums; flossing teeth; caring for lips; and caring for dentures (Fig. 6-32). When giving oral care, NAs must wear gloves. They should follow Standard Precautions.

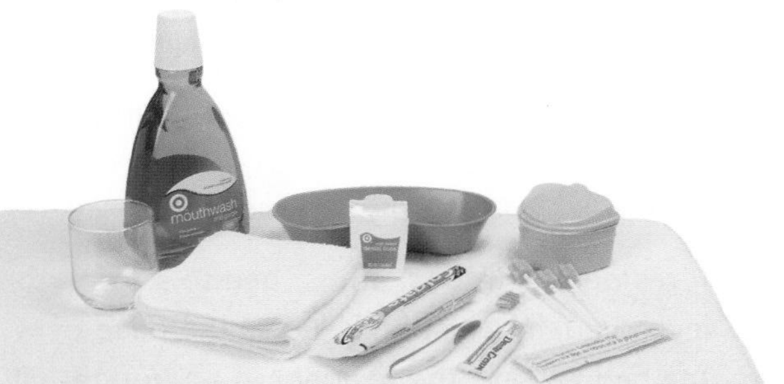

Fig. 6-32. *Some supplies needed for oral care.*

Observing and Reporting: Oral Care

When performing oral care, observe the resident's mouth carefully. Report any of these to the nurse:

- O/R Irritation
- O/R Raised areas
- O/R Coated or swollen tongue
- O/R Ulcers, such as canker sores or small, painful, white sores
- O/R Flaky, white spots
- O/R Dry, cracked, bleeding, or chapped lips
- O/R Loose, chipped, broken or decayed teeth
- O/R Swollen, irritated, bleeding, or whitish gums
- O/R Breath that smells bad or fruity
- O/R Resident reports of mouth pain

Providing oral care

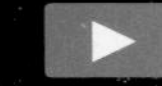

Equipment: toothbrush; toothpaste; emesis basin; gloves; clothing protector, towel, or washcloth; cup of water; lip moisturizer

1. Identify yourself by name. Identify the resident by name.
   Resident has right to know identity of his or her caregiver. Addressing resident by name shows respect and establishes correct identification.
2. Wash your hands.
   Provides for infection prevention.

3. Explain procedure to resident. Speak clearly, slowly, and directly. Maintain face-to-face contact whenever possible.
   Promotes understanding and independence.

4. Provide for resident's privacy with curtain, screen, or door.
   Maintains resident's right to privacy and dignity.

5. If resident is in bed, adjust bed to a safe level, usually waist high. Raise the head of the bed to have the resident in an upright sitting position. Lock bed wheels.
   Prevents injury to you and to resident. Prevents fluids from running down resident's throat, causing choking.

6. Put on gloves.
   Brushing may cause gums to bleed.

7. Place a clothing protector, towel, or washcloth across the resident's chest.
   Protects resident's clothing and bed linen.

8. Wet the toothbrush. Put on small amount of toothpaste.
   Water helps distribute toothpaste.

9. Clean the entire mouth, including the tongue and all surfaces of the teeth and gumline. Use gentle strokes. First brush the inner, outer, and chewing surfaces of the upper teeth. Then do the same with the lower teeth. Use short strokes. Brush back and forth. Brush the tongue.
   Brushing upper teeth first lessens production of saliva in lower part of mouth.

10. Give the resident water to rinse the mouth. Place the emesis basin under the resident's chin, with the inward curve under the chin. Have the resident spit water into the basin (Fig. 6-33). Wipe his mouth and remove the towel. Apply lip moisturizer.

11. Rinse the toothbrush and place in proper container. Empty, rinse, and dry basin. Place basin in designated dirty supply area or return to storage, depending on facility policy.

12. Place soiled clothing and linens in proper containers.

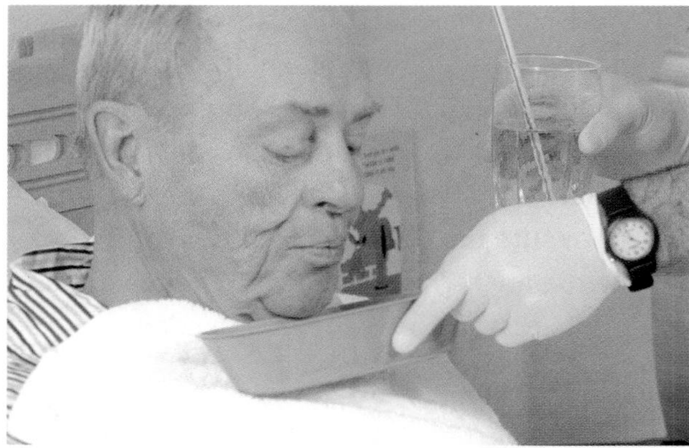

Fig. 6-33. *Rinsing and spitting removes food particles and toothpaste.*

13. Remove and discard gloves. Wash your hands.
    Provides for infection prevention.

14. Return bed to lowest position. Remove privacy measures.
    Lowering the bed provides for safety.

15. Place call light within resident's reach.
    Allows resident to communicate with staff as necessary.

16. Report any problems with teeth, mouth, tongue, or lips to the nurse. This includes odor, cracking, sores, bleeding, and any discoloration.
    Provides nurse with information to assess resident.

17. Document procedure using facility guidelines.
    If you do not document the care, legally it did not happen.

Even though a person who is unconscious cannot eat, breathing through the mouth causes saliva to dry in the mouth. Oral care needs to be performed more often to keep the mouth clean and moist. For a resident who is unconscious, the NA must use as little liquid as possible when giving mouth care. Because the person's swallowing reflex is weak, he is at risk for aspiration. **Aspiration** is the inhalation of food, fluid, or foreign material into the lungs. Aspiration can cause pneumonia or death. Turning an unconscious resident on his side before giving oral care can also help prevent aspiration. Only swabs soaked in tiny amounts of fluid should be used to clean the mouth.

Providing oral care for the unconscious resident 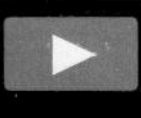

Equipment: sponge swabs, tongue depressor, towel, emesis basin, gloves, cup of water, lip moisturizer, cleaning solution (check the care plan)

1. Identify yourself by name. Identify the resident by name. Even residents who are unconscious may be able to hear you. Always speak to them as you would to any resident.
   Resident has right to know identity of his or her caregiver. Addressing resident by name shows respect and establishes correct identification.
2. Wash your hands.
   Provides for infection prevention.
3. Explain procedure to resident. Speak clearly, slowly, and directly. Maintain face-to-face contact whenever possible.
   Promotes understanding. The resident may be able to hear and understand even though he is unconscious.
4. Provide for resident's privacy with curtain, screen, or door.
   Maintains resident's right to privacy and dignity.
5. Adjust bed to a safe level, usually waist high. Lock bed wheels.
   Prevents injury to you and to resident.
6. Put on gloves.
   Protects you from coming into contact with body fluids.
7. Turn resident onto his side. Place a towel under his cheek and chin. Place an emesis basin next to the cheek and chin for excess fluid.
   Protects resident's clothing and bed linen.
8. Hold the mouth open with the tongue depressor. (You can also use gentle pressure on the chin to open the mouth. Follow facility policy.)
   Enables you to safely clean mouth.
9. Dip the sponge swab in the cleaning solution. Squeeze excess solution to prevent aspiration. Wipe the teeth, gums, tongue, and inside surfaces of the mouth. Remove debris with the swab. Change the swab often. Repeat this until the mouth is clean.
   Stimulates gums and removes mucus.
10. Rinse with clean swab dipped in water. Squeeze swab first to remove excess water.
    Removes solution from mouth.
11. Remove the towel and basin. Pat lips or face dry if needed. Apply lip moisturizer.
    Prevents lips from drying and cracking. Improves resident's comfort.
12. Empty, rinse, and dry basin. Place basin in designated dirty supply area or return to storage, depending on facility policy.
13. Place soiled linens in the proper container.
14. Remove and discard gloves. Wash your hands.
    Provides for infection prevention.
15. Return bed to lowest position. Remove privacy measures.
    Lowering the bed provides for safety.
16. Place call light within resident's reach.
    Allows resident to communicate with staff as necessary.
17. Report any problems with teeth, mouth, tongue, or lips to the nurse. This includes odor, cracking, sores, bleeding, and any discoloration.
    Provides nurse with information to assess resident.
18. Document procedure using facility guidelines.
    If you do not document the care, legally it did not happen.

Flossing the teeth removes plaque and tartar buildup around the gumline and between the teeth. Teeth may be flossed immediately after or before they are brushed, as the resident prefers. NAs should follow the care plan's instructions for flossing.

Flossing teeth

Equipment: dental floss, cup of water, emesis basin, gloves, towel

1. Identify yourself by name. Identify the resident by name.
   Resident has right to know identity of his or her caregiver. Addressing resident by name shows respect and establishes correct identification.
2. Wash your hands.
   Provides for infection prevention.
3. Explain procedure to resident. Speak clearly, slowly, and directly. Maintain face-to-face contact whenever possible.
   Promotes understanding and independence.
4. Provide for resident's privacy with curtain, screen, or door.
   Maintains resident's right to privacy and dignity.
5. If resident is in bed, adjust bed to a safe level, usually waist high. Raise the head of the bed to have the resident in an upright sitting position. Lock bed wheels.
   Prevents fluids from running down resident's throat, causing choking.
6. Put on gloves.
   Flossing may cause gums to bleed.
7. Wrap the ends of the floss securely around each index finger (Fig. 6-34).

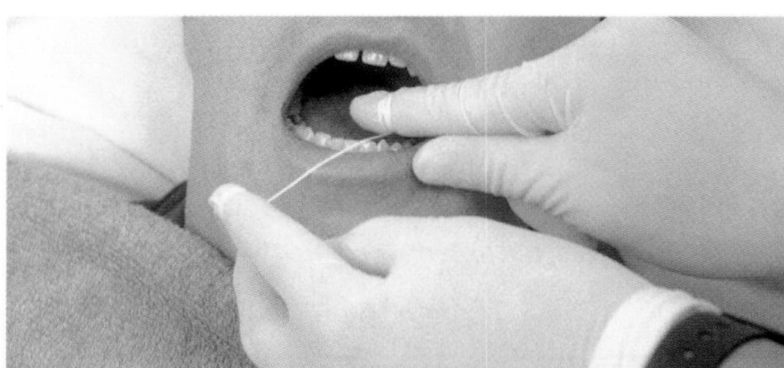

Fig. 6-34. *Before beginning, wrap floss securely around each index finger.*

8. Start with the back teeth. Place the floss between the teeth. Move it down the surface of the tooth. Use a gentle sawing motion (Fig. 6-35).

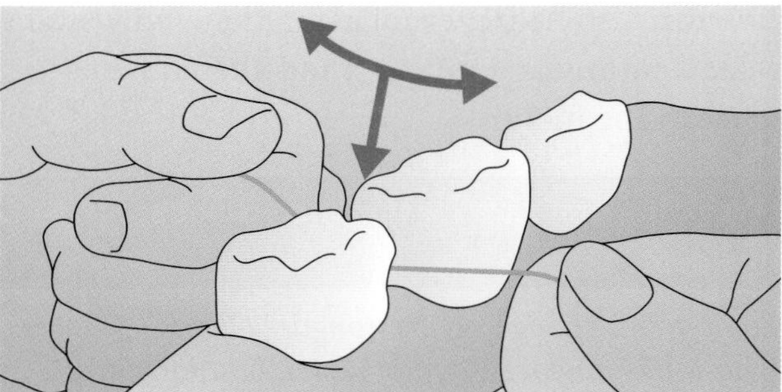

Fig. 6-35. *Being gentle protects the gums.*

   Continue to the gumline. At the gumline, curve the floss. Slip it gently into the space between the gum and tooth. Then go back up, scraping that side of the tooth (Fig. 6-36). Repeat this on the side of the other tooth.
   Removes food and prevents tooth decay.

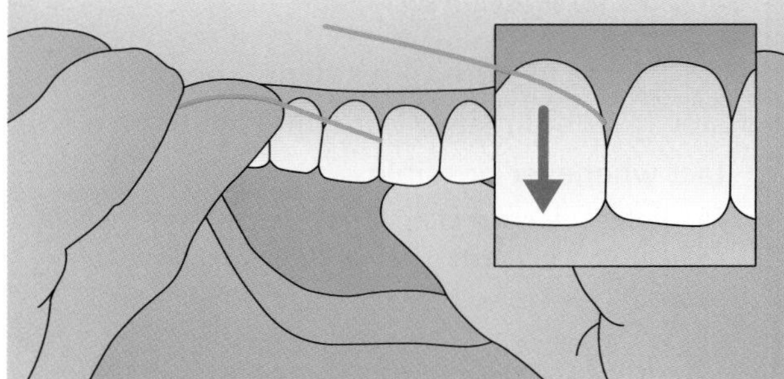

Fig. 6-36. *Floss gently in the space between the gum and tooth.*

9. After every two teeth, unwind the floss from your fingers. Move it so you are using a clean area. Floss all teeth.
10. Occasionally offer water so that the resident can rinse debris from his mouth into the basin.
    Flossing loosens food. Rinsing removes it.
11. Offer resident a face towel when done flossing all teeth.
    Promotes dignity.
12. Discard the floss. Discard the water and rinse and dry the basin. Place basin in designated dirty supply area or return to storage, depending on facility policy.
13. Place soiled linen in the proper container.

14. Remove and discard gloves. Wash your hands.
Provides for infection prevention.

15. Return bed to lowest position. Remove privacy measures.
Lowering the bed provides for safety.

16. Place call light within resident's reach.
Allows resident to communicate with staff as necessary.

17. Report any problems with teeth, mouth, tongue, or lips to the nurse. This includes odor, cracking, sores, bleeding, and any discoloration.
Provides nurse with information to assess resident.

18. Document procedure using facility guidelines.
If you do not document the care, legally it did not happen.

Dentures are artificial teeth. They are expensive. Dentures must be handled carefully to avoid breaking or chipping them. If a resident's dentures break, he or she cannot eat. The NA should notify the nurse if a resident's dentures do not fit properly, are chipped, or are missing.

The NA must wear gloves when handling and cleaning dentures. Dentures and denture brushes should not be placed on contaminated surfaces. Once dentures are cleaned, they should either be returned to the resident or stored in denture solution or in clean, moderate/cool water (not hot water) so that they do not dry out and warp. Dentures may crack if left uncovered. Dentures should be stored in a denture cup labeled with the resident's name and room number when not being worn. They should not be removed from the resident's room.

Residents' Rights

Denture Care

Denture care is very personal. The NA should pull the privacy curtain and close the door before beginning. Many people who have dentures do not want to be seen without their teeth in place. After teeth are removed, they should be cleaned and returned immediately.

Cleaning and storing dentures

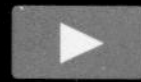

Equipment: denture brush or toothbrush, denture cleanser, labeled denture cup, 2 towels, gloves

1. Wash your hands.
Provides for infection prevention.

2. Put on gloves.
Prevents you from coming into contact with body fluids.

3. Line the sink or basin with a towel(s) and partially fill the sink with water.
Prevents dentures from breaking if dropped.

4. Handle dentures carefully. Hold them over the sink. Rinse dentures in clean, moderate/cool running water before brushing them. Do not use hot water.
Hot water may warp dentures.

5. Apply cleanser to the brush.

6. Brush dentures on all surfaces (Fig. 6-37). This includes the inner, outer, and chewing surfaces of dentures, as well as the groove that will touch gum surfaces.

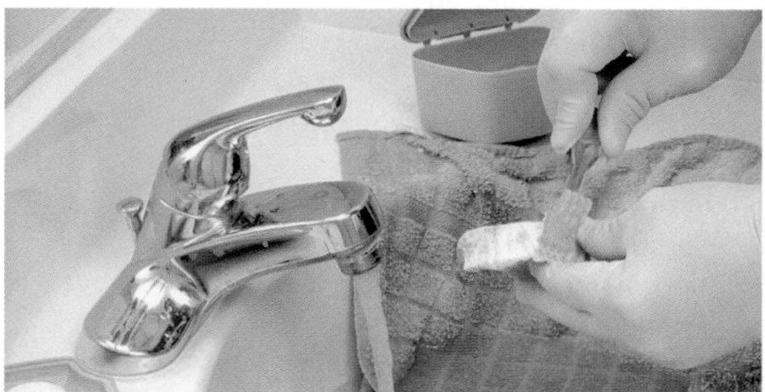

Fig. 6-37. *Brush dentures on all surfaces to properly clean them.*

7. Rinse all surfaces of dentures under clean, moderate/cool running water. Do not use hot water.
Hot water may warp dentures.

8. Rinse the denture cup and lid before placing clean dentures in the cup.
Removes pathogens.

9. Place dentures in clean, labeled denture cup with solution or moderate/cool water.

Dentures should be completely covered with solution. Place the lid on the cup. Return the cup to where it is stored. Some residents will want to wear their dentures all of the time. They will only remove them for cleaning. If the resident wants to continue wearing dentures, return them to her. Do not place them in the denture cup.

10. Rinse the brush. Clean, dry, and return equipment to storage. Drain the sink. Place soiled linens in the proper container.

11. Remove and discard gloves. Wash your hands.
Provides for infection prevention.

12. Document procedure using facility guidelines. Report any change in appearance of dentures to the nurse.
If you do not document the care, legally it did not happen.

Removing and Reinserting Dentures

If a resident cannot remove her dentures, the NA must do it if trained and allowed to do so. The resident should be sitting upright before beginning. The NA should first don gloves. The lower denture should be removed first. The lower denture is easier to remove because it floats on the gumline of the lower jaw. The NA should grasp the lower denture with a gauze square (for a good grip) and remove it. She should place it in a denture cup filled with solution or moderate/cool water.

The upper denture is sealed by suction. The NA should firmly grasp the upper denture with a gauze square and give a slight downward pull to break the suction. She should turn it at an angle to take it out of the mouth. When inserting dentures, the NA should ask the resident to sit upright, then she should don gloves. If needed, she should apply denture cream or adhesive to the dentures. When the resident's mouth is open, the upper denture should be placed into the mouth by turning it at an angle. The NA should straighten it and press it onto the upper gumline firmly and evenly. She should insert the lower denture onto the gumline of the lower jaw and press firmly.

7. Explain guidelines for assisting with toileting

Residents who are unable to get out of bed to use the toilet may be given a standard bedpan, a fracture pan, or a urinal. A **fracture pan** is a bedpan that is flatter than the regular bedpan. It is used for residents who cannot assist with raising their hips onto a regular bedpan (Fig. 6-38). Women will generally use a bedpan for urination and bowel movements. Men will generally use a urinal for urination and a bedpan for bowel movements (Fig. 6-39).

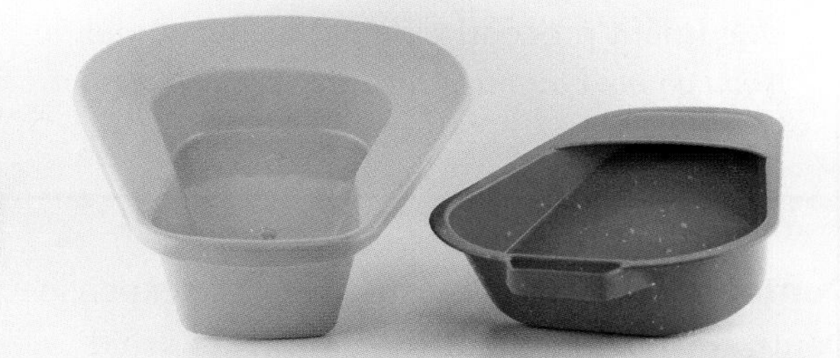

Fig. 6-38. *On the left is a standard pan, and a fracture pan is on the right.*

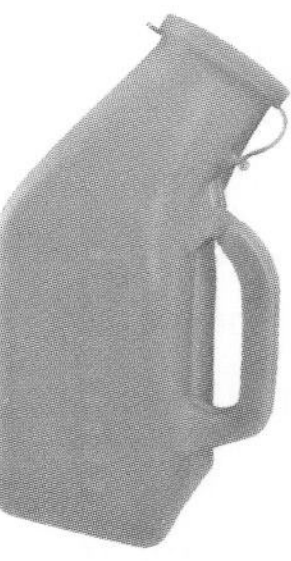

Fig. 6-39. *A urinal.* (PHOTO COURTESY OF NOVA MEDICAL PRODUCTS, WWW.NOVAMEDICALPRODUCTS.COM)

Elimination equipment is usually kept in the bathroom between uses. Residents who share bathrooms may need to have urinals and bedpans labeled. This equipment must never be placed on overbed tables or on top of side tables.

Urine and feces are considered infectious wastes. NAs must always wear gloves when handling bedpans, urinals, or basins that contain wastes, including dirty bath water. NAs should be careful not to spill or splash wastes, and wastes should be discarded in the toilet. Immediately after use, containers used for elimination should be placed in the proper area for cleaning, or they should be cleaned and stored according to facility policy.

Assisting a resident with the use of a bedpan

Equipment: bedpan, bedpan cover, disposable bed protector, bath blanket, toilet paper, disposable wipes, 2 towels, 2 pairs of gloves, supplies for perineal care

1. Identify yourself by name. Identify the resident by name.
   Resident has right to know identity of his or her caregiver. Addressing resident by name shows respect and establishes correct identification.
2. Wash your hands.
   Provides for infection prevention.
3. Explain procedure to resident. Speak clearly, slowly, and directly. Maintain face-to-face contact whenever possible.
   Promotes understanding and independence.
4. Provide for resident's privacy with curtain, screen, or door.
   Maintains resident's right to privacy and dignity.
5. Adjust bed to a safe level, usually waist high. Before placing bedpan, lower the head of the bed. Lock bed wheels.
   When bed is flat, resident can be moved without working against gravity.
6. Put on gloves.
   Prevents contact with body fluids.
7. Cover the resident with the bath blanket. Ask him to hold it while you pull down the top covers underneath. Do not expose more of the resident than you need to. Keep the resident covered from the chest down except when placing or removing the bedpan. Keeping him covered, ask the resident to remove his undergarments, or help him do so.
   Maintains resident's right to privacy and dignity.
8. Ask the resident to raise his hips by pushing with his feet and hands at the count of three. If he needs help, place your arm under the small of his back and tell him to push with his heels and hands on your signal as you raise his hips. Place the bed protector under the resident's buttocks and hips. Slide the bedpan in the correct position under his hips (Fig. 6-40). A **standard bedpan** should be positioned with the wider end aligned with the resident's buttocks. A **fracture pan** should be positioned with the handle toward the foot of bed.
   Prevents linen from being soiled.

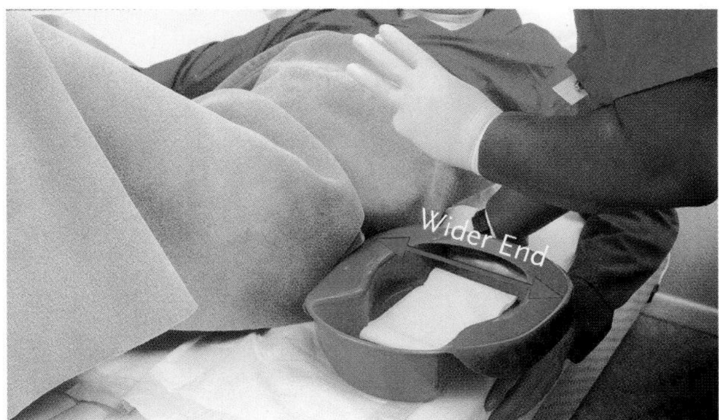

Fig. 6-40. *On the count of three, slide the bedpan under the buttocks after placing the bed protector. The wider end of the bedpan should be aligned with the buttocks.*

   If the resident cannot assist in getting on the bedpan, raise the far side rail (if used). Help the resident to turn toward the raised rail. Place the protective pad on the area where the resident will lie on his back. Place the bedpan firmly against the resident's buttocks (Fig. 6-41). Holding the bedpan securely, gently roll the resident back onto the bedpan. Keep the bedpan centered underneath.

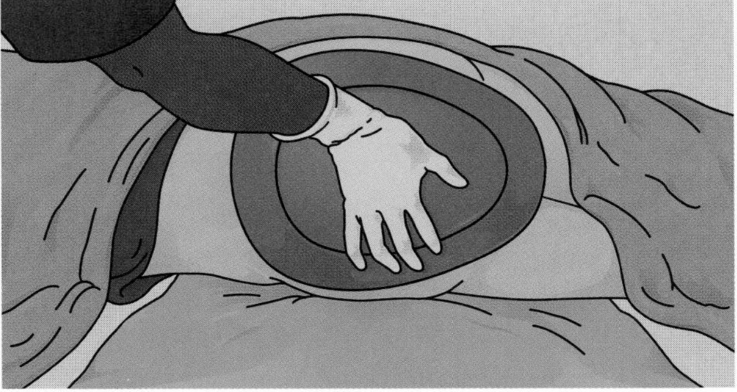

Fig. 6-41. *Placing the bedpan firmly against the resident's buttocks, gently roll him back onto the bedpan.*

9. Remove and discard gloves. Wash your hands.
   Provides for infection prevention.

10. Raise the head of the bed. Prop the resident into a semi-sitting position using pillows. Leave side rails up (if used). Return bed to its lowest position.
Puts resident in comfortable position for voiding.

11. Make sure the bath blanket is still covering the resident. Place toilet paper and disposable wipes within the resident's reach. Ask the resident to clean his hands with a wipe when finished if he is able.

12. Place the call light within resident's reach. Ask the resident to signal when done. Leave the room and close the door.
Ensures ability to communicate need for help.

13. When called by the resident, return and wash your hands. Put on clean gloves.

14. Raise bed to a safe level. Lower the head of the bed. Make sure the resident is still covered.
Places resident in proper position to remove pan. Promotes dignity.

15. Remove the bedpan carefully and cover it with a bedpan cover or towel.
Promotes infection prevention and odor control. Provides dignity for resident.

16. Give perineal care if help is needed. Wipe from front to back. Dry the perineal area. Help the resident put on an undergarment. Cover resident and remove the bath blanket.
Wiping from front to back prevents spread of pathogens that may cause urinary tract infection.

17. Remove and discard the bed protector. Discard disposable supplies. Place the towel and bath blanket in a hamper or bag.

18. Return bed to lowest position. Leave side rails in ordered position. Remove privacy measures.
Lowering the bed provides for resident's safety.

19. Take the bedpan to the bathroom. Note color, odor, and consistency of contents. Empty contents carefully into the toilet unless a specimen is needed or urine is being measured for intake/output monitoring. If you notice anything unusual about the stool or urine (for example, the presence of blood), do not discard it. Inform the nurse.
Changes may be the first sign of a medical problem.

20. Turn the faucet on with a paper towel. Rinse the bedpan with cold water and empty it into the toilet. Flush the toilet. Place bedpan in proper area for cleaning or clean it according to policy.

21. Remove and discard gloves. Wash your hands.
Provides for infection prevention.

22. Place call light within resident's reach.
Allows resident to communicate with staff as necessary.

23. Report any changes in resident to the nurse.
Provides nurse with information to assess resident.

24. Document procedure using facility guidelines.
If you do not document the care, legally it did not happen.

Assisting a male resident with a urinal

Equipment: urinal, disposable bed protector, disposable wipes, 2 pairs of gloves

1. Identify yourself by name. Identify the resident by name.
Resident has right to know identity of his caregiver. Addressing resident by name shows respect and establishes correct identification.

2. Wash your hands.
Provides for infection prevention.

3. Explain procedure to resident. Speak clearly, slowly, and directly. Maintain face-to-face contact whenever possible.
Promotes understanding and independence.

4. Provide for resident's privacy with curtain, screen, or door.
Maintains resident's right to privacy and dignity.

5. Adjust bed to a safe level, usually waist high. Lock bed wheels.
   Prevents injury to you and to resident.

6. Put on gloves.
   Prevents you from coming into contact with body fluids.

7. Place the bed protector under the resident's buttocks and hips, as in earlier procedure.
   Prevents linen from being soiled.

8. Hand the urinal to the resident. If the resident is not able to help himself, place urinal between his legs and position the penis inside the urinal (Fig. 6-42). Replace covers.
   Promotes independence, dignity, and privacy.

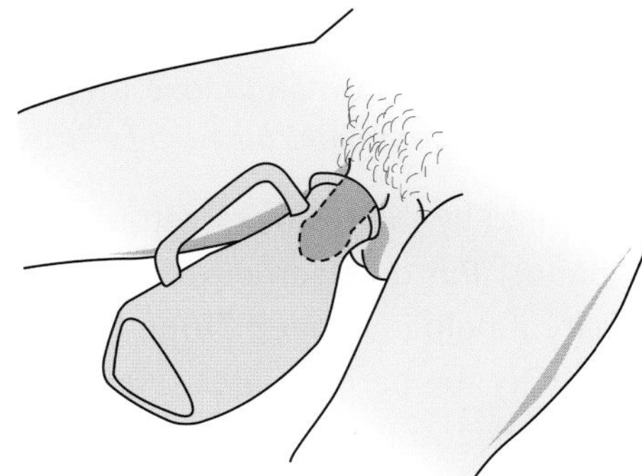

Fig. 6-42. *Position the penis inside the urinal if the resident cannot do it himself.*

9. Remove and discard gloves. Wash your hands.

10. Raise the head of the bed. Return bed to its lowest position. Place disposable wipes within resident's reach. Ask the resident to clean his hands with a hand wipe when finished if he is able.
    Lowering the bed provides for resident's safety.

11. Place the call light within resident's reach. Ask the resident to signal when done. Leave the room and close the door.
    Ensures ability to communicate need for help.

12. When called by the resident, return and wash your hands. Put on clean gloves.

13. Discard disposable wipes.

14. Remove urinal or have resident hand it to you. Note color, odor, and qualities (for example, cloudiness) of contents. Empty contents into the toilet unless specimen is needed or urine is being measured for intake/output monitoring.
    Changes may be the first sign of a medical problem.

15. Turn the faucet on with a paper towel. Rinse the urinal with cold water and empty it into the toilet. Flush the toilet. Place urinal in proper area for cleaning or clean it according to facility policy.

16. Remove and discard the bed protector. Remove and discard gloves. Wash your hands.

17. Leave bed in its lowest position. Remove privacy measures.
    Lowering the bed provides for resident's safety.

18. Place call light within resident's reach.
    Allows resident to communicate with staff as necessary.

19. Report any changes in resident to the nurse.
    Provides nurse with information to assess resident.

20. Document procedure using facility guidelines.
    If you do not document the care, legally it did not happen.

Some residents are able to get out of bed, but may still need help walking to the bathroom and using the toilet. Others who are able to get out of bed but cannot walk to the bathroom may use a portable commode, or bedside commode (BSC). A **portable commode** is a chair with a toilet seat and a removable container underneath (Fig. 6-43).

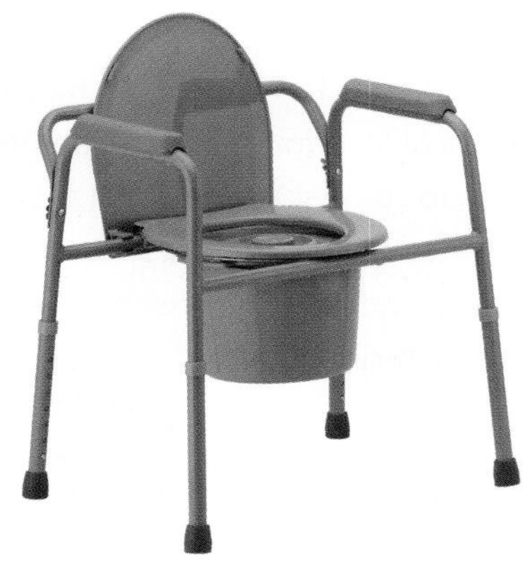

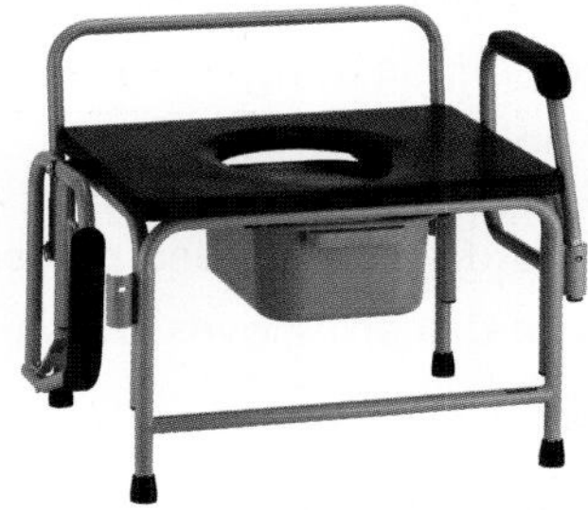

Fig. 6-43. *The top photo shows a regular portable commode, and the bottom photo shows a bariatric portable commode, which can be used for people who are overweight or obese.* (PHOTO COURTESY OF NOVA MEDICAL PRODUCTS, WWW.NOVAMEDICALPRODUCTS.COM)

Assisting a resident to use a portable commode or toilet

Equipment: portable commode with basin, toilet paper, disposable wipes, towel, 3 pairs of gloves, supplies for perineal care

1. Identify yourself by name. Identify the resident by name.
   Resident has right to know identity of his or her caregiver. Addressing resident by name shows respect and establishes correct identification.

2. Wash your hands.
   Provides for infection prevention.

3. Explain procedure to resident. Speak clearly, slowly, and directly. Maintain face-to-face contact whenever possible.
   Promotes understanding and independence.

4. Provide for resident's privacy with curtain, screen, or door.
   Maintains resident's right to privacy and dignity.

5. Lock commode wheels. Adjust bed to lowest position. Lock bed wheels. Make sure resident is wearing nonskid shoes and that the laces are tied. Help resident out of bed and to the portable commode or bathroom.

6. Put on gloves.
   Prevents contact with body fluids.

7. If needed, help the resident remove clothing and sit comfortably on the toilet seat. Put toilet paper and disposable wipes within reach. Ask resident to clean his hands with a wipe when finished if he is able.

8. Remove and discard gloves. Wash your hands.

9. Provide privacy. Place the call light within resident's reach. Ask resident to signal when done. Leave the room and close the door.
   Ensures ability to communicate need for help.

10. When called by the resident, return and wash your hands. Put on clean gloves. Give perineal care if help is needed. Wipe from front to back. Dry the perineal area. Help the resident put on clothing.
    Wiping from front to back prevents spread of pathogens that may cause urinary tract infection.

11. Place the towel in a hamper or bag. Discard disposable supplies.

12. Remove and discard gloves. Wash your hands.

13. Help the resident back to bed.

14. Put on clean gloves.

15. If using a portable commode, remove the waste container. Note color, odor, and consistency of contents. Empty contents into the toilet unless a specimen is needed or the urine is being measured for intake/output monitoring.
    Changes may be the first sign of a medical problem.

16. Turn the faucet on with a paper towel. Rinse the container with cold water and empty it into the toilet. Flush the toilet. Place con-

tainer in proper area for cleaning or clean it according to facility policy.

17. Remove and discard gloves. Wash your hands.
    Provides for infection prevention.

18. Make sure bed is in its lowest position. Remove privacy measures.

19. Place call light within resident's reach.
    Allows resident to communicate with staff as necessary.

20. Report any changes in resident to the nurse.
    Provides nurse with information to assess resident.

21. Document procedure using facility guidelines.
    If you do not document the care, legally it did not happen.

8. Explain guidelines for safely positioning and moving residents

Residents who spend a lot of time in bed often need help getting into comfortable positions. They also need to change positions periodically to avoid muscle stiffness and skin breakdown. Too much pressure on one area for too long can cause a decrease in circulation. This can lead to pressure injuries and other problems like muscle contractures. **Positioning** means helping residents into positions that promote comfort and health. Bedbound residents should be repositioned at least every two hours. Residents in wheelchairs or chairs should be repositioned at least every hour. Each time there is a change, the NA should document the position and the time. The NA should also check the skin for signs of irritation each time a resident is repositioned. These are the five basic body positions:

1. **Supine** or lying flat on the back (Fig. 6-44)

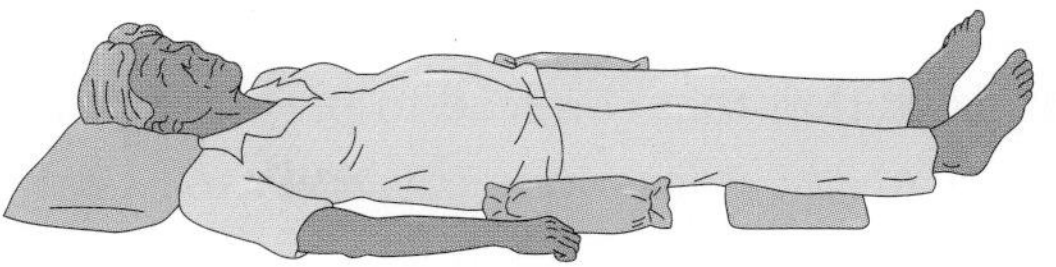

Fig. 6-44. *A person in the supine position is lying flat on her back.*

2. **Lateral** or lying on either side (Fig. 6-45)

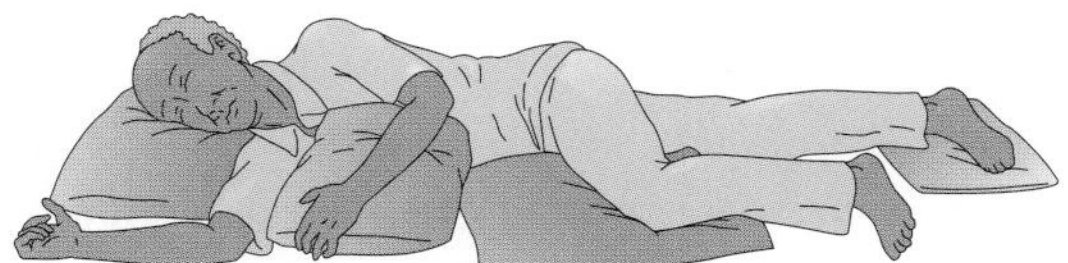

Fig. 6-45. *A person in the lateral position is lying on his side.*

3. **Prone** or lying on the stomach (Fig. 6-46)

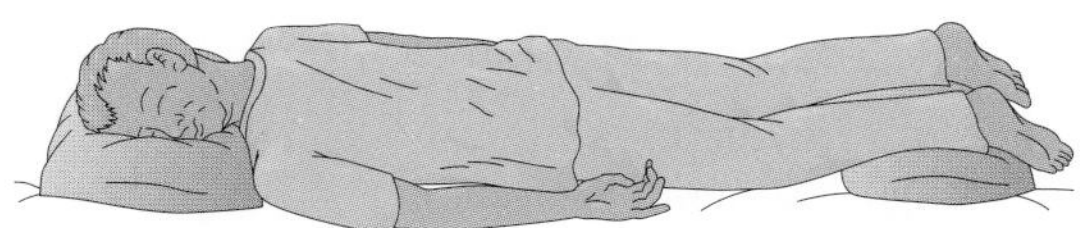

Fig. 6-46. *A person in the prone position is lying on his stomach.*

4. **Fowler's** or semi-sitting position (45 to 60 degrees) (Fig. 6-47)

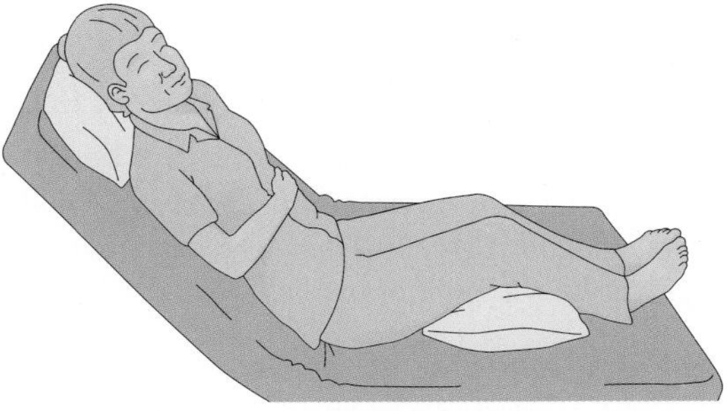

Fig. 6-47. *A person in the Fowler's position is partially reclined.*

5. **Sims'** or left side-lying position (Fig. 6-48)

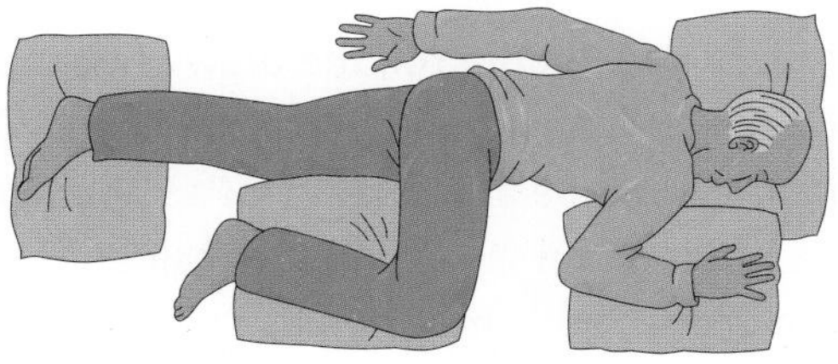

Fig. 6-48. *A person lying in the Sims' position is lying on his left side with one leg drawn up.*

Helping a resident move up in bed helps prevent skin irritation that can lead to pressure injuries. An NA needs at least one coworker to assist to perform this procedure safely.

Moving a resident up in bed

Equipment: draw sheet or other device, coworker

1. Identify yourself by name. Identify the resident by name.
   Resident has right to know identity of his or her caregiver. Addressing resident by name shows respect and establishes correct identification.
2. Wash your hands.
   Provides for infection prevention.
3. Explain procedure to resident. Speak clearly, slowly, and directly. Maintain face-to-face contact whenever possible.
   Promotes understanding and independence.
4. Provide for resident's privacy with curtain, screen, or door.
   Maintains resident's right to privacy and dignity.
5. Adjust bed to a safe level, usually waist high. Lock bed wheels.
   Prevents injury to you and to resident.
6. Lower the head of the bed to make it flat. Move the pillow to the head of the bed.
   When bed is flat, resident can be moved without working against gravity. Pillow prevents injury should resident hit the head of the bed.
7. Stand on one side of the bed with your feet shoulder-width apart. Face the head of the bed. The foot that is closer to the head of the bed should be pointed toward the head of the bed. Your coworker should be standing on the other side of the bed.
8. Both of you should roll the draw sheet up to the resident's side and grasp the sheet. One hand should be at the resident's shoulders, the other about level with the resident's hips. Use proper body mechanics.
9. Let resident know you will be moving her on the count of three. On three, both of you shift your body weight to your front leg. Help move the resident.
   Communicating helps resident help you.
10. Place the pillow under the resident's head.
    Provides for resident's comfort.
11. Return bed to lowest position. Remove privacy measures.
    Lowering the bed provides for resident's safety.
12. Place call light within resident's reach.
    Allows resident to communicate with staff as necessary.
13. Wash your hands.
    Provides for infection prevention.
14. Report any changes in resident to the nurse.
    Provides nurse with information to assess resident.
15. Document procedure using facility guidelines.
    If you do not document the care, legally it did not happen.

Moving a resident to the side of the bed

Equipment: draw sheet or other device

1. Identify yourself by name. Identify the resident by name.
   Resident has right to know identity of his or her caregiver. Addressing resident by name shows respect and establishes correct identification.
2. Wash your hands.
   Provides for infection prevention.
3. Explain procedure to resident. Speak clearly, slowly, and directly. Maintain face-to-face contact whenever possible.
   Promotes understanding and independence.
4. Provide for resident's privacy with curtain, screen, or door.
   Maintains resident's right to privacy and dignity.
5. Adjust the bed to a safe level, usually waist high. Lock bed wheels.
   Prevents injury to you and to resident.
6. Lower the head of the bed.

When bed is flat, resident can be moved without working against gravity.

7. Stand on the side of the bed to which you are moving the resident. Stand with feet shoulder-width apart and bend your knees.

8. **With a draw sheet**: Roll the draw sheet up to the resident's side and grasp the sheet. One hand should be at the resident's shoulders, the other about level with the resident's hips. Apply one knee against the side of the bed, and lean back with your body. On the count of three, slowly pull the draw sheet and resident toward you.

   Without a draw sheet: Gently slide your hands under the resident's head and shoulders and move them toward you (Fig. 6-49). Gently slide your hands under her midsection and move it toward you. Gently slide your hands under the hips and legs and move them toward you (Fig. 6-50).
   Being gentle while sliding helps protect resident's skin.

9. Return bed to lowest position. Remove privacy measures.
   Lowering the bed provides for resident's safety.

10. Place call light within resident's reach.
    Allows resident to communicate with staff as necessary.

11. Wash your hands.
    Provides for infection prevention.

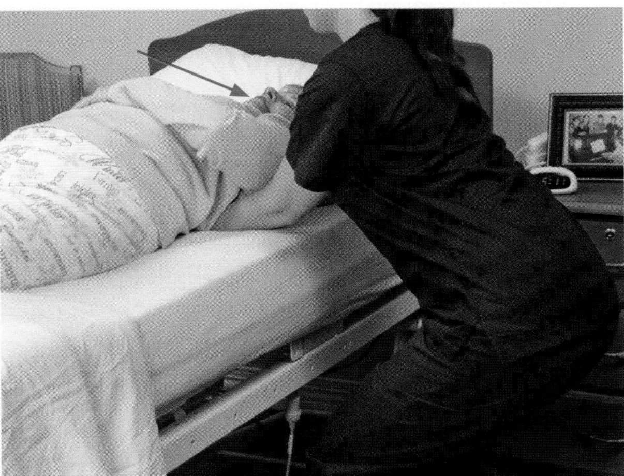

Fig. 6-49. *Gently move the resident's head and shoulders toward you.*

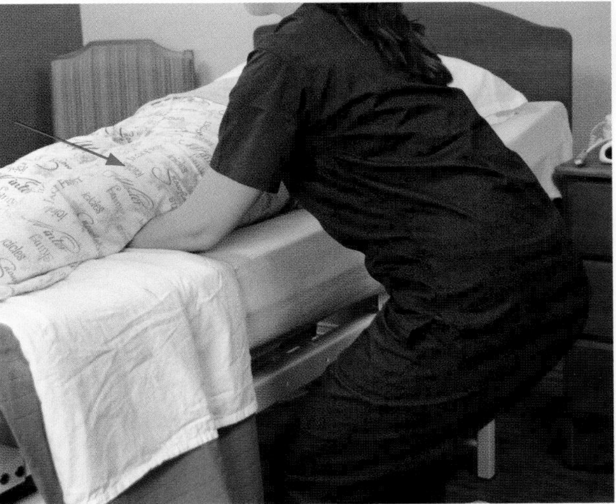

Fig. 6-50. *Gently move the hips and legs toward you.*

12. Report any changes in resident to the nurse.
    Provides nurse with information to assess resident.

13. Document procedure using facility guidelines.
    If you do not document the care, legally it did not happen.

Residents may be turned on their sides in preparation for sitting up or to change position and to take pressure off their backs. This helps prevent skin irritation and pressure injuries.

Positioning a resident on his side 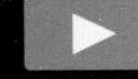

1. Identify yourself by name. Identify the resident by name.
   Resident has right to know identity of his or her caregiver. Addressing resident by name shows respect and establishes correct identification.

2. Wash your hands.
   Provides for infection prevention.

3. Explain procedure to resident. Speak clearly, slowly, and directly. Maintain face-to-face contact whenever possible.
   Promotes understanding and independence.

4. Provide for resident's privacy with curtain, screen, or door.
   Maintains resident's right to privacy and dignity.

5. Adjust bed to a safe level, usually waist high. Lock bed wheels.
   Prevents injury to you and to resident.

6. Lower the head of the bed to make it flat.
   When bed is flat, resident can be moved without working against gravity.

7. Move the resident to the side of the bed near you, using previous procedure.
   Positions resident for turn.

8. Raise the far side rail (if used).

Turning a resident away from you:

a. Cross the resident's arms over his chest. Cross the near leg over the far leg.

b. Stand with feet shoulder-width apart. Bend your knees.
   Reduces your risk of injury. Promotes proper body mechanics.

c. Place one hand on the resident's shoulder. Place the other hand on the near hip.

d. While supporting the body, gently roll the resident onto his side as one unit, toward the raised side rail.

Turning a resident toward you:

a. Cross the resident's far arm over his chest. Move the arm on the side the resident is being turned to out of the way. Cross the far leg over the near leg.

b. Stand with feet shoulder-width apart. Bend your knees.
   Reduces your risk of injury. Promotes proper body mechanics.

c. Place one hand on the resident's far shoulder. Place the other hand on the far hip.

d. While supporting the body, gently roll the resident onto his side as one unit, toward you. Use your body to block the resident to prevent him from rolling out of bed.

9. Position the resident properly:
   - Head supported by a pillow (resident's face should not be obstructed by the pillow)
   - Shoulder adjusted so the resident is not lying on his arm or hand
   - Top arm supported by pillow
   - Back supported by supportive device
   - Top knee flexed
   - Supportive device between legs with top knee flexed; knee and ankle supported
   - Pillow under bottom foot so that toes and ankle are not touching the bed

10. Return bed to lowest position. Leave side rails in ordered position. Remove privacy measures.
    Lowering the bed provides for resident's safety.

11. Place call light within resident's reach.
    Allows resident to communicate with staff as necessary.

12. Wash your hands.
    Provides for infection prevention.

13. Report any changes in resident to the nurse.
    Provides nurse with information to assess resident.

14. Document procedure using facility guidelines.
    If you do not document the care, legally it did not happen.

Some residents' spinal columns must be kept in alignment. To turn these residents in bed, they have to be logrolled. **Logrolling** means moving a resident as a unit, without disturbing the alignment of the body. The head, back, and legs must be kept in a straight line. This is necessary in cases of neck or back problems, spinal cord injuries, or after back or hip surgeries. It is safer for two people to perform this procedure together. A draw sheet helps with moving.

Logrolling a resident

Equipment: draw sheet or other device, coworker

1. Identify yourself by name. Identify the resident by name.
   Resident has right to know identity of his or her caregiver. Addressing resident by name shows respect and establishes correct identification.
2. Wash your hands.
   Provides for infection prevention.
3. Explain procedure to resident. Speak clearly, slowly, and directly. Maintain face-to-face contact whenever possible.
   Promotes understanding and independence.
4. Provide for resident's privacy with curtain, screen, or door.
   Maintains resident's right to privacy and dignity.
5. Adjust bed to a safe level, usually waist high. Lock bed wheels.
   Prevents injury to you and to resident.
6. Lower the head of the bed to make it flat.
   When bed is flat, resident can be moved without working against gravity.
7. Both of you stand on the same side of the bed. One person stands at the resident's head and shoulders. The other stands near the resident's midsection.
8. Place a pillow under the resident's head to support the neck during the move.
9. Place the resident's arms across his chest. Place a pillow between the knees.
10. Stand with feet shoulder-width apart. Bend your knees.
    Reduces your risk of injury. Promotes good body mechanics.
11. Grasp the draw sheet on the far side (Fig. 6-51).

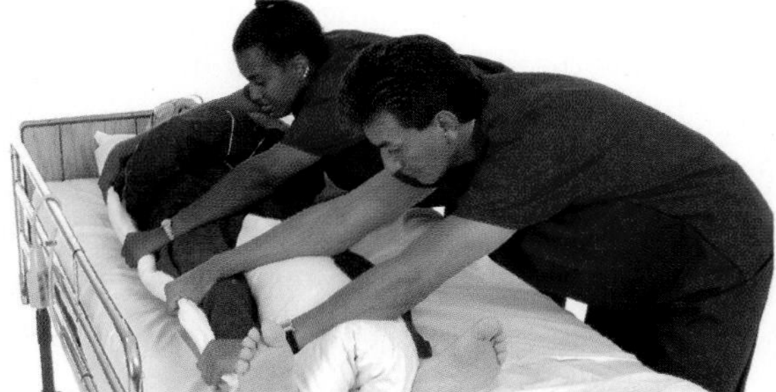

***Fig. 6-51.** Both of you grasp the draw sheet on the far side.*

12. On the count of three, gently roll the resident toward you. Turn the resident as a unit (Fig. 6-52). Use your bodies to block the resident to prevent him from rolling out of bed.
    Work together for your safety and the resident's.

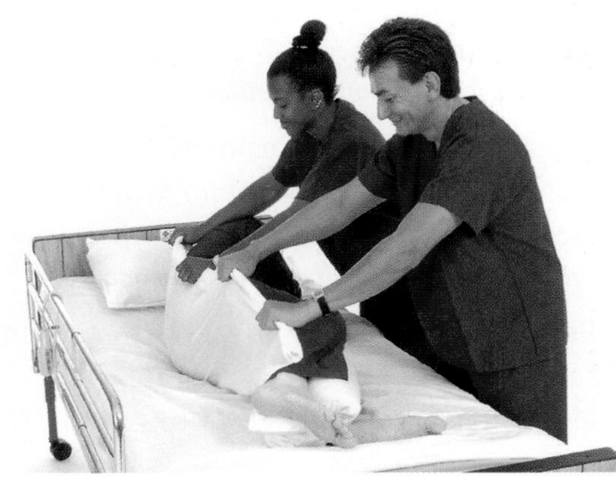

***Fig. 6-52.** On the count of three, both workers should roll the resident toward them, turning him as a unit.*

13. Reposition resident comfortably.
    Maintains alignment.
14. Return bed to lowest position.
    Lowering the bed provides for resident's safety.
15. Place call light within resident's reach.
    Allows resident to communicate with staff as necessary.
16. Wash your hands.
    Provides for infection prevention.
17. Report any changes in resident to the nurse.
    Provides nurse with information to assess resident.
18. Document procedure using facility guidelines.
    If you do not document the care, legally it did not happen.

Before a resident who has been lying down stands up, he should dangle. To **dangle** means to sit up on the side of the bed with the legs hanging over the side. This helps residents regain balance. It allows blood pressure to stabilize. It helps prevent dizziness and lightheadedness that can cause fainting.

Assisting resident to sit up on side of bed: dangling

1. Identify yourself by name. Identify the resident by name.
   Resident has right to know identity of his or her caregiver. Addressing resident by name shows respect and establishes correct identification.
2. Wash your hands.
   Provides for infection prevention.
3. Explain procedure to resident. Speak clearly, slowly, and directly. Maintain face-to-face contact whenever possible.
   Promotes understanding and independence.
4. Provide for resident's privacy with curtain, screen, or door.
   Maintains resident's right to privacy and dignity.
5. Adjust bed to lowest position. Lock bed wheels.
   Allows resident's feet to touch floor when sitting. Reduces chance of injury if resident falls.
6. Raise the head of the bed to a sitting position.
   Resident can move without working against gravity.
7. Stand with feet shoulder-width apart. Bend your knees.
   Reduces your risk of injury. Promotes proper body mechanics.
8. Place one arm under the resident's shoulder blades. Place the other arm under the resident's thighs (Fig. 6-53).
   Placing your arm under the resident's neck may cause injury.

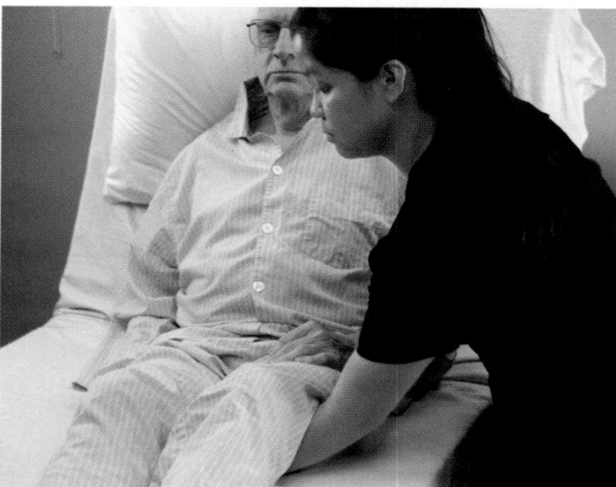

Fig. 6-53. *One arm should be under the resident's shoulder blades and the other arm should be under the thighs.*

9. On the count of three, slowly move the resident into sitting position with the legs dangling over the side of the bed (Fig. 6-54).
   Communicating helps resident help you.

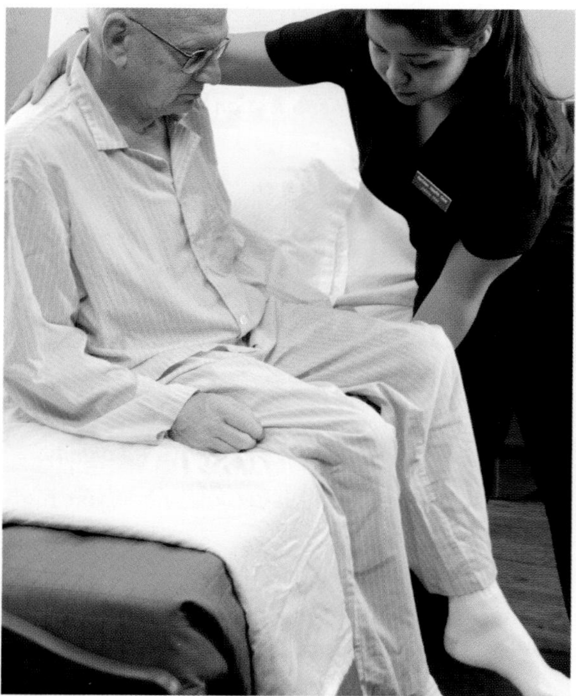

Fig. 6-54. *The weight of the resident's legs hanging down from the bed helps the resident sit up.*

10. Ask resident to sit up straight and hold onto the edge of the mattress with both hands. Help resident to put on nonskid shoes.
    Prevents sliding on floor and protects resident's feet from contamination.
11. Have resident dangle as long as ordered. The care plan may direct you to allow the resident to dangle for several minutes and then return him to lying down, or it may direct you to allow the resident to dangle in preparation for walking or a transfer. Follow the care plan. Do not leave the resident alone. If the resident is dizzy for more than a minute, have him lie down again and report to the nurse. Count his pulse and respiration rates and report to the nurse (you will learn how to measure vital signs in Chapter 7).
    Change of position may cause dizziness due to a drop in blood pressure.
12. Remove the resident's shoes.

13. Gently assist the resident back into bed. Place one arm around his shoulders. Place the other arm under his knees. Slowly swing the resident's legs onto the bed.
14. Leave bed in lowest position. Remove privacy measures.
Lowering the bed provides for resident's safety.
15. Place call light within resident's reach.
Allows resident to communicate with staff as necessary.
16. Wash your hands.
Provides for infection prevention.
17. Report any changes in resident to the nurse.
Provides nurse with information to assess resident.
18. Document procedure using facility guidelines.
If you do not document the care, legally it did not happen.

Transferring a resident means that an NA is moving him from one place to another. Transfers can move residents from a bed to a chair or wheelchair, from a wheelchair to a shower or toilet, and so on.

Safety is one of the most important things to consider during transfers. The Occupational Safety and Health Administration (OSHA, osha.gov) sets specific ergonomic guidelines to help avoid injuries during transfers. **Ergonomics** is the science of designing equipment, areas, and work tasks to make them safer and to suit the worker's abilities. OSHA states that manual lifting and transferring of residents should be reduced and eliminated when possible. Manual lifting, transferring, and repositioning of residents may increase risks of injury.

To reduce injuries, many facilities have adopted *no-lift, zero-lift,* or *lift-free* policies. These policies set strict guidelines for lifting and transferring of residents. Lift-free policies vary. Some facilities do not allow lifting at all and require that equipment always be used when lifting and moving residents. The more restrictions placed on lifting, the less chance there is of injury. NAs must follow facility policies on lifting and use equipment properly. They should ask for help and always get help when they need it.

A **transfer belt** is a safety device used to transfer residents who are weak, unsteady, or uncoordinated. It is called a **gait belt** when it is used to help residents walk. The belt is made of canvas or other heavy material. It has a buckle and sometimes has handles. It fits around the resident's waist, outside the clothing. It should never be placed on bare skin. The belt gives the NA something firm to hold on to when helping with transfers. The NA should grasp the belt securely on both sides, with hands in an upward position. Transfer belts cannot be used if a resident has fragile bones, fractures, or has had certain kinds of surgery recently.

A slide or transfer board may be used to help transfer residents who are unable to bear weight on their legs. Slide boards can be used for almost any transfer that involves moving from one sitting position to another (Fig. 6-55). Slide boards should not be used against bare skin.

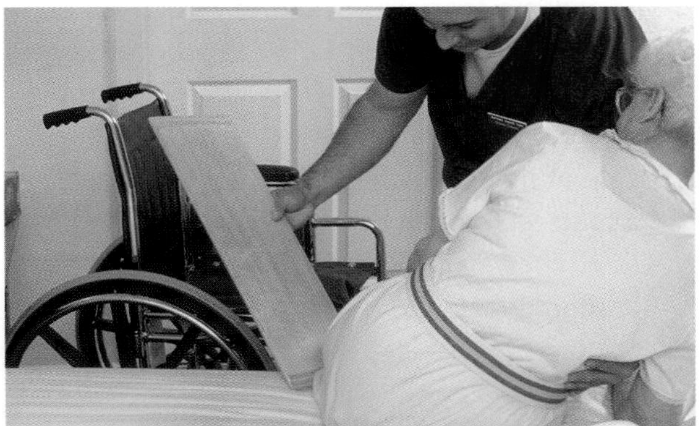

Fig. 6-55. *A slide board can help with bed-to-chair transfers. Before beginning the transfer, the NA should make sure that the resident's fingers are not under the board.*

Guidelines: Wheelchairs

G Learn how each wheelchair works. Residents may use manual (require human power to move) or electric wheelchairs. Know how to apply and release the brake and how to work the armrests and footrests. Always lock a wheelchair before helping a resident into or out of it (Fig. 6-56). After a transfer, unlock the wheelchair.

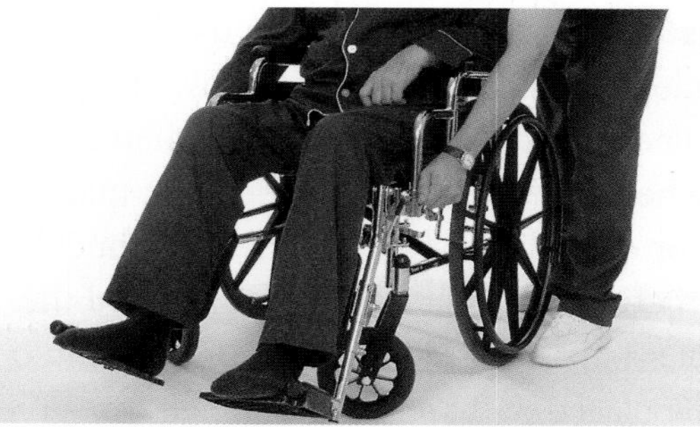

Fig. 6-56. *Always lock the wheelchair before a resident gets into or out of it.*

- G To unfold a standard wheelchair, tilt the chair slightly to raise the wheels on the opposite side. Press down on one or both seat rails until the chair opens and the seat is flat. To fold a standard wheelchair, lift up under the center edge of the seat.
- G To remove an armrest, release the arm lock by the armrest, and lift the arm from the center. To replace the armrest, simply reverse the procedure.
- G To move a footrest out of the way, press or pull the release lever. Swing the footrest out toward the side of the wheelchair. To remove the footrest, lift it off when it is toward the side of the wheelchair (Fig. 6-57). To replace a footrest, simply put it back in the side position. Then swing it back to the front position. It should lock into place.

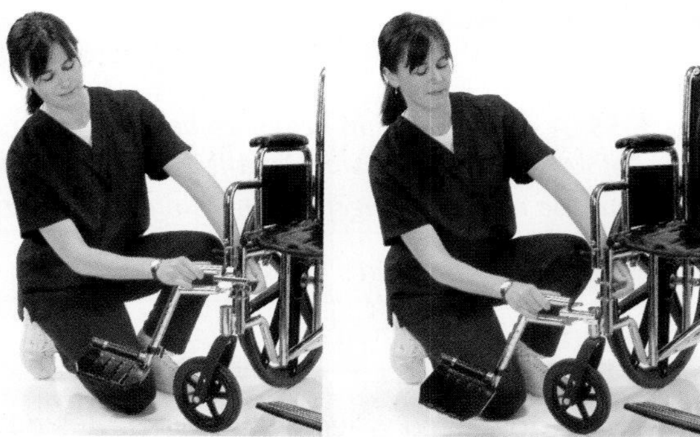

Fig. 6-57. *To remove a footrest, swing the footrest toward the side of the wheelchair and lift it off.*

- G To lift or lower a footrest, support the leg or foot. Squeeze the lever and pull up or push down.
- G To transfer to or from a wheelchair, the resident must use the side of the body that can bear weight to support and lift the side that cannot bear weight. Residents who can bear no weight with their legs may use leg braces or overhead trapezes to support themselves.
- G Before any transfer, make sure the resident is wearing nonskid footwear that is securely fastened. This promotes residents' safety and reduces the risk of falls.
- G During wheelchair transfers, make sure the resident is safe and comfortable. Ask the resident how you can help. Some may only want you to bring the chair to the bedside. Others may want you to be more involved. Be sure the chair is as close as possible to the resident and is locked in place. Use a transfer belt if you are going to help with the transfer. Be sure the transfer is done slowly, allowing time for the resident to rest. Upon standing, check to see if the resident is dizzy. If he is, help him sit back down. Check vital signs as ordered and report to the nurse.
- G Keep the resident's body in proper alignment while in a wheelchair or chair. Special cushions and pillows can be used for support. The hips should be well positioned back in the chair.
- G When a resident is in a wheelchair or any chair, he or she should be repositioned at least every hour. The reasons for doing this are as follows:
    - It promotes comfort.
    - It reduces pressure.
    - It increases circulation.
    - It exercises the joints.
    - It improves muscle tone.

Falls

If a resident starts to fall during a transfer, the NA should do the following:

- Widen his stance.
- Bring the resident's body close to him to break the fall.

- Bend his knees and support the resident as he lowers the resident to the floor (Fig. 6-58). If needed, the NA can drop to the floor with the resident to avoid injury to himself or the resident.

The NA should not try to reverse or stop a fall. The NA or the resident can suffer worse injuries if he tries to stop, rather than break, a fall. If a resident has fallen, the NA should call for help. He should not try to get the resident up after the fall.

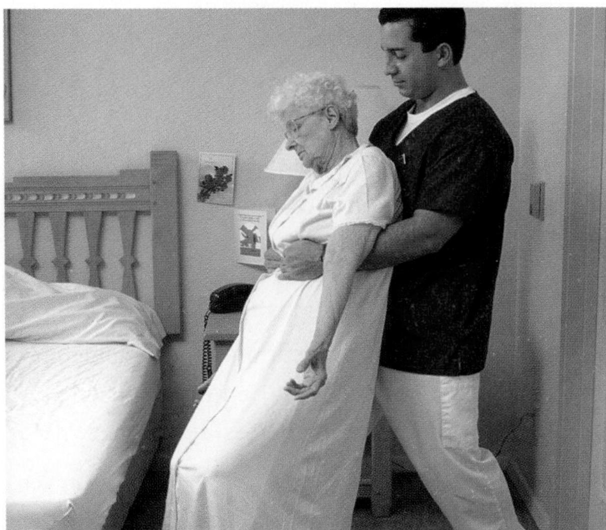

Fig. 6-58. *A nursing assistant should not try to reverse or stop a fall. Instead, he should bend his knees and support the resident as he lowers her to the floor.*

This procedure may need to be done with two workers, depending on the resident's abilities. The NA should follow the care plan.

Transferring a resident from bed to wheelchair

Equipment: wheelchair, transfer belt, nonskid footwear, and robe or folded blanket

1. Identify yourself by name. Identify the resident by name.
   Resident has right to know identity of his or her caregiver. Addressing resident by name shows respect and establishes correct identification.
2. Wash your hands.
   Provides for infection prevention.
3. Explain procedure to resident. Speak clearly, slowly, and directly. Maintain face-to-face contact whenever possible.
   Promotes understanding and independence.
4. Provide for resident's privacy with curtain, screen, or door. Check the area to be certain it is uncluttered and safe.
   Maintains resident's right to privacy and dignity. Keeping area free from clutter promotes safety.
5. Place the wheelchair at the head of the bed, facing the foot of the bed, or at the foot of the bed, facing the head of the bed. The arm of the wheelchair should be almost touching the bed. It should be placed on the resident's stronger, or unaffected, side.
   Unaffected side supports weight.
6. Remove both wheelchair footrests close to the bed.
7. Lock wheelchair wheels.
   Wheel locks prevent chair from moving.
8. Raise the head of the bed. Adjust bed to its lowest position. Lock bed wheels.
   Prevents injury to you and to resident.
9. Assist the resident into a sitting position. Make sure his feet are flat on the floor. Adjust the bed height if needed. Let resident sit for a few minutes to adjust to the change in position.
   Prevents injury and promotes stability.
10. Put nonskid footwear on the resident and fasten securely.
    Promotes resident's safety. Reduces risk of falls.
11. Stand in front of and face the resident. Place your feet about shoulder-width apart.
    Reduces your risk of injury. Promotes proper body mechanics.
12. Place the transfer belt around the resident's waist over his clothing (not on bare skin). Tighten the buckle until it is snug. Leave enough room to insert flat fingers/hand comfortably under the belt. Check to make sure that skin or skin folds (for example, breasts) are not caught under the belt. Grasp the belt securely on both sides, with hands in an upward position.

13. Provide instructions to allow the resident to help with the transfer. Instructions may include: "When you start to stand, push with your hands against the bed." "Once standing, if you're able, you can take small steps in the direction of the chair." "Once standing, reach for the chair with your stronger hand."

14. With your legs, brace (support) the resident's lower legs to prevent slipping (Fig. 6-59). This can be done by placing one or both of your knees against the resident's knees. Or you can stand toe to toe with the resident. Bend your knees. Keep your back straight.

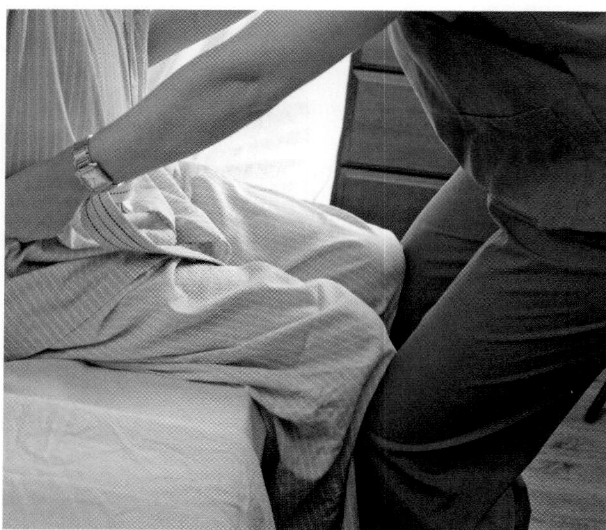

Fig. 6-59. *Brace the resident's lower legs to prevent slipping by placing either one or two knees (shown) against the resident's knees.*

15. Count to three to alert the resident. If possible, have the resident rock while counting to three. On three, with hands still grasping the transfer belt on both sides and moving upward, slowly help the resident to stand.
Communicating helps resident help you.

16. Tell the resident to take small steps in the direction of the chair while turning his back toward it. If more help is needed, help the resident pivot (turn) to stand in front of the wheelchair with back of the resident's legs against the wheelchair (Fig. 6-60).
Pivoting is safer than twisting.

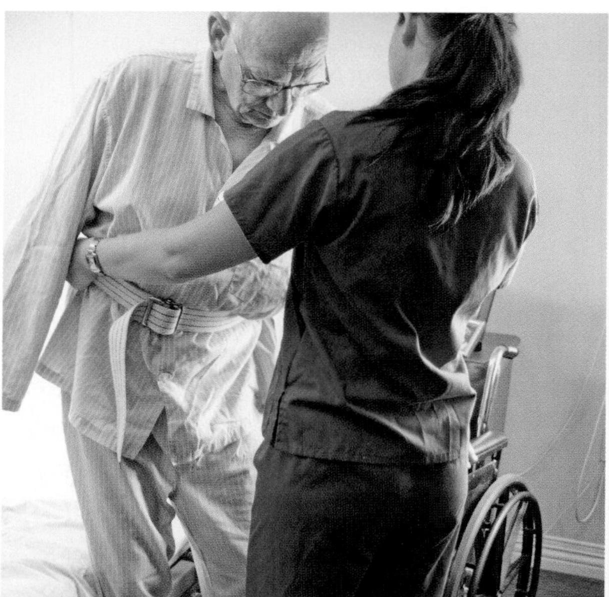

Fig. 6-60. *Help him pivot to the front of the wheelchair.*

17. Ask the resident to put hands on wheelchair armrests if he is able. When the chair is touching the back of the resident's legs, help him lower himself into the chair.

18. Reposition the resident so that his hips touch the back of the wheelchair seat.
Using full seat of chair is safest.

19. Attach footrests. Place the resident's feet on the footrests. Check that the resident is in proper alignment. Gently remove the transfer belt. Place a robe or folded blanket over the resident's lap as appropriate.
Protects feet and ankles.

20. Remove privacy measures.

21. Place call light within resident's reach.
Allows resident to communicate with staff as necessary.

22. Wash your hands.
Provides for infection prevention.

23. Report any changes in resident to the nurse.
Provides nurse with information to assess resident.

24. Document procedure using facility guidelines.
If you do not document the care, legally it did not happen.

Mechanical Lifts

Facilities often have mechanical (also called *hydraulic, power,* or *standing*) lifts available to transfer residents. This equipment helps prevent injury to residents and staff members. NAs may assist residents with many types of transfers using a mechanical lift. Using these lifts requires special training. NAs should not use equipment they have not been trained to use, as this could cause injury. There are many different types of mechanical lifts (Fig. 6-61). NAs should always ask for help if there is anything they do not understand about lift equipment.

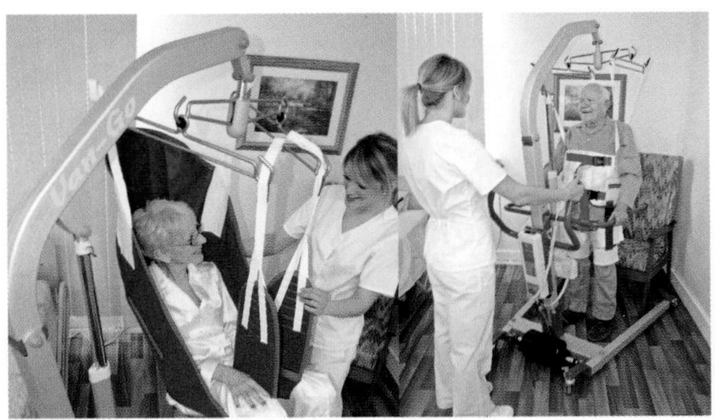

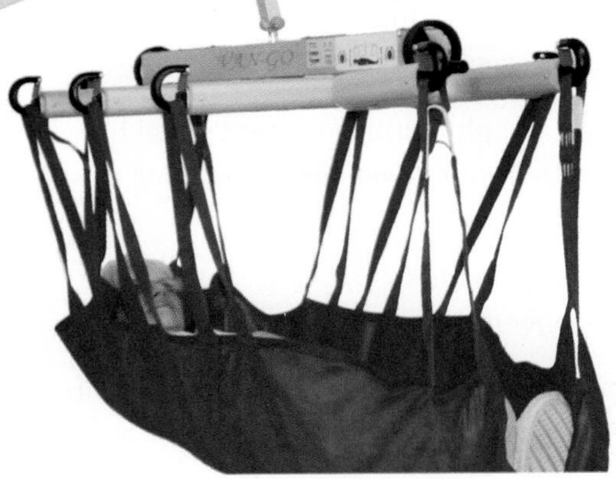

Fig. 6-61. *There are different types of lifts for transferring completely dependent residents and residents who can bear some weight.* (PHOTOS COURTESY OF VANCARE INC., 800-694-4525)

Guidelines: Mechanical or Hydraulic Lifts

- **G** Be careful when moving a resident using a mechanical lift. Have another person help you when using these lifts. It is safer for at least two people to do these types of transfers.
- **G** Keep the chair to which the resident is to be moved close to the bed so that the resident is only moved a short distance in the lift. Lock the wheels on the chair if it has wheels.
- **G** Check that the valves on the lift are working before using it.
- **G** Use the correct sling for the lift that is being used. Using an incorrect sling may result in serious injury or death. If you have questions about the sling, talk to the nurse.
- **G** Check the sling and straps for any fraying or tears. Do not use the lift if there are tears or holes.
- **G** Open the legs of the stand to the widest position before helping the resident into the lift.
- **G** Once the resident is in the sling and the straps are connected, pump up the lift only to the point where the resident's body clears the bed or chair.
- **G** Electric/battery-powered lifts have emergency releases. Be aware of where the release is located and how to operate this function. Talk to the nurse if you do not know how to do this.

Transferring a resident using a mechanical lift

Equipment: wheelchair or chair, coworker, mechanical or hydraulic lift

This is a basic procedure for transferring using a mechanical lift. Ask someone to help you before starting.

1. Identify yourself by name. Identify the resident by name.
   Resident has right to know identity of his or her caregiver. Addressing resident by name shows respect and establishes correct identification.
2. Wash your hands.
   Provides for infection prevention.
3. Explain procedure to resident. Speak clearly, slowly, and directly. Maintain face-to-face contact whenever possible.
   Promotes understanding and independence.

4. Provide for resident's privacy with curtain, screen, or door.
   Maintains resident's right to privacy and dignity.

5. Lock bed wheels.
   Wheel locks prevent bed from moving.

6. Position wheelchair next to bed. Lock brakes.
   Wheel locks prevent chair from moving.

7. Help the resident turn toward you, as described in previous procedure. Go to the far side of the bed. Position the sling under the resident, with the edge next to the resident's back. Fanfold if necessary. Make the bottom of the sling even with the resident's knees. Help the resident roll back to the middle of the bed. Spread out the fanfolded edge of the sling.

8. Roll the mechanical lift to bedside. Make sure the base is opened to its widest point. Push the base of the lift under the bed.

9. Place the overhead bar directly over the resident.

10. With the resident lying on his back, attach one set of straps to each side of the sling. Attach one set of straps to the overhead bar. Have coworker support the resident's head, shoulders, and knees while being lifted. The resident's arms should be folded across his chest (Fig. 6-62). If the device has S hooks, they should face away from the resident. Make sure all straps are connected properly and are smooth and straight.

11. Following manufacturer's instructions, raise the resident two inches above the bed. Pause a moment for the resident to gain balance.

12. Have coworker help support and guide the resident's body. You can then roll the lift so that the resident is positioned over the chair or wheelchair.
    Having another person help promotes safety during the transfer and lessens chance of injury.

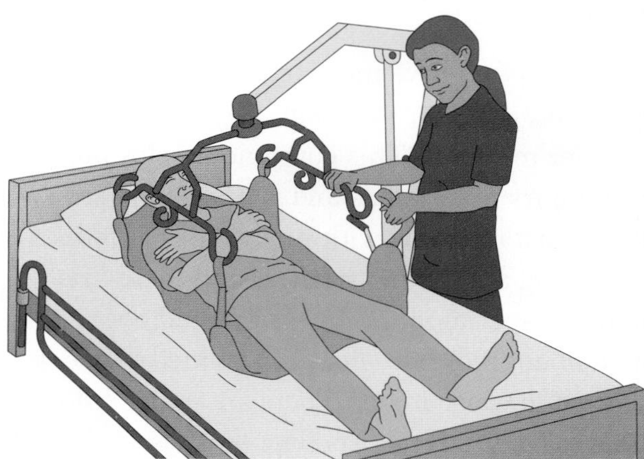

Fig. 6-62. *With the resident's arms folded across his chest, attach the straps to the sling.*

13. Slowly lower the resident into the chair or wheelchair. Push down gently on the resident's knees to help him into a sitting, rather than reclining, position.

14. Undo the straps from the overhead bar to the sling. Remove the sling or leave in place; follow facility policy.

15. Be sure the resident is seated comfortably and correctly in the chair or wheelchair. Remove privacy measures.

16. Place call light within resident's reach.
    Allows resident to communicate with staff as necessary.

17. Wash your hands.
    Provides for infection prevention.

18. Report any changes in resident to the nurse.
    Provides nurse with information to assess resident.

19. Document procedure using facility guidelines.
    If you do not document the care, legally it did not happen.

7 Basic Nursing Skills

1. Explain admission, transfer, and discharge of a resident

Moving always requires an adjustment, but as a person ages, it can be even harder. This is especially true if illness, disability, and mobility problems are present. Nursing assistants play an important role in helping residents make a successful transition to long-term care facilities. By giving emotional support such as listening and being kind, compassionate, and helpful, NAs can help residents feel better about their new homes.

Residents' Rights

New LGBTQ Residents

Entering a long-term care facility can be especially difficult for residents who are lesbian, gay, bisexual, transgender, or queer (LGBTQ). These residents may fear that they will not be accepted by staff or other residents. They may worry that their partner will not receive the same welcome the spouse or partner of a heterosexual resident would receive. NAs must not judge residents. Every resident deserves professional, caring service from facility staff. The facility is the resident's home. All staff members should make every effort to make all residents feel comfortable and welcome.

Admission is often the first time an NA meets a new resident. This is a time of first impressions. The NA should try to make sure the resident has a positive impression of him and his facility. Because change is difficult, staff must communicate with new residents. NAs can explain what to expect during the process. They can answer any questions that are within their scope of practice. If residents or their families have questions that an NA cannot answer, he should find the nurse. It is a good idea for the NA to ask a new resident questions to find out their personal preferences and routines. NAs can also ask residents' families about personal preferences if residents are not able to respond.

Guidelines: Admission

- G Prepare the room before the resident arrives. This helps her to feel expected and welcome. Make sure the bed is made and the room is tidy. Restock supplies that are low. Make sure there is an admission kit available if used. Admission kits often contain personal care items, such as a bath basin, an emesis basin, a water pitcher and drinking glass, toothpaste, soap, a comb, lotion, and tissues (Fig. 7-1). The kit may also contain a urine specimen cup, label, and transport bag.
- G When a new resident arrives at the facility, note the time and her condition. Is she using a wheelchair, on a stretcher, or walking? Who is with her? Observe the new resident for level of consciousness and signs of confusion. Look for signs of nervousness. Note any tubes she has, such as IVs or catheters.
- G Introduce yourself. State your position. Smile and be friendly. Always call the person by her formal name until she tells you what she wants to be called.

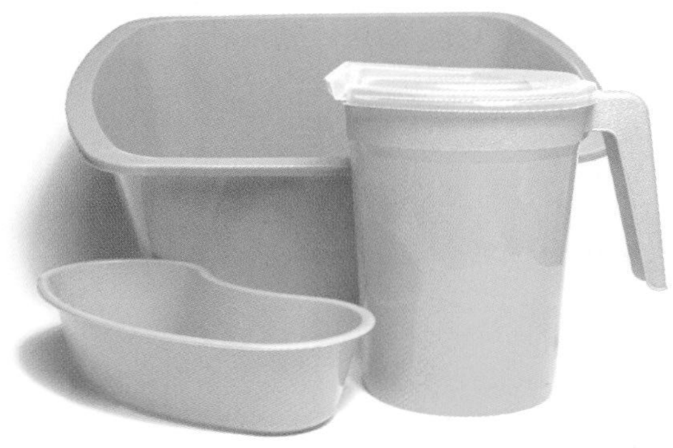

Fig. 7-1. An admission kit is usually placed in a resident's room before he or she is admitted. It may contain personal care items that the resident will need.

G Never rush the process or the new resident. She should not feel like she is an inconvenience. Make sure that the new resident feels welcome and wanted.

G Explain day-to-day life in the facility. Offer to take the resident and her family on a tour. Show the resident important areas. When showing the resident where the dining room is, review the posted dining schedules. During the tour, introduce the resident to other residents and staff members you see. Introduce the roommate if there is one.

G Handle personal items with care and respect. A resident has a legal right to have her personal items treated carefully. When setting up the room, place personal items where the resident wants them (Fig. 7-2).

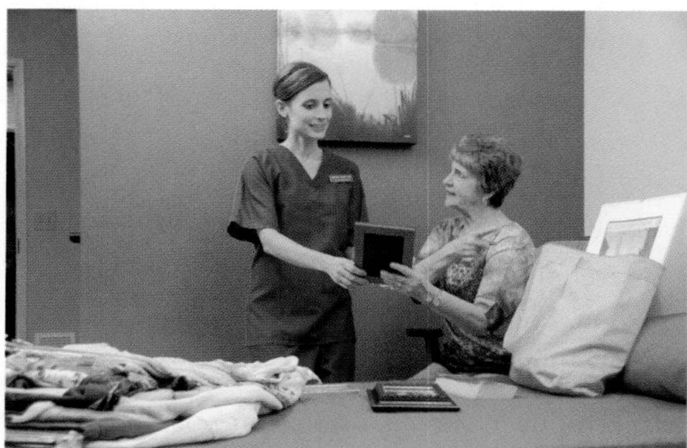

Fig. 7-2. Handle personal items carefully, and set up the room as the resident prefers.

G Admission is a stressful time. Observe the resident, as there could be something important that was missed. Report to the nurse if you notice any of the following:

- Disconnected tubing
- Resident seems confused, combative, and/or unaware of surroundings
- Resident is having difficulty breathing, pain, or any other signs of distress
- Resident has bruises or wounds
- Resident has missed a meal during the admission process
- Resident has valuables, medications, hearing aids, eyeglasses, or dentures

G Follow facility policy on any other tasks that are required during admission.

G New residents may have good days followed by difficult days. Let residents adapt to their new homes at their own pace. However, report signs of confusion or depression to the nurse.

Residents' Rights

Admission

OBRA requires that on admission, residents must be told of their legal rights. They must be provided with a written copy of these rights. This includes rights about their funds and the right to file a complaint with the state survey agency. Residents must also be provided with information about their rights related to advance directives.

Admitting a resident

Equipment: may include admission paperwork (checklist and inventory form), gloves, vital signs equipment

1. Identify yourself by name. Identify the resident by name.
   Resident has right to know identity of his or her caregiver. Addressing resident by name shows respect and establishes correct identification.
2. Wash your hands.
   Provides for infection prevention.

3. Explain procedure to resident. Speak clearly, slowly, and directly. Maintain face-to-face contact whenever possible.
   Promotes understanding and independence.

4. Provide for resident's privacy with curtain, screen, or door (Fig. 7-3). If the family is present, ask them to step outside until the admission process is over. Show them where they can wait. Let them know approximately how long the process will take.
   Maintains resident's right to privacy and dignity.

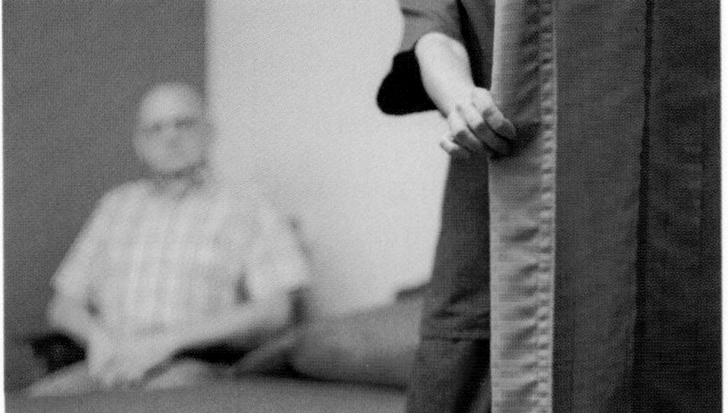

***Fig. 7-3.** All residents have a legal right to privacy, and providing privacy is part of doing your job professionally. Your professional, respectful behavior can help put a new resident at ease.*

5. If part of facility procedure, do these things:
   - Measure the resident's height and weight.
   - Measure the resident's baseline vital signs. Baseline signs are initial values that can then be compared to future measurements.
   - Obtain a urine specimen if required.
   - Complete the paperwork. Take an inventory of all the personal items.
   - Help the resident put personal items away. Label personal items according to facility policy.
   - Provide fresh water.

6. Show the resident the room and bathroom. Explain how to work the bed controls and the call light. Show the resident the telephone, lights, and television controls.
   Promotes resident's safety.

7. Introduce the resident to his roommate if there is one. Introduce other residents and staff.
   Makes resident feel more comfortable.

8. Make sure resident is comfortable. Remove privacy measures. Bring the family back inside if they were outside.

9. Place call light within resident's reach.
   Allows resident to communicate with staff as necessary.

10. Wash your hands.
    Provides for infection prevention.

11. Document procedure using facility guidelines.
    If you do not document the care, legally it did not happen.

Residents may be transferred to a different area of the facility. In cases of acute illness, they may be transferred to a hospital. Change is difficult. This is especially true when a person has an illness or her condition gets worse. Staff should make the transfer as smooth as possible for the resident. A resident should be informed of the transfer as soon as possible so that she can begin to adjust to the idea. The nurse will tell the resident about the transfer and should explain how, where, when, and why the transfer will occur. Any questions the resident has should be answered.

NAs help residents pack their personal items before transferring. Residents often worry about losing their belongings. NAs can involve them in the packing process. For example, the NA can let the resident see the empty closet, drawer, etc.

Transferring a resident

Equipment: may include a wheelchair, cart for belongings, the medical record, all of the resident's personal care items and packed personal items

1. Identify yourself by name. Identify the resident by name.
   Resident has right to know identity of his or her caregiver. Addressing resident by name shows respect and establishes correct identification.
2. Wash your hands.
   Provides for infection prevention.
3. Explain procedure to resident. Speak clearly, slowly, and directly. Maintain face-to-face contact whenever possible.
   Promotes understanding and independence.
4. Collect items to be moved onto the cart. Take them to the new location. If the resident is going into the hospital, they may be placed in temporary storage.
5. Help the resident into the wheelchair (or onto a stretcher if one is used). Take him or her to proper area.
6. Introduce new residents and staff.
   Makes resident feel more comfortable.
7. Help the resident to put personal items away.
8. Make sure that the resident is comfortable.
9. Place call light within resident's reach.
   Allows resident to communicate with staff as necessary.
10. Wash your hands.
    Provides for infection prevention.
11. Report any changes in resident to the nurse.
    Provides nurse with information to assess resident.
12. Document procedure using facility guidelines.
    If you do not document the care, legally it did not happen.

To discharge a resident from a facility, a doctor must give the discharge order. The nurse then completes instructions for the resident to follow after discharge. The nurse will review these instructions and information with the resident and her family and friends. Some of these areas may be discussed:

- Future doctor or physical, speech, and occupational therapy appointments
- Home care, skilled nursing care
- Medications
- Ambulation instructions
- Medical equipment needed
- Medical transportation
- Any restrictions on activities
- Special exercises to keep the resident functioning at the highest level
- Special nutrition or dietary requirements
- Community resources

NAs help by collecting the resident's belongings and packing them carefully. The NA should know what the resident's condition is at the time of discharge and find out if the resident will be using a wheelchair or stretcher.

The day of discharge is often a happy day for residents who are going home. However, some residents may feel uncertainty or fear about leaving the facility. They may be concerned that their health will suffer. NAs can help by being positive. They can remind residents that their doctors believe they are ready to leave. However, if a resident has specific questions about care, the NA should inform the nurse.

Residents' Rights

Transfers or Discharges

OBRA requires that residents have the right to receive advance notice before being transferred or discharged from a facility. The written notice must contain the specifics of where and why they are being transferred or discharged. It must be in a language residents can understand. Staff must provide proper preparation for the transfer or discharge.

Discharging a resident

Equipment: may include a wheelchair, cart for belongings, discharge paperwork (including the inventory list from admission), resident's care items, vital signs equipment

1. Identify yourself by name. Identify the resident by name.
   Resident has right to know identity of his or her caregiver. Addressing resident by name shows respect and establishes correct identification.
2. Wash your hands.
   Provides for infection prevention.
3. Explain procedure to resident. Speak clearly, slowly, and directly. Maintain face-to-face contact whenever possible.
   Promotes understanding and independence.
4. Provide for resident's privacy with curtain, screen, or door.
   Maintains resident's right to privacy and dignity.
5. Measure the resident's vital signs.
6. Compare the checklist to the items there. If all items are there, ask the resident to sign.
7. Put the personal items to be taken onto the cart and take them to the pick-up area.
8. Help the resident dress and then into the wheelchair or onto the stretcher if used.
9. Help the resident to say his goodbyes to the staff and residents.
10. Take resident to the pick-up area. Help him into the vehicle. You are responsible for the resident until he is safely in the vehicle and the door is closed.
11. Wash your hands.
    Provides for infection prevention.
12. Document procedure using facility guidelines. Include the following:
    - The vital signs at discharge
    - Time of discharge
    - Method of transport
    - Who was with the resident
    - What items the resident took with her (inventory checklist)

    If you do not document the care, legally it did not happen.

2. Explain the importance of monitoring vital signs

Nursing assistants monitor, document, and report residents' **vital signs**. Vital signs are important. They show how well the vital organs of the body, such as the heart and lungs, are working. They consist of the following:

- Measuring body temperature
- Counting the pulse rate
- Counting the rate of respirations
- Measuring blood pressure
- Observing and reporting the level of pain

Watching for changes in vital signs is very important. Changes can indicate a resident's condition is worsening. An NA should always notify the nurse if

- The resident has a fever (temperature is above average for the resident or outside the normal range)
- The resident has a respiratory or pulse rate that is too rapid or too slow
- The resident's blood pressure changes
- The resident's pain is worse or is not relieved by pain management

Ranges for Adult Vital Signs

Temp. Site	**Fahrenheit**	**Celsius**
Mouth (oral)	97.6°–99.6°	36.5°–37.5°
Rectum (rectal)	98.6°–100.6°	37.0°–38.1°
Armpit (axilla)	96.6°–98.6°	35.9°–37.0°
Ear (tympanic)	96.6°–99.7°	35.9°–37.6°
Temporal Artery (forehead)	97.2°–100.1°	36.2°–37.8°

Normal Pulse Rate: 60–100 beats per minute
Normal Respiratory Rate: 12–20 respirations per minute

Blood Pressure

Normal	Systolic–less than 120 Diastolic–less than 80
Low	Less than 90/60
High	Systolic of 130 or higher or Diastolic of 80 or higher

Basic Nursing Skills

Temperature

Body temperature is normally very close to 98.6°F (Fahrenheit) or 37°C (Celsius). Body temperature is a balance between the heat created by the body and the heat lost to the environment. Many factors affect body temperature, such as age, illness, stress, environment, exercise, and the circadian rhythm. The circadian rhythm is the 24-hour day-night cycle. Average temperature readings change throughout the day. People tend to have lower temperatures in the morning. Increases in body temperature may indicate an infection or disease.

There are different sites for measuring body temperature: the mouth (oral), the rectum (rectal), the armpit (axilla), the ear (tympanic), and the temporal artery (the artery just under the skin of the forehead). The different sites require different thermometers. Common types of thermometers are as follows:

- Digital (Fig. 7-4)
- Electronic (Fig. 7-5)
- Tympanic (Fig. 7-6)
- Temporal artery (Fig. 7-7)
- Mercury-free (Fig. 7-8)

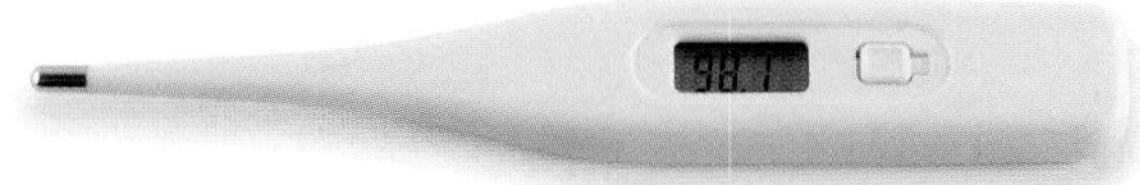

Fig. 7-4. *A digital thermometer.*

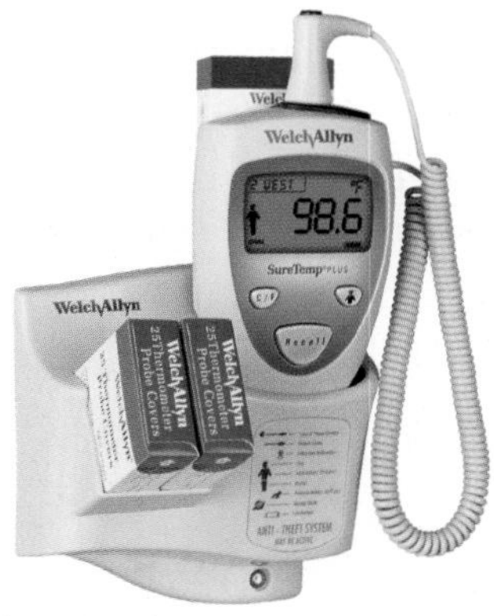

Fig. 7-5. *An electronic thermometer.* (PHOTO COURTESY OF WELCH ALLYN, WWW.WELCHALLYN.COM, 800-535-6663)

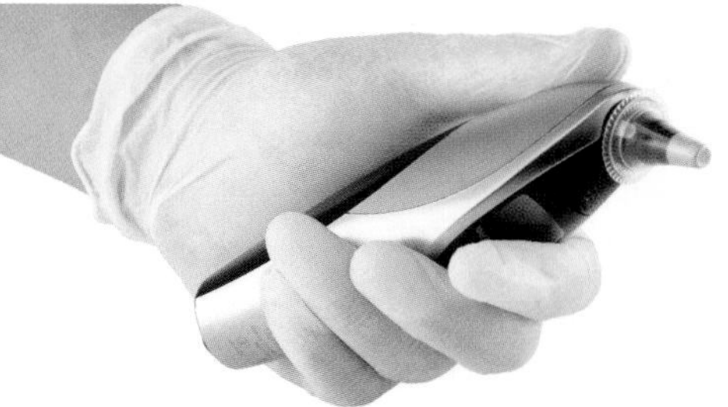

Fig. 7-6. *A tympanic thermometer.*

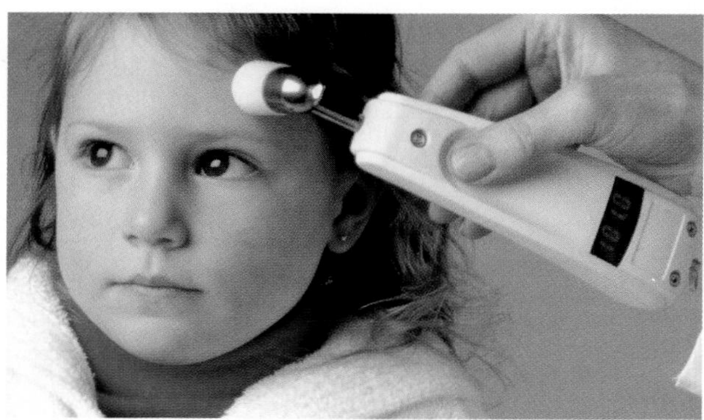

Fig. 7-7. *A temporal artery thermometer.* (PHOTO COURTESY OF EXERGEN CORPORATION, WWW.EXERGEN.COM, 800-422-3006)

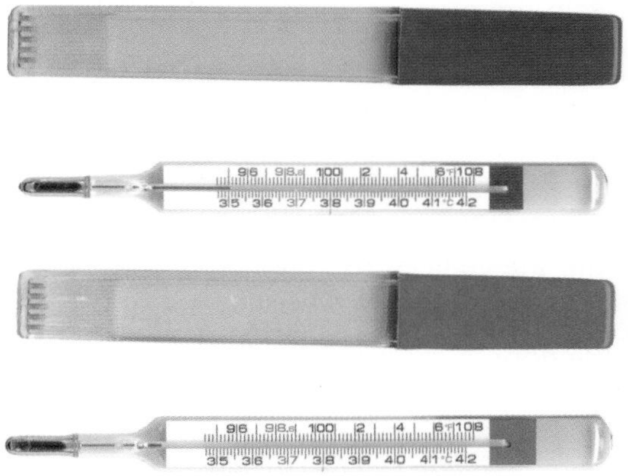

Fig. 7-8. *A mercury-free oral thermometer and a mercury-free rectal thermometer. Oral thermometers are usually green or blue; rectal thermometers are usually red.* (PHOTOS COURTESY OF RG MEDICAL DIAGNOSTICS OF WIXOM, MI, RGMD.COM)

Numbers on the thermometer allow the temperature to be read after it registers. Most thermometers show the temperature in degrees Fahrenheit (F). Each long line represents one degree. Each short line represents two-tenths of a degree. Some thermometers show the temperature in degrees Celsius (C). The long lines represent one degree. The short lines represent one-tenth of a degree. Small arrows or highlighted numbers show the normal temperature: 98.6°F and 37°C (Fig. 7-9).

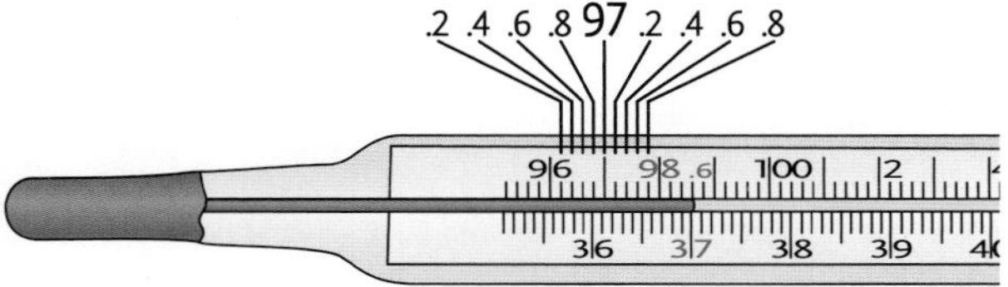

Fig. 7-9. This shows a normal temperature reading: 98.6°F and 37°C.

There is a range of normal temperatures. Some people's temperatures normally run low. Others in good health will run slightly higher. Normal temperature readings also vary by the method used to take the temperature. A rectal temperature is generally considered to be the most accurate. However, measuring a rectal temperature on an uncooperative person, such as a resident with dementia, can be dangerous. An axillary temperature is considered the least accurate.

An NA should not measure an oral temperature on a person who

- Is unconscious
- Has recently had facial or oral surgery
- Is younger than 5 years old
- Is confused or disoriented
- Is heavily sedated
- Is likely to have a seizure
- Is coughing
- Is using oxygen
- Has facial paralysis
- Has a nasogastric tube (a feeding tube that is inserted through the nose and goes into the stomach)
- Has sores, redness, swelling, or pain in the mouth
- Has an injury to the face or neck

Measuring and recording an oral temperature

Equipment: clean digital, electronic, or mercury-free thermometer, gloves, disposable sheath/cover for thermometer, tissues, pen and paper

Do not take an oral temperature if the resident has smoked, eaten or drunk fluids, chewed gum, or exercised in the last 10 to 20 minutes.

1. Identify yourself by name. Identify the resident by name.
   Resident has right to know identity of his or her caregiver. Addressing resident by name shows respect and establishes correct identification.
2. Wash your hands.
   Provides for infection prevention.
3. Explain procedure to resident. Speak clearly, slowly, and directly. Maintain face-to-face contact whenever possible.
   Promotes understanding and independence.
4. Provide for resident's privacy with curtain, screen, or door.
   Maintains resident's right to privacy and dignity.
5. Put on gloves.
6. **Digital thermometer**: Put on the disposable sheath. Turn on the thermometer and wait until the ready sign appears.

   Electronic thermometer: Remove the probe from the base unit. Put on the probe cover.

   Mercury-free thermometer: Hold the thermometer by the stem. Before inserting it in the resident's mouth, shake thermometer down to below the lowest number (at least below 96°F or 35°C). To shake the thermometer down, hold it at the end opposite the bulb with the thumb and two fingers. With a snapping motion of the wrist, shake the thermometer (Fig. 7-10). Stand away from furniture and walls while doing so.
   Holding the stem end prevents contamination of the bulb end. The thermometer reading must be below the resident's actual temperature.

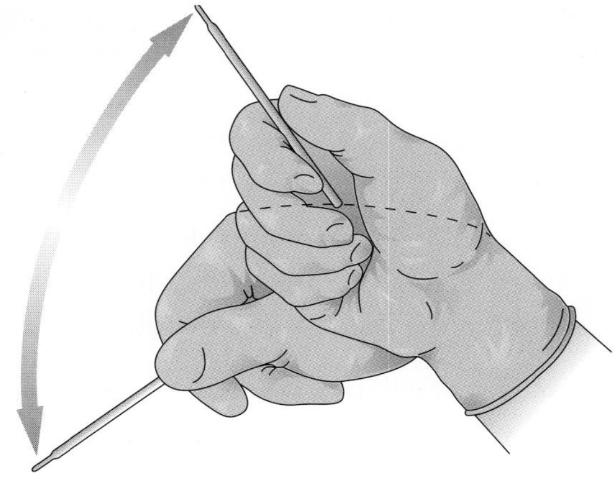

Fig. 7-10. Shake thermometer down to below the lowest number before inserting it into a resident's mouth.

7. **Digital thermometer**: Insert the end of the thermometer into the resident's mouth, under the tongue and to one side.
   The thermometer measures heat from blood vessels under the tongue.

   Electronic thermometer: Insert the end of the thermometer into the resident's mouth, under the tongue and to one side.

   Mercury-free thermometer: Put on disposable sheath if available. Insert bulb end of the thermometer into the resident's mouth, under the tongue and to one side.

8. **For all thermometers:** Tell the resident to hold the thermometer in her mouth with her lips closed (Fig. 7-11). Assist as necessary. The resident should breathe through her nose. Ask the resident not to bite down or talk.
   The lips hold the thermometer in position. If it is broken, injury to the mouth may occur. More time may be required if resident opens mouth to talk.

   Digital thermometer: Leave in place until the thermometer blinks or beeps.

   Electronic thermometer: Leave in place until you hear a tone or see a flashing or steady light.

   Mercury-free thermometer: Leave in place for at least three minutes.

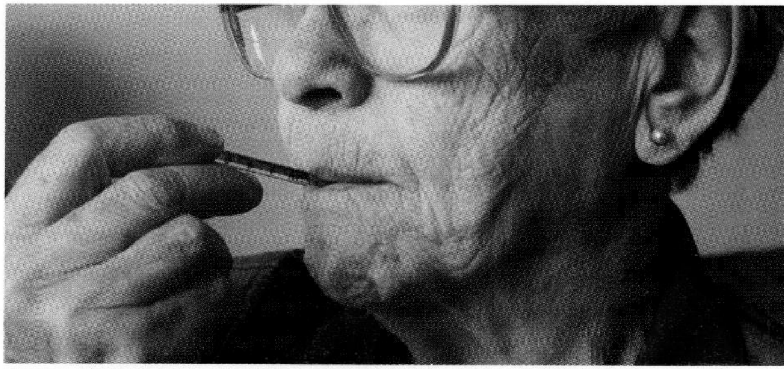

Fig. 7-11. While the thermometer is in the resident's mouth, she should keep her lips closed.

9. **Digital thermometer**: Remove the thermometer. Read the temperature on the display screen. Remember the temperature reading.

   Electronic thermometer: Read the temperature on the display screen. Remember the temperature reading. Remove the probe.

   Mercury-free thermometer: Remove the thermometer. Wipe it with a tissue from stem to bulb or remove the sheath. Discard the tissue or sheath. Hold the thermometer at eye level. Rotate until the line appears, rolling the thermometer between your thumb and forefinger. Read the temperature. Remember the temperature reading.

10. **Digital thermometer**: Using a tissue, remove and discard the sheath. Replace the thermometer in the case.

    Electronic thermometer: Press the eject button to discard the cover. Return the probe to the holder.

    Mercury-free thermometer: Clean thermometer according to facility guidelines. Rinse with clean water and dry. Return it to case.

11. Remove and discard gloves.

12. Wash your hands.
    Provides for infection prevention.

13. Immediately record the temperature, date, time, and method used (oral).
    Record temperature immediately so you won't forget. Care plans are made based on your report.

14. Place call light within resident's reach.
    Allows resident to communicate with staff as necessary.

15. Report any changes in resident to the nurse.
Provides nurse with information to assess resident.

The NA must always explain what she will do before starting to measure a rectal temperature. The NA needs the resident's cooperation. She should ask the resident to hold still and reassure him that the task will only take a few minutes. It is important to hold on to the thermometer at all times while the thermometer is in the rectum.

Measuring and recording a rectal temperature

Equipment: clean rectal digital, electronic, or mercury-free thermometer, lubricant, gloves, tissue, disposable sheath/cover, pen and paper

1. Identify yourself by name. Identify resident by name.
Resident has right to know identity of his or her caregiver. Addressing resident by name shows respect and establishes correct identification.

2. Wash your hands.
Provides for infection prevention.

3. Explain procedure to resident. Speak clearly, slowly, and directly. Maintain face-to-face contact whenever possible.
Promotes understanding and independence.

4. Provide for resident's privacy with curtain, screen, or door.
Maintains resident's right to privacy and dignity.

5. Adjust bed to a safe level, usually waist high. Lock bed wheels.
Promotes safety.

6. Help the resident to the left-lying (Sims') position (Fig. 7-12).

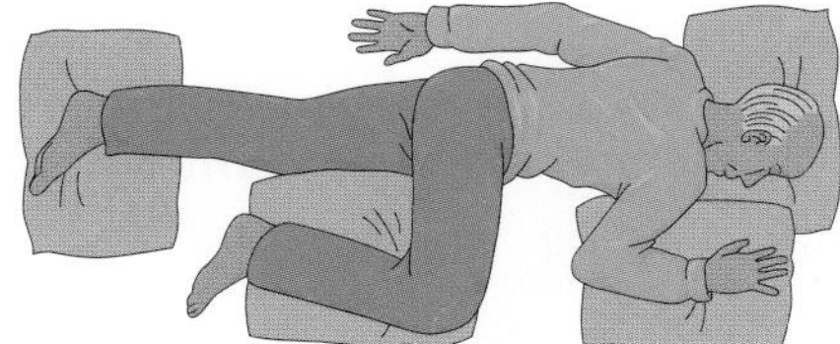

Fig. 7-12. *The resident must be in the left-lying (Sims') position.*

7. Fold back the linens to expose only the rectal area.

8. Put on gloves.

9. **Digital thermometer**: Put on the disposable sheath. Turn on the thermometer and wait until the ready sign appears.

   Electronic thermometer: Remove the probe from the base unit. Put on the probe cover.

   Mercury-free thermometer: Hold the thermometer by the stem. Shake the thermometer down to below the lowest number.

10. Apply a small amount of lubricant to the tip of the bulb or probe cover (or apply pre-lubricated cover).

11. Separate the buttocks. Gently insert the thermometer into the rectum 1/2 to 1 inch. Stop if you meet resistance. Do not force the thermometer into the rectum (Fig. 7-13).

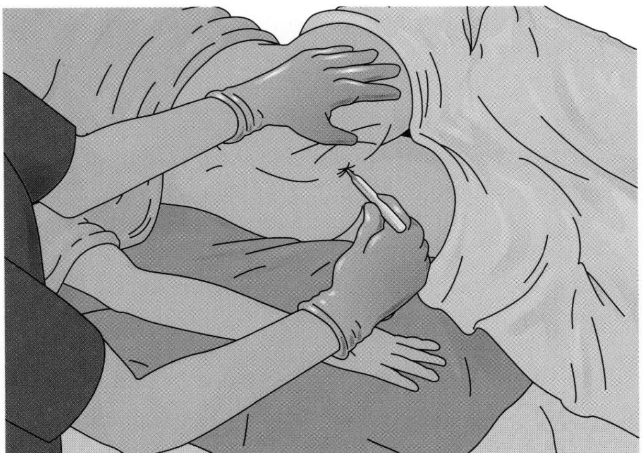

Fig. 7-13. *Gently insert a rectal thermometer one-half to one inch into the rectum.*

12. Replace the sheet over the buttocks. Hold on to the thermometer at all times.

13. **Digital thermometer**: Leave in place until the thermometer blinks or beeps.

   Electronic thermometer: Leave in place until you hear a tone or see a flashing or steady light.

   Mercury-free thermometer: Leave in place for at least three minutes.

14. Gently remove the thermometer. Wipe it with a tissue from stem to bulb or remove the sheath. Discard the tissue or sheath.

15. Read the thermometer at eye level as you would for an oral temperature. Remember the temperature reading.

16. **Digital thermometer**: Clean the thermometer according to policy and replace it in the case.

    Electronic thermometer: Press the eject button to discard the cover. Return the probe to the holder.

    Mercury-free thermometer: Clean thermometer according to facility guidelines. Rinse with clean water and dry. Return it to case.

17. Remove and discard gloves.

18. Assist the resident to a comfortable and safe position. Return bed to lowest position.

19. Wash your hands.
    Provides for infection prevention.

20. Immediately record the temperature, date, time, and method used (rectal).
    Record temperature immediately so you won't forget. Care plans are made based on your report.

21. Place call light within resident's reach.
    Allows resident to communicate with staff as necessary.

22. Report any changes in resident to the nurse.
    Provides nurse with information to assess resident.

Tympanic thermometers can take a fast temperature reading. The NA should tell the resident that she will be placing a thermometer in the ear canal. She should reassure the resident that this is painless. The short tip of the thermometer will only go into the ear 1/4 to 1/2 inch.

Measuring and recording a tympanic temperature

Equipment: tympanic thermometer, gloves, disposable probe sheath/cover, pen and paper

1. Identify yourself by name. Identify the resident by name.
   Resident has right to know identity of his or her caregiver. Addressing resident by name shows respect and establishes correct identification.

2. Wash your hands.
   Provides for infection prevention.

3. Explain procedure to resident. Speak clearly, slowly, and directly. Maintain face-to-face contact whenever possible.
   Promotes understanding and independence.

4. Provide for resident's privacy with curtain, screen, or door.
   Maintains resident's right to privacy and dignity.

5. Put on gloves.

6. Put a disposable sheath over the earpiece of the thermometer.
   Protects equipment. Reduces risk of contamination.

7. Position the resident's head so that the ear is in front of you. Straighten the ear canal by gently pulling up and back on the outside edge of the ear (Fig. 7-14). Insert the covered probe into the ear canal. Press the button.

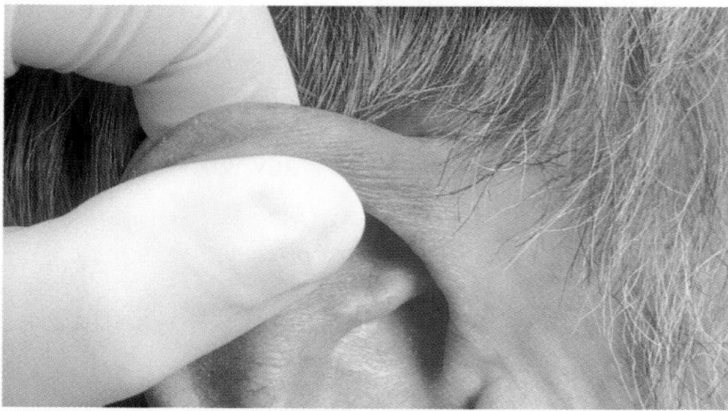

Fig. 7-14. *Straighten the ear canal by gently pulling up and back on the outside edge of the ear.*

8. Hold the thermometer in place until it blinks or beeps.

9. Read the temperature. Remember the temperature reading.

10. Discard sheath. Return thermometer to storage or to the battery charger if thermometer is rechargeable.

11. Remove and discard gloves.
12. Wash your hands.
    Provides for infection prevention.
13. Immediately record the temperature, date, time, and method used (tympanic).
    Record temperature immediately so you won't forget. Care plans are made based on your report.
14. Place call light within resident's reach.
    Allows resident to communicate with staff as necessary.
15. Report any changes in resident to the nurse.
    Provides nurse with information to assess resident.

Axillary temperatures are not as accurate as temperatures taken at other sites. However, they can be safer if a resident is confused, disoriented, uncooperative, or has dementia.

Measuring and recording an axillary temperature

Equipment: clean digital, electronic, or mercury-free thermometer, gloves, tissues, disposable sheath/cover, pen and paper

1. Identify yourself by name. Identify resident by name.
   Resident has right to know identity of his or her caregiver. Addressing resident by name shows respect and establishes correct identification.
2. Wash your hands.
   Provides for infection prevention.
3. Explain procedure to resident. Speak clearly, slowly, and directly. Maintain face-to-face contact whenever possible.
   Promotes understanding and independence.
4. Provide for resident's privacy with curtain, screen, or door.
   Maintains resident's right to privacy and dignity.
5. Put on gloves.
6. Remove the resident's arm from the sleeve of gown to allow skin contact with the end of the thermometer. Wipe the axillary area with tissues before placing the thermometer.
7. **Digital thermometer**: Put on the disposable sheath. Turn on the thermometer and wait until the *ready* sign appears.

   Electronic thermometer: Remove the probe from the base unit. Put on the probe cover.

   Mercury-free thermometer: Hold the thermometer by the stem. Shake the thermometer down to below the lowest number.
8. Position the thermometer (bulb end for mercury-free) in the center of the armpit. Fold the resident's arm over his chest.
9. **Digital thermometer**: Leave in place until the thermometer blinks or beeps.

   Electronic thermometer: Leave in place until you hear a tone or see a flashing or steady light.

   Mercury-free thermometer: Leave in place, with the arm close against the side, for 8 to 10 minutes (Fig. 7-15).

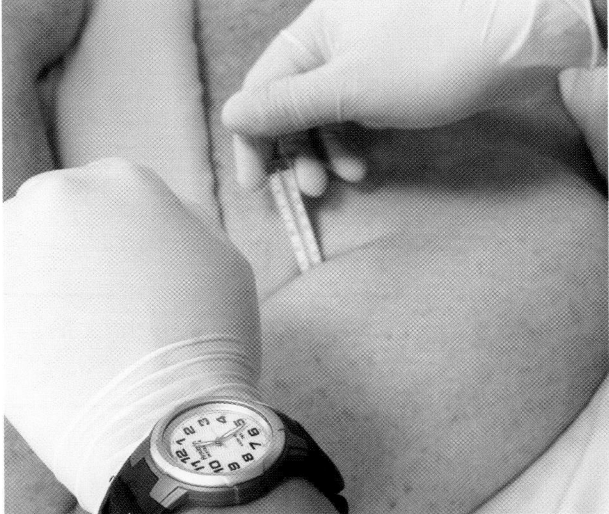

Fig. 7-15. *After inserting the thermometer, fold the resident's arm over his chest and hold it in place for 8 to 10 minutes.*

10. **Digital thermometer**: Remove the thermometer. Read the temperature on the display screen. Remember the temperature reading.

Electronic thermometer: Read the temperature on the display screen. Remember the temperature reading. Remove the probe.

Mercury-free thermometer: Remove the thermometer. Wipe it with a tissue from stem to bulb or remove the sheath. Discard the tissue or sheath. Read the thermometer at eye level as you would for an oral temperature. Remember the temperature reading.

11. **Digital thermometer**: Using a tissue, remove and discard the sheath. Replace the thermometer in the case.

    Electronic thermometer: Press the eject button to discard the cover. Return the probe to the holder.

    Mercury-free thermometer: Clean thermometer according to facility guidelines. Rinse with clean water and dry. Return it to case.

12. Remove and discard gloves.
13. Wash your hands.
    Provides for infection prevention.
14. Put resident's arm back into sleeve of gown.
15. Immediately record the temperature, date, time and method used (axillary).
    Record temperature immediately so you won't forget. Care plans are made based on your report.
16. Place call light within resident's reach.
    Allows resident to communicate with staff as necessary.
17. Report any changes in resident to the nurse.
    Provides nurse with information to assess resident.

Pulse

The pulse is the number of heartbeats per minute. The beat that is felt at certain pulse points in the body represents the wave of blood moving as a result of the heart pumping. The most common site for checking the pulse is on the inside of the wrist, where the radial artery runs just beneath the skin. This is called the **radial pulse**.

The **brachial pulse** is the pulse inside the elbow. It is about one to one-and-a-half inches above the elbow. The radial and brachial pulses are involved in taking blood pressure. Blood pressure is explained later in this chapter. Common pulse sites are shown in Figure 7-16 below.

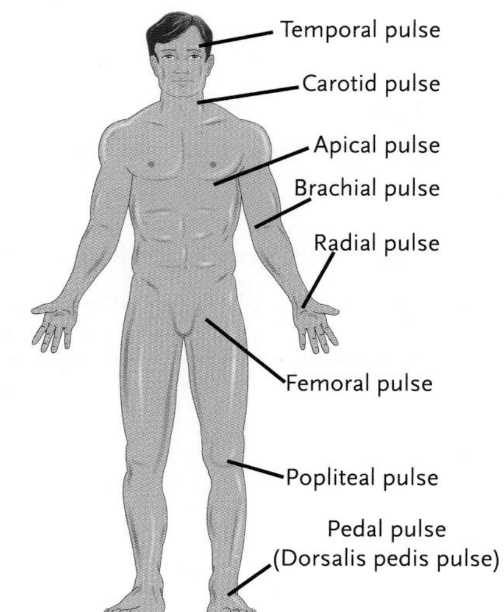

Fig. 7-16. *Common pulse sites.*

For adults, the normal pulse rate is 60 to 100 beats per minute. Small children have faster pulses, in the range of 100 to 120 beats per minute. A newborn baby's pulse may be as high as 120 to 180 beats per minute. Many things can affect the pulse rate. These include exercise, fear, anger, anxiety, heat, infection, illness, medications, and pain. A high or low rate may not indicate disease. However, sometimes the pulse rate can signal that illness exists. For example, a rapid pulse may result from fever, dehydration, or heart failure. A slow or weak pulse may indicate infection.

Respirations

Respiration is the process of inhaling air into the lungs, or **inspiration**, and exhaling air out of the lungs, or **expiration**. Each respiration consists of an inspiration and an expiration. The chest rises during inspiration and falls during expiration.

The normal respiration rate for adults ranges from 12 to 20 breaths per minute. Infants and children have a faster respiratory rate. Infants normally breathe at a rate of 30 to 40 respirations per minute. Respirations are usually counted directly after counting the pulse rate. This is because people may breathe more quickly if they know they are being observed. The NA should keep her fingers on the resident's wrist or on the stethoscope over the heart. She should not make it obvious that she is watching the resident's breathing. She should not mention she is counting respirations.

Counting and recording radial pulse and counting and recording respirations

Equipment: watch with a second hand, pen and paper

1. Identify yourself by name. Identify the resident by name.
   Resident has right to know identity of his or her caregiver. Addressing resident by name shows respect and establishes correct identification.
2. Wash your hands.
   Provides for infection prevention.
3. Explain procedure to resident. Speak clearly, slowly, and directly. Maintain face-to-face contact whenever possible.
   Promotes understanding and independence.
4. Provide for resident's privacy with curtain, screen, or door.
   Maintains resident's right to privacy and dignity.
5. Place the tips of your index finger and middle finger on the thumb side of the resident's wrist. Locate the radial pulse (Fig. 7-17).

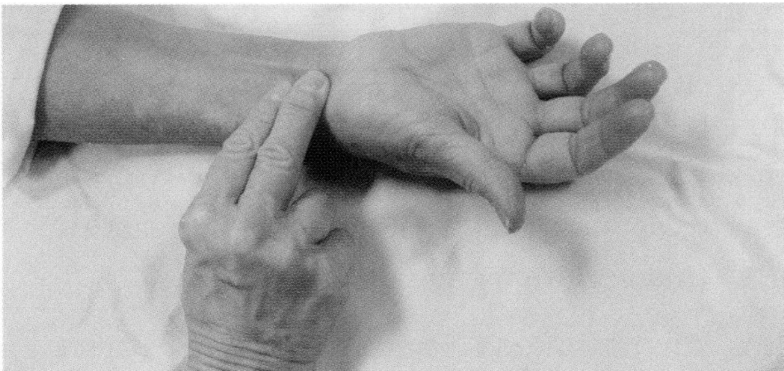

Fig. 7-17. *Count the radial pulse by placing the tips of your index finger and middle finger on the thumb side of the wrist.*

6. Count the beats for one full minute.
7. Keep your fingertips on the resident's wrist. Count respirations for one full minute. Observe the pattern and character of the resident's breathing. Normal breathing is smooth and quiet. If you see signs of troubled, shallow, or noisy breathing, such as wheezing, report it.
   Count will be more accurate if resident does not know you are counting his respirations.
8. Wash your hands.
   Provides for infection prevention.
9. Immediately record the pulse rate, date, time, and method used (radial). Record the respiratory rate and the pattern or character of breathing.
   Record pulse and respiration rate immediately so you won't forget. Care plans are made based on your report.
10. Place call light within resident's reach.
    Allows resident to communicate with staff as necessary.
11. Report any changes in resident to the nurse. Report to the nurse if the pulse is less than 60 beats per minute, over 100 beats per minute, if the rhythm is irregular, or if breathing is irregular.
    Provides nurse with information to assess resident.

Blood Pressure

Blood pressure is an important indicator of health. The measurement shows how well the heart is working. Blood pressure is measured in millimeters of mercury (mm Hg). It is recorded as a fraction—for example, 120/80. There are two parts of blood pressure: the systolic measurement and the diastolic measurement.

In the **systolic** phase, which is the top number of the reading, the heart is at work. It contracts and pushes blood from the left ventricle of the heart. The reading shows the pressure on the walls of the arteries as blood is pumped through the body. The normal range for systolic blood pressure is below 120 mm Hg.

The second measurement reflects the **diastolic** phase, which is the bottom number of the reading. This is when the heart relaxes. The diastolic measurement is always lower than the systolic measurement. It shows the pressure in the arteries when the heart is at rest. The normal range for adults is below 80 mm Hg.

People with consistently high blood pressure, or hypertension, have elevated systolic and/or diastolic blood pressures. In late 2017, the American Heart Association and American College of Cardiology released new joint guidelines for blood pressure. A systolic reading of 130 mm Hg or higher or a diastolic reading of 80 mm Hg or higher is now considered high blood pressure. Previously a person was considered to have high blood pressure when the blood pressure reading was 140/90 or above. Systolic and diastolic readings do not both need to be high for a reading to be considered high. A systolic reading of 130 mm Hg or higher or a diastolic reading of 80 mm Hg or higher should be reported.

Blood pressure is affected by many factors. These include aging, exercise, stress, pain, medications, illness, obesity, alcohol intake, tobacco products, and the volume of blood in circulation.

Blood pressure is measured with either a manual or digital sphygmomanometer (Fig. 7-18). A manual sphygmomanometer requires the use of a stethoscope to determine the blood pressure reading. With a digital sphygmomanometer, the systolic and diastolic pressure readings are displayed digitally. The use of a stethoscope is not required with a digital sphygmomanometer.

When measuring blood pressure, the first sound heard is the systolic pressure (top number). When the sound changes to a soft muffled thump or disappears, this is the diastolic pressure (bottom number).

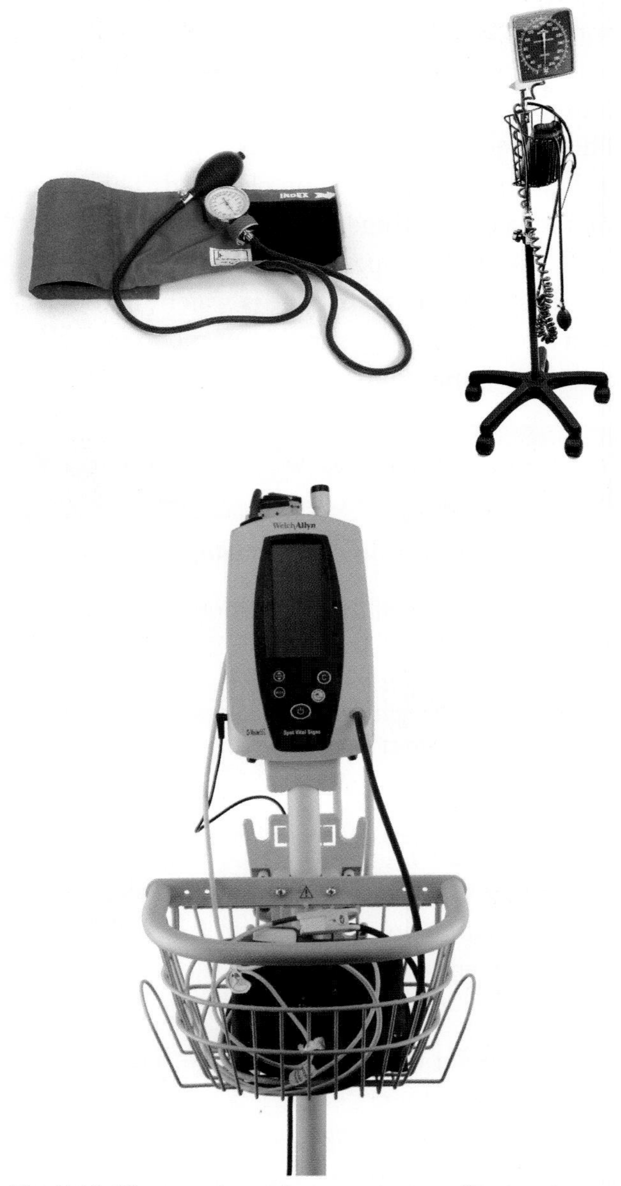

Fig. 7-18. *The top photo shows two types of manual sphygmomanometers. The bottom photo shows a type of digital sphygmomanometer that measures blood pressure, as well as other vital signs.*

Blood pressure should not be measured on an arm that has an IV, a dialysis shunt, or any medical equipment. A side that has a cast, recent trauma, paralysis, burns, or has had breast surgery (mastectomy) should be avoided.

It is important to use a cuff that is the correct size when measuring blood pressure. Available sizes for adults include small adult, adult, large adult, and thigh.

Measuring and recording blood pressure (one-step method)

Equipment: sphygmomanometer, stethoscope, alcohol wipes, pen and paper

1. Identify yourself by name. Identify the resident by name.
   Resident has right to know identity of his or her caregiver. Addressing resident by name shows respect and establishes correct identification.
2. Wash your hands.
   Provides for infection prevention.
3. Explain procedure to the resident. Speak clearly, slowly, and directly. Maintain face-to-face contact whenever possible.
   Promotes understanding and independence.
4. Provide for resident's privacy with curtain, screen, or door.
   Maintains resident's right to privacy and dignity.
5. Before using the stethoscope, wipe the diaphragm and earpieces with alcohol wipes.
   Reduces pathogens, prevents ear infections, and prevents spread of infection.
6. Ask the resident to roll up his sleeve so that the upper arm is exposed. Do not measure blood pressure over clothing.
7. Position the resident's arm with his palm up. The arm should be level with the heart.
   A false low reading is possible if arm is above heart level.
8. With the valve open, squeeze the cuff. Make sure it is completely deflated.
9. Place the blood pressure cuff snugly on the resident's upper arm. The center of the cuff with sensor/arrow is placed over the brachial artery (1–1½ inches above the elbow, toward the inside of the elbow) (Fig. 7-19).
   Cuff must be proper size and put on arm correctly so amount of pressure on artery is correct. If not, reading will be falsely high or low.
10. Locate the brachial pulse with your fingertips.
11. Place the earpieces of the stethoscope in your ears.

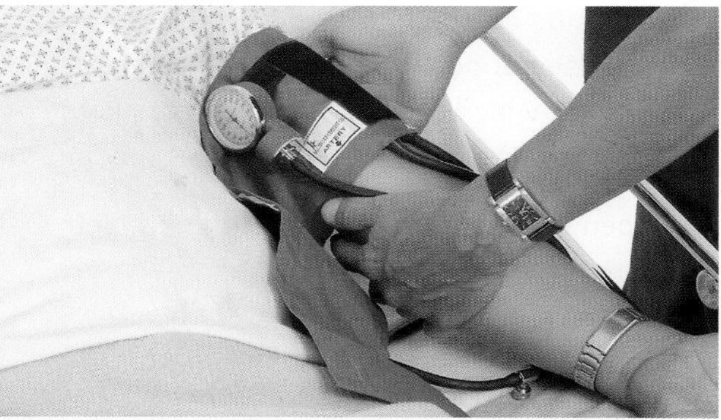

Fig. 7-19. *Place the center of the cuff over the brachial artery.*

12. Place the diaphragm of the stethoscope over the brachial artery.
13. Close the valve (clockwise) until it stops. Do not overtighten it (Fig. 7-20).
    Tight valves are hard to release.

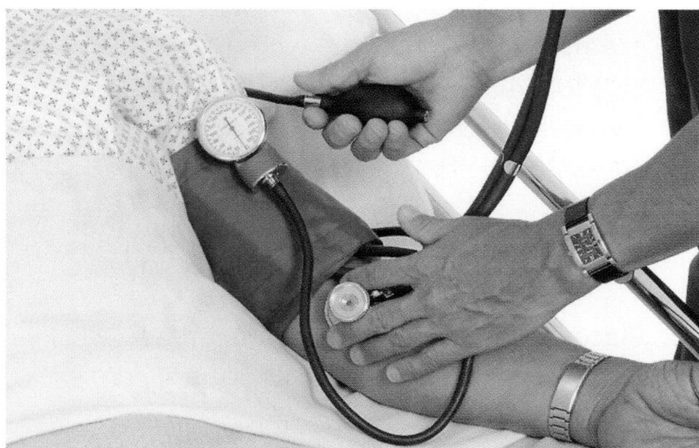

Fig. 7-20. *Close the valve by turning it clockwise until it stops. Do not overtighten it.*

14. Inflate the cuff to between 160 mm Hg to 180 mm Hg. If a beat is heard immediately upon cuff deflation, completely deflate the cuff. Reinflate the cuff to no more than 200 mm Hg.
15. Open the valve slightly with the thumb and index finger. Deflate the cuff slowly.
    Releasing the valve slowly allows you to hear beats accurately.
16. Watch the gauge. Listen for the sound of the pulse.
17. Remember the reading at which the first pulse sound is heard. This is the systolic pressure.

18. Continue listening for a change or muffling of pulse sound. The point of a change or the point at which the sound disappears is the diastolic pressure. Remember this reading.

19. Open the valve. Deflate the cuff completely. Remove the cuff.
An inflated cuff left on resident's arm can cause numbness and tingling. If you must take blood pressure again, completely deflate cuff and wait 30 seconds. Never partially deflate a cuff and then pump it up again. Blood vessels will be damaged and reading will be falsely high or low.

20. Wash your hands.
Provides for infection prevention.

21. Immediately record both the systolic and diastolic pressures. Record the numbers like a fraction, with the systolic reading on top and the diastolic reading on the bottom (for example: 120/80). Note which arm was used. Use RA for right arm and LA for left arm.
Record readings immediately so you won't forget. Care plans are made based on your report.

22. Wipe diaphragm and earpieces of stethoscope with alcohol wipes. Store equipment.

23. Place call light within resident's reach.
Allows resident to communicate with staff as necessary.

24. Wash your hands.
Provides for infection prevention.

25. Report any changes in resident to the nurse.
Provides nurse with information to assess resident.

If using a digital sphygmomanometer, the NA will place the cuff on the resident's upper arm, with the center of the cuff over the brachial artery. A start button may need to be pressed. Usually the cuff inflates on its own and then deflates once the blood pressure measurement has been obtained. The reading will appear on the screen.

In addition to other vital sign measurements, some NAs may be asked to obtain a pulse oximeter reading. A pulse oximeter is a device that uses a light to determine the amount of oxygen in the blood. A pulse oximeter also measures a person's pulse rate (Fig. 7-21).

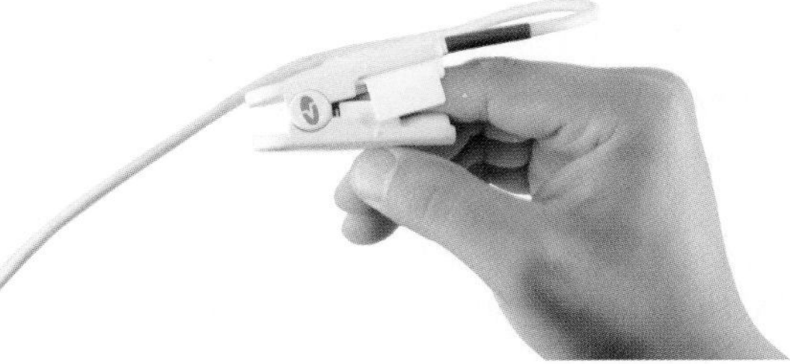

***Fig. 7-21.** A pulse oximeter sensor is usually clipped on a person's finger to measure the amount of oxygen in the blood, as well as pulse rate.*

A pulse oximeter may be used when residents have had surgery, are on oxygen, are in intensive care, or have cardiac or respiratory problems. When asked to obtain this reading, the NA should report the oxygen percentage to the nurse. The nurse will determine if the level is adequate for the resident.

Pain Management

Pain is sometimes referred to as the fifth vital sign because it is as important to monitor as the other vital signs. However, pain is different in that it is subjective (something reported by the person). The other vital signs are objective measurements (information collected by using the senses). Pain is also a personal experience, which means it is different for each person.

Pain is uncomfortable. It can quickly drain energy and hope. NAs spend the most time with residents. They play an important role in pain monitoring, management, and prevention. Care plans are made based on NAs' reports.

Pain is **not** a normal part of aging. Chronic pain may lead to withdrawal, depression, and isolation. NAs must treat residents' complaints of pain seriously. They should listen to what residents are saying about the way they feel. They should take action to help them. The following are questions that nurses may ask residents to assess their pain. A nurse may ask an NA to ask these questions and then immediately report the information to the nurse:

- Where is the pain?
- When did the pain start?
- How long does the pain last, and how often does it occur?
- How severe is the pain? To help find out, the resident may be asked to rate the pain on a scale of 0 to 10, with 0 being no pain and 10 being the worst pain (Fig. 7-22).

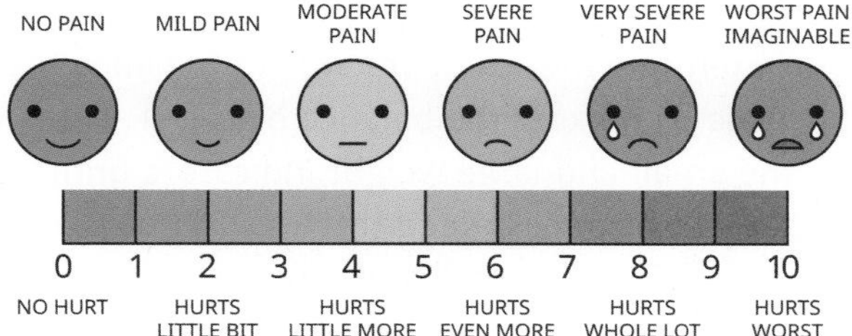

Fig. 7-22. *This is one type of pain scale that nurses may use to assess pain levels.*

- Can you describe the pain? The NA should use the resident's words when reporting to the nurse.
- What makes the pain better? What makes the pain worse?
- What were you doing when the pain started?

Residents may have concerns about their pain. These concerns may make them hesitant to report their pain. Barriers to managing pain include the following:

- Fear of addiction to pain medication
- Feeling that pain is a normal part of aging
- Worrying about constipation and fatigue from pain medication
- Feeling that caregivers are too busy to deal with their pain
- Feeling that too much pain medication will cause death

NAs should be patient and caring when helping residents who are in pain. If residents are worried about the effects of pain medication or have questions about it, the NA should tell the nurse. Some people do not feel comfortable saying that they are in pain. A person's culture affects how he or she responds to pain. In some cultures, there is a belief that it is best not to react to pain. In other cultures, people are encouraged to express pain freely. Body language or other messages that a resident may be in pain are important for the NA to observe.

Guidelines: Pain Management

G Report complaints of pain or unrelieved pain immediately.

G Gently position the body in proper alignment. Use pillows for support. Help with changes of position if the resident wishes.

G Give back rubs.

G Ask if the resident would like to take a warm bath or shower.

G Help the resident to the bathroom or commode or offer the bedpan or urinal.

G Encourage slow, deep breathing.

G Provide a calm and quiet environment. Soft music may distract the resident.

G Be patient, caring, gentle, and responsive.

Observing and Reporting: Pain

Report any of these to the nurse:

O/R Increased pulse, respirations, blood pressure

O/R Sweating

O/R Nausea

O/R Vomiting

O/R Tightening the jaw

O/R Squeezing eyes shut

- O/R Holding or guarding a body part
- O/R Frowning
- O/R Grinding teeth
- O/R Increased restlessness
- O/R Agitation or tension
- O/R Change in behavior
- O/R Crying
- O/R Sighing
- O/R Groaning
- O/R Breathing heavily
- O/R Rocking
- O/R Pacing
- O/R Repetitive movements
- O/R Difficulty moving or walking

3. Explain how to measure weight and height

NAs measure weight and height as part of regular care. Height is checked less often than weight. Weight changes can be signs of illness. NAs must report **any** weight loss or gain, no matter how small. Weight will be measured using pounds or kilograms. A pound is a unit of weight equal to 16 ounces. A kilogram is a unit of mass equal to 1000 grams; one kilogram equals 2.2 pounds.

Measuring and recording weight of an ambulatory resident

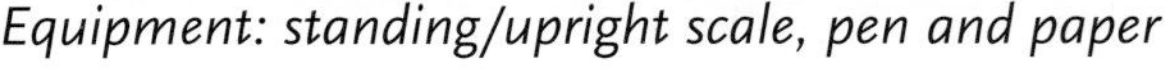

Equipment: standing/upright scale, pen and paper

1. Identify yourself by name. Identify the resident by name.
   Resident has right to know identity of his or her caregiver. Addressing resident by name shows respect and establishes correct identification.

2. Wash your hands.
   Provides for infection prevention.

3. Explain procedure to resident. Speak clearly, slowly, and directly. Maintain face-to-face contact whenever possible.
   Promotes understanding and independence.

4. Provide for resident's privacy with curtain, screen, or door.
   Maintains resident's right to privacy and dignity.

5. Make sure the resident is wearing nonskid shoes that are fastened before walking to the scale.

6. Start with the scale balanced at zero before weighing the resident.
   Scale must be balanced on zero for weight to be accurate.

7. Help the resident to step onto the center of the scale. Be sure she is not holding, touching, or leaning against anything.
   This interferes with weight measurement.

8. Determine the resident's weight. Balance the scale by making the balance bar level. Move the small and large weight indicators until the bar balances. Read the two numbers shown (on the small and large weight indicators) when the bar is balanced. Add these two numbers together. This is the resident's weight (Fig. 7-23).

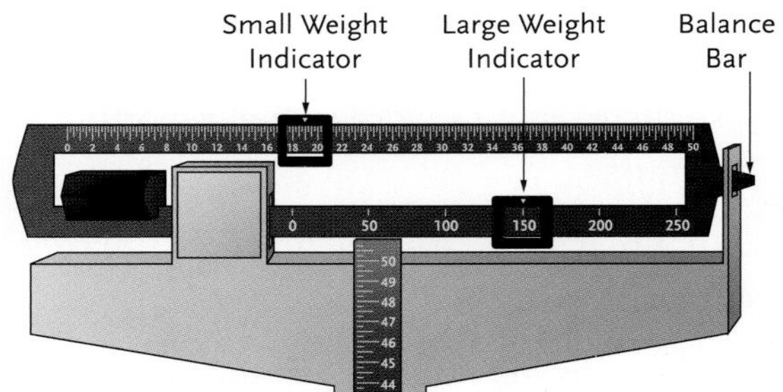

***Fig. 7-23.** Move the small and large weight indicators until the bar balances. The weight shown in the illustration is 169 pounds.*

9. Help the resident to safely step off the scale before recording weight.
   Protects against falls.

10. Wash your hands.
    Provides for infection prevention.

11. Immediately record the resident's weight in pounds (lb) or kilograms (kg), depending on facility policy.
    Record weight immediately so you won't forget. Care plans are made based on your report.

12. Place call light within resident's reach.
    Allows resident to communicate with staff as necessary.

13. Report any changes in resident to the nurse.
    Provides nurse with information to assess resident.

Some residents will not be able to get out of wheelchairs easily. These residents may be weighed on a wheelchair scale. With this scale, wheelchairs are rolled directly onto the scale (Fig. 7-24). On some wheelchair scales, the NA will need to subtract the weight of the wheelchair from a resident's weight. If the wheelchair weight is not listed on the chair, the NA should weigh the empty wheelchair first. The footrests should be attached if they will be attached when the resident is in the chair. Then the NA should subtract the wheelchair's weight from the total.

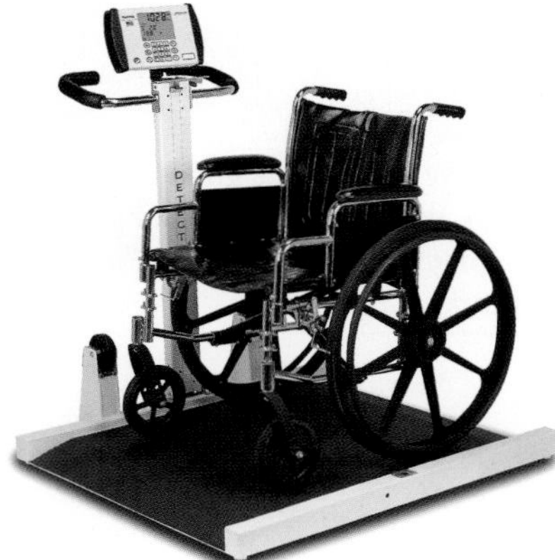

Fig. 7-24. *Wheelchairs can be rolled directly onto wheelchair scales to determine weight.* (PHOTO COURTESY OF DETECTO, WWW.DETECTO.COM, 800-641-2008)

When residents are not able to get out of bed, they are weighed on special bed scales (Fig. 7-25). Before using a bed scale, the NA should know how to use it properly and safely.

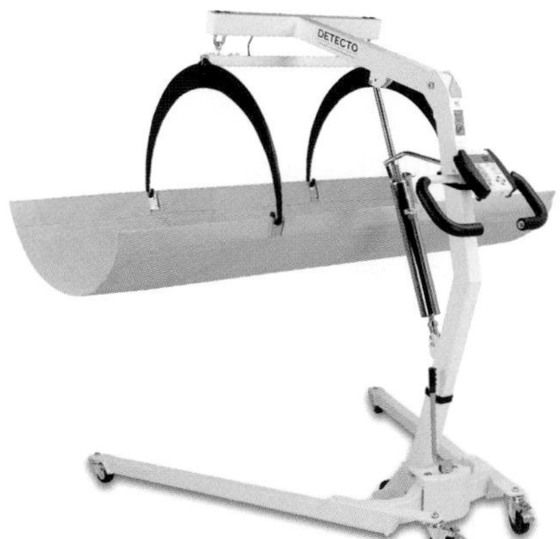

Fig. 7-25. *A type of bed scale.* (PHOTO COURTESY OF DETECTO, WWW.DETECTO.COM, 800-641-2008)

For measuring height, there is a rod attached to the scale. The rod measures in inches and fractions of inches. The NA should record the total number of inches. If inches need to be converted into feet, there are 12 inches in one foot.

Measuring and recording height of an ambulatory resident

For residents who can get out of bed, you will measure height using a standing scale.

Equipment: standing scale, pen, and paper

1. Identify yourself by name. Identify the resident by name.
   Resident has right to know identity of his or her caregiver. Addressing resident by name shows respect and establishes correct identification.
2. Wash your hands.
   Provides for infection prevention.
3. Explain procedure to resident. Speak clearly, slowly, and directly. Maintain face-to-face contact whenever possible.
   Promotes understanding and independence.
4. Provide for resident's privacy with curtain, screen, or door.
   Maintains resident's right to privacy and dignity.
5. Make sure the resident is wearing nonskid shoes that are securely fastened before walking to the scale.
6. Help the resident to step onto the scale, facing away from the scale.
7. Ask the resident to stand straight if possible. Help as needed.
   Ensures accurate reading.
8. Pull up the measuring rod from the back of the scale. Gently lower the rod until it rests flat on the resident's head (Fig. 7-26).
9. Determine the resident's height.
10. Help the resident to step off the scale before recording height. Make sure the measuring

rod does not hit the resident in the head while doing so.

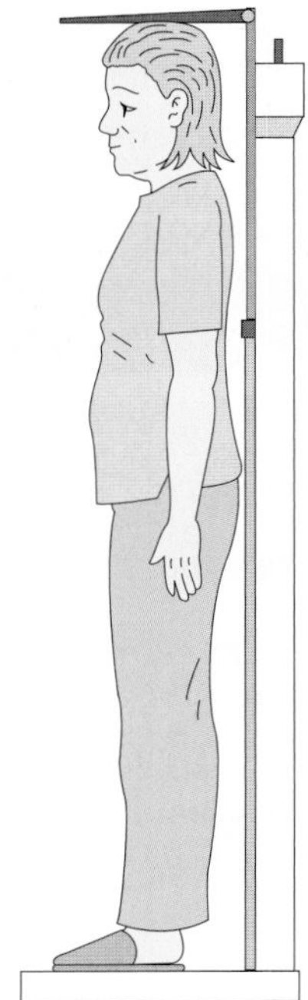

Fig. 7-26. To determine height on a standing scale, gently lower the measuring rod until it rests flat on the resident's head.

11. Wash your hands.
    Provides for infection prevention.
12. Immediately record the resident's height.
    Record height immediately so you won't forget. Care plans are made based on your report.
13. Place call light within resident's reach.
    Allows resident to communicate with staff as necessary.
14. Report any changes in resident to the nurse.
    Provides nurse with information to assess resident.

Some residents will be unable to get out of bed. Height can be measured by using a tape measure and making two pencil marks on the sheet that is underneath the resident. The NA makes a mark at the top of the resident's head and one at his feet and measures the distance between the marks (Figs. 7-27 and 7-28). Height of a resident who is bedridden can also be measured using other methods. NAs should follow the procedures used at their facilities.

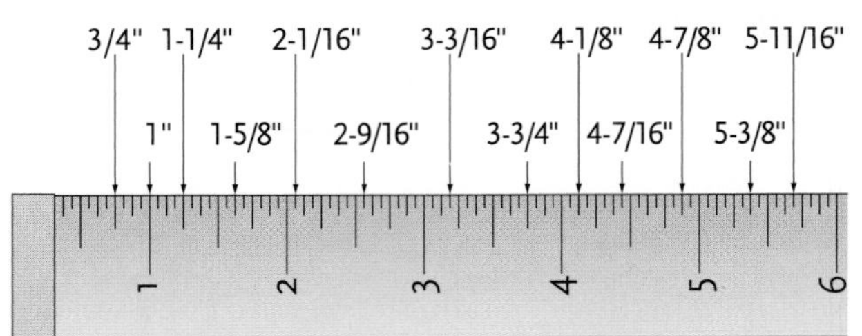

Fig. 7-27. Height can be measured in bed using a tape measure.

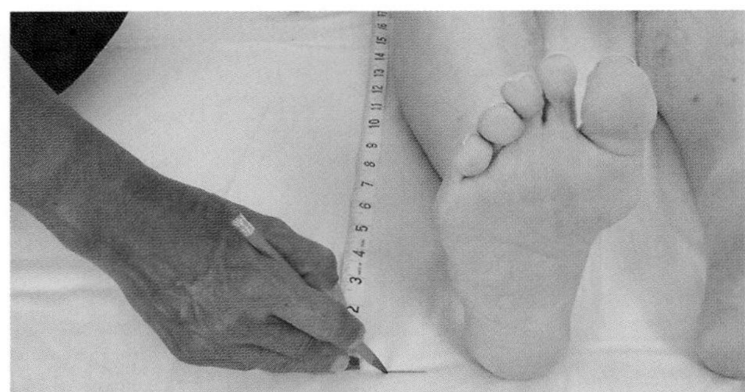

Fig. 7-28. One way that the height of a resident who is bedridden can be measured is by making marks on the sheet at the resident's head and heel. Then the distance between the marks is measured.

4. Explain restraints and how to promote a restraint-free environment

A **restraint** is a physical or chemical way to restrict voluntary movement or behavior. A *physical restraint* is any method, device, material, or equipment that restricts a person's freedom of movement. Types of physical restraints include vest restraints, belt restraints, wrist/ankle restraints, and mitt restraints. *Chemical restraints* are medications used to control a person's mood or behavior.

An *enabler* is equipment or a device that promotes a resident's safety, comfort, independence, and mobility. Wheelchairs, geriatric chairs, cushions and pillows, and certain types of assistive devices, such as special utensils, are examples of enablers. However, if a person cannot remove an enabler independently, it may be considered a restraint. Raised side rails on beds and geriatric chairs with tray tables attached may be considered enablers or physical restraints. This depends upon their intended use and the resident's condition or abilities (Figs. 7-29 and 7-30).

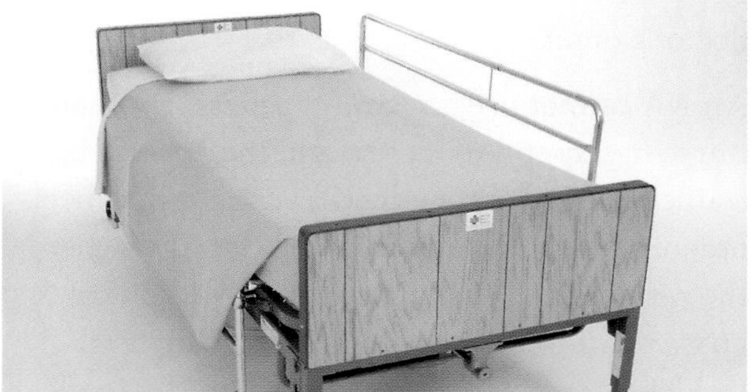

Fig. 7-29. *Raised side rails may be considered restraints. It depends on their intended use and on the resident's abilities.*

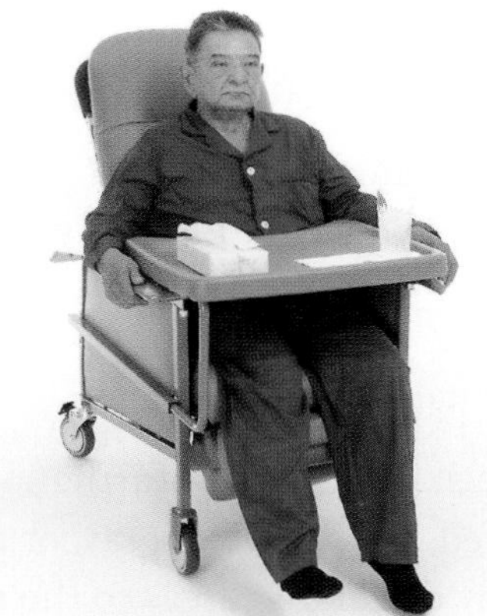

Fig. 7-30. *If a resident cannot remove an attached tray table, a geriatric chair may be considered a restraint.*

In the past, restraints were commonly used to prevent confused people from wandering or to prevent falls. They were used to keep people from injuring themselves or others or to prevent people from pulling out tubing needed for treatment. Restraints were often overused by caregivers. Residents were injured. This led to new laws restricting the use of restraints.

Today, long-term care facilities are prohibited from using restraints unless they are medically necessary. They are only used as a last resort. They are only used after other measures have been tried. If a restraint is needed, a doctor must order it. Very specific guidelines apply to carrying out a restraint order. This includes frequent monitoring of the resident. This is important because residents have been severely injured and have died due to improper restraint use and lack of monitoring. NAs cannot use a physical restraint unless a doctor has ordered it in the care plan and they have been trained in the restraint's use. It is against the law for staff to apply a restraint for convenience or to discipline a resident. NAs can check with their supervisor for policies regarding restraints.

There are many serious problems that occur with restraint use. They include the following:

- Pressure injuries
- Pneumonia
- Risk of suffocation (suffocation is the stoppage of breathing from a lack of oxygen or excess of carbon dioxide in the body; it may result in unconsciousness or death)
- Reduced blood circulation
- Stress on the heart
- Incontinence
- Constipation
- Weakened muscles and bones
- Muscle atrophy (weakening or wasting away of the muscle)
- Loss of bone mass
- Poor appetite and malnutrition
- Depression and/or withdrawal
- Sleep disorders
- Loss of dignity
- Loss of independence
- Stress and anxiety
- Increased agitation (anxiety, restlessness)
- Loss of self-esteem
- Severe injury
- Death

Restraint usage has significantly decreased in facilities. State and federal agencies encourage facilities to take steps to create restraint-free environments. **Restraint-free care** means that restraints are not kept or used for any reason. Creative ideas that help avoid the need for restraints are being used instead. **Restraint alternatives** are measures used in place of a restraint or that reduce the need for a restraint. Examples of restraint alternatives include the following:

- Make sure call lights are within reach. Respond to call lights promptly.
- Improve safety measures to prevent accidents and falls. Improve lighting.
- Ambulate the resident when he is restless. The doctor or nurse may add exercise into the care plan.
- Provide activities for those who wander at night.
- Encourage activities and independence. Escort the resident to social activities. Increase visits and social interaction.
- Give frequent help with elimination needs. Help with cleaning immediately after an episode of incontinence.
- Offer food or drink. Offer reading materials.
- Distract or redirect interest. Give the resident a repetitive task.
- Decrease the noise level. Listen to soothing music. Offer massage or use relaxation techniques.
- Reduce pain levels through medication. The resident should be monitored closely. Complaints of pain should be reported immediately.
- Provide familiar caregivers. Increase the number of caregivers by using family and volunteers.
- Use a team approach to meeting needs. Offer training to teach gentle approaches to difficult people.

There are also several types of pads, belts, special chairs, and alarms that can be used instead of restraints. If a resident is ordered to have an alarm on his bed or chair, the NA should make sure it is there and is turned on.

OBRA sets specific rules for restraint use. Restraints are used only after everything else has been ruled out and can only be applied with a doctor's order.

An NA cannot use a restraint unless the charge nurse has approved its use and the NA has been trained to use it properly. If a restraint has been ordered, the NA must place the call light where the resident can easily access it. She should answer call lights immediately. A restrained resident must be monitored constantly. He must be checked at least every 15 minutes, following facility policy. At a minimum, the restraint must be released every two hours and the resident must be given proper care:

- Help with elimination needs. Check for episodes of incontinence. Provide skin care.
- Offer fluids and food.
- Measure vital signs.
- Check the skin for signs of irritation. Report any red, purple, blue, gray, or pale skin or any discolored areas to the nurse immediately.
- Check for swelling of body parts and report any swelling immediately.
- Reposition the resident.
- Ambulate the resident if he is able.

If any problems occur with the restraint, especially injury, the NA should notify the nurse and complete an incident report as soon as possible.

5. Define *fluid balance* and explain intake and output (I&O)

To maintain health, the body must take in a certain amount of fluid each day. Fluid comes in the form of liquids that a person drinks. It is also found in semi-liquid foods like gelatin, soup, ice cream, pudding, and yogurt. The fluid a person consumes is called **intake**, or **input**. A general recommendation for daily fluid intake is 64 ounces (or eight 8-ounce glasses) for a healthy person. However, that is not necessarily a firm guideline for health. Some people may need more than 64 ounces, while others may need less. The amount needed depends on factors such as activity, heat, and overall health. All fluid taken in each day cannot stay in the body. It must be eliminated as **output**. Output includes urine, feces (including diarrhea), and vomitus. It also includes perspiration, moisture in the air that a person exhales, and wound drainage.

Fluid balance is maintaining equal input and output, or taking in and eliminating equal amounts of fluids. Most people do this naturally. But some residents must have their intake and output, or I&O, monitored and recorded. To do this, the NA will need to measure and document all food and fluids the resident takes by mouth, as well as all urine and vomitus produced. This is recorded on an Intake and Output (I&O) sheet (Fig. 7-31).

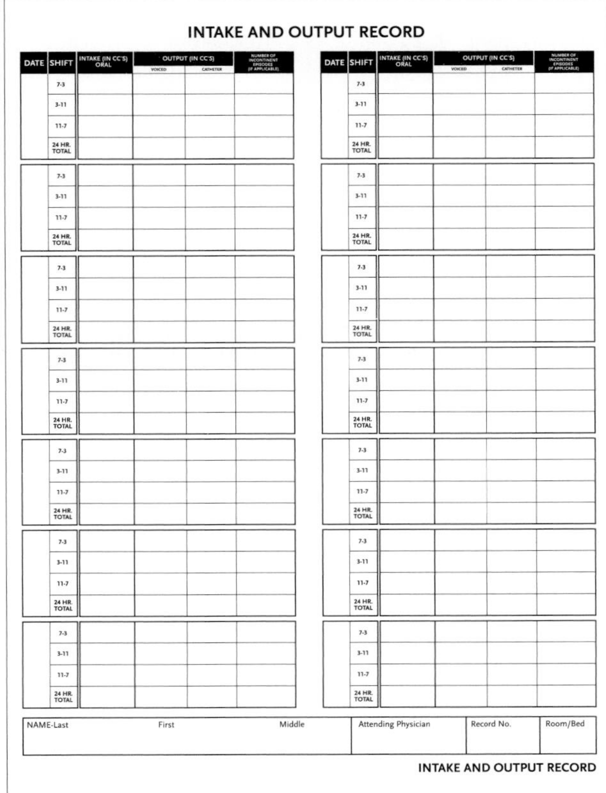

INTAKE AND OUTPUT RECORD

DATE	SHIFT	INTAKE (IN CC'S) ORAL	OUTPUT (IN CC'S) VOIDED	OUTPUT (IN CC'S) CATHETER	NUMBER OF INCONTINENT EPISODES (IF APPLICABLE)	DATE	SHIFT	INTAKE (IN CC'S) ORAL	OUTPUT (IN CC'S) VOIDED	OUTPUT (IN CC'S) CATHETER	NUMBER OF INCONTINENT EPISODES (IF APPLICABLE)
	7-3						7-3				
	3-11						3-11				
	11-7						11-7				
	24 HR. TOTAL						24 HR. TOTAL				
	7-3						7-3				
	3-11						3-11				
	11-7						11-7				
	24 HR. TOTAL						24 HR. TOTAL				
	7-3						7-3				
	3-11						3-11				
	11-7						11-7				
	24 HR. TOTAL						24 HR. TOTAL				
	7-3						7-3				
	3-11						3-11				
	11-7						11-7				
	24 HR. TOTAL						24 HR. TOTAL				
	7-3						7-3				
	3-11						3-11				
	11-7						11-7				
	24 HR. TOTAL						24 HR. TOTAL				
	7-3						7-3				
	3-11						3-11				
	11-7						11-7				
	24 HR. TOTAL						24 HR. TOTAL				
	7-3						7-3				
	3-11						3-11				
	11-7						11-7				
	24 HR. TOTAL						24 HR. TOTAL				

NAME-Last	First	Middle	Attending Physician	Record No.	Room/Bed

INTAKE AND OUTPUT RECORD

Fig. 7-31. *This is one type of intake/output sheet.*

Conversions

Milliliters (mL) are units of measurement in the metric system. One milliliter is 1/1000 of a liter. Ounces (oz) are converted to milliliters. One ounce equals 30 milliliters. To convert ounces to milliliters, the number of ounces must be multiplied by 30.

1 oz = 30 mL

2 oz = 60 mL

3 oz = 90 mL

4 oz = 120 mL

5 oz = 150 mL

6 oz = 180 mL

7 oz = 210 mL

8 oz = 240 mL

¼ cup = 2 oz = 60 mL

½ cup = 4 oz = 120 mL

1 cup = 8 oz = 240 mL

Measuring and recording urinary output 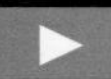

Equipment: I&O sheet, graduate (measuring container), gloves, pen and paper

1. Wash your hands.
   Provides for infection prevention.
2. Put on gloves before handling bedpan/urinal.
3. Pour the contents of the bedpan or urinal into the graduate. Do not spill or splash any of the urine.
4. Place the graduate on a flat surface. Measure the amount of urine at eye level. Keep the container level (Fig. 7-32). Note the amount on paper, converting to mL if necessary. (If the amount is between measurement lines, you may need to round up to the nearest 25 mL. Follow policy.)
   A flat surface helps get an accurate reading.

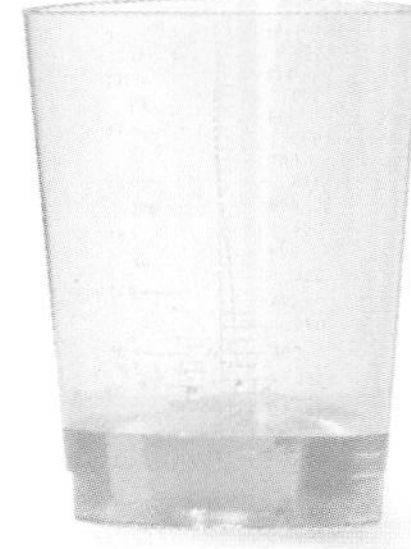

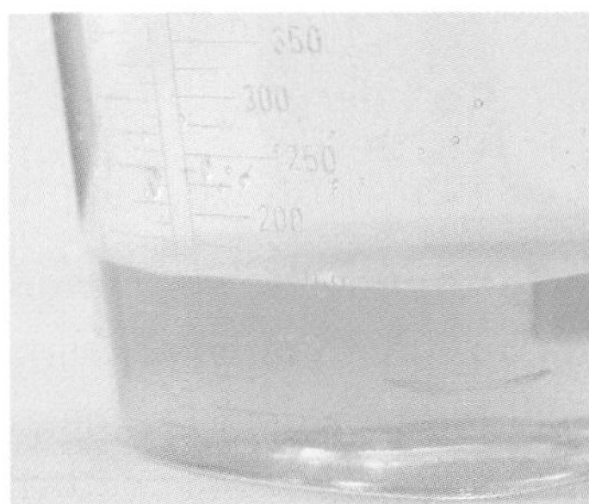

Fig. 7-32. *Keep the container level on a flat surface while measuring output.*

5. After measuring urine, empty the graduate into the toilet. Do not splash urine.
   Reduces risk of contamination.

6. Rinse the graduate. Pour rinse water into the toilet.

7. Rinse the bedpan/urinal. Pour rinse water into the toilet. Flush the toilet.

8. Place graduate and bedpan/urinal in area for cleaning or clean and store according to facility policy.

9. Remove and discard gloves.

10. Wash hands before recording output.
    Provides for infection prevention.

11. Immediately document the time and amount of urine in output column on sheet. For example: 1545 hours, 200 mL urine.
    Record amount immediately so you won't forget. Care plans are made based on your report. If you do not document the care, legally it did not happen.

12. Report any changes in resident to the nurse.
    Provides nurse with information to assess resident.

Collecting Specimens

NAs may need to collect a specimen from a resident. A **specimen** is a sample that is used for analysis in order to try to make a diagnosis. Different types of specimens are used for different tests. Different types of specimens that NAs may be asked to collect include the following:

- Urine (routine, clean-catch/mid-stream, or 24-hour)
- Stool (feces)
- Sputum (mucus coughed up from the lungs)

A **routine urine specimen** is collected anytime the resident **voids**, or urinates. The resident will void into a bedpan, urinal, commode, or hat. A **hat** is a plastic collection container sometimes put into a toilet bowl to collect and measure urine or stool (Fig. 7-33). Some residents will be able to collect their own specimens. Others will need help. The seal must be intact on specimen containers before they are used. This helps avoid specimen contamination. All specimens must be labeled with the resident's first and last name, date of birth, room number, and the date and time the specimen was collected.

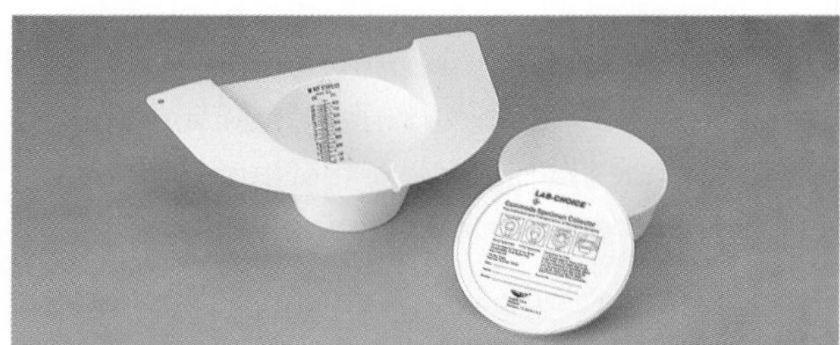

Fig. 7-33. *A hat is a container that is sometimes placed under the toilet seat to collect a specimen. Hats should be labeled. They must be cleaned after each use.*

Residents' Rights

Specimens

Body wastes and elimination needs are very private matters for most people. Having another person handle their body wastes may make residents embarrassed. NAs should be sensitive to this. They should empathize with residents. When collecting specimens, the NA should be professional. If she feels that this is an unpleasant task, she should not make it known. She should not make faces or frown. She should not use words that let the resident know she feels uncomfortable. Remaining professional when collecting specimens can help put residents at ease.

Collecting a routine urine specimen

Equipment: urine specimen container and lid, completed label (labeled with resident's name, date of birth, room number, date, and time), specimen bag, 2 pairs of gloves, bedpan or urinal (if resident cannot use portable commode or toilet), hat for toilet (if resident uses portable commode or toilet), plastic bag, toilet paper, disposable wipes, paper towels, supplies for perineal care, lab slip

1. Identify yourself by name. Identify the resident by name.
   Resident has right to know identity of his or her caregiver. Addressing resident by name shows respect and establishes correct identification.

2. Wash your hands.
   Provides for infection prevention.

3. Explain procedure to the resident. Speak clearly, slowly, and directly. Maintain face-to-face contact whenever possible.
   Promotes understanding and independence.

4. Provide for resident's privacy with curtain, screen, or door.
   Maintains resident's right to privacy and dignity.

5. Put on gloves.
   Prevents you from coming into contact with body fluids.

6. Fit the hat to toilet or commode, or provide resident with bedpan or urinal.

7. Ask the resident to void into the hat, urinal, or bedpan. Ask the resident not to put toilet paper in with the sample. Provide a plastic bag to discard toilet paper separately.
   Paper ruins the sample.

8. Make sure bed is in its lowest position. Place toilet paper and disposable wipes within resident's reach. Ask the resident to clean his hands with a wipe when finished if he is able.

9. Remove and discard gloves. Wash your hands.

10. Place the call light within resident's reach. Ask the resident to signal when done. Leave the room and close the door.
    Promotes resident's privacy and dignity.

11. When called by the resident, return and wash your hands. Put on clean gloves. Give perineal care if help is needed.

12. Take bedpan, urinal, or hat to the bathroom.

13. Pour urine into the specimen container. Specimen container should be at least half full.

14. Cover the urine container with its lid. Do not touch the inside of the container. Wipe off the outside with a paper towel. Discard the paper towel.
    Prevents contamination.

15. Apply label. Place the container in a clean specimen bag (Fig. 7-34). Seal the bag.
    Provides for safe transport.

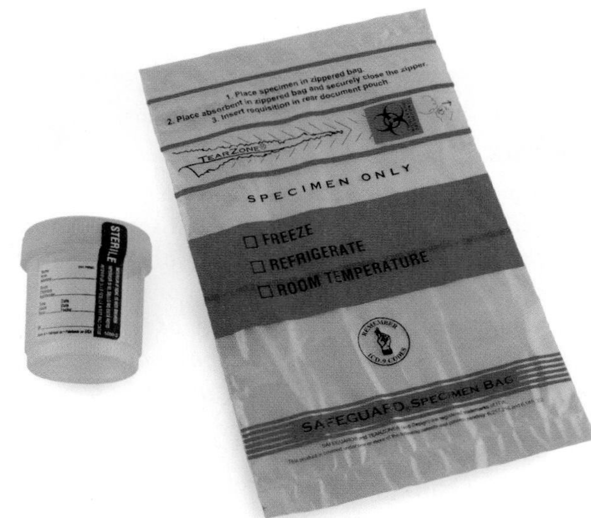

Fig. 7-34. *Specimens must always be labeled with the resident's name, date of birth, room number, the date, and time, before being taken to the lab. A specimen may need to be placed in a clean specimen bag before transporting it.*

16. Discard extra urine in the toilet. Turn the faucet on with a paper towel. Rinse the bedpan, urinal, or hat with cold water and empty it into the toilet. Flush the toilet. Place equipment in proper area for cleaning or clean it according to facility policy.

17. Remove and discard gloves.

18. Wash your hands.
    Provides for infection prevention.

19. Place call light within resident's reach.
    Allows resident to communicate with staff as necessary.

20. Report any changes in resident to the nurse.
    Provides nurse with information to assess resident.

21. Take specimen and lab slip to proper area. Document procedure using facility guidelines. Note amount and characteristics of urine.
    If you do not document the care, legally it did not happen.

A **clean-catch specimen**, or mid-stream specimen (CCMS), does not include the first and last urine in the sample. Its purpose is to determine the presence of bacteria in the urine.

Collecting a clean-catch (mid-stream) urine specimen

Equipment: specimen kit with container and lid, completed label (labeled with resident's name, date of birth, room number, date, and time), specimen bag, cleansing wipes, gloves, bedpan or urinal (if resident cannot use portable commode or toilet), plastic bag, toilet paper, disposable wipes, paper towels, towels, supplies for perineal care, lab slip

1. Identify yourself by name. Identify the resident by name.
   Resident has right to know identity of his or her caregiver. Addressing resident by name shows respect and establishes correct identification.
2. Wash your hands.
   Provides for infection prevention.
3. Explain procedure to resident. Speak clearly, slowly, and directly. Maintain face-to-face contact whenever possible.
   Promotes understanding and independence.
4. Provide for resident's privacy with curtain, screen, or door.
   Maintains resident's right to privacy and dignity.
5. Put on gloves.
   Prevents you from coming into contact with body fluids.
6. Open the specimen kit. Do not touch the inside of the container or the inside of the lid.
   Prevents contamination.
7. If the resident cannot clean his or her perineal area, you will do it. Use the cleansing wipes to do this. Be sure to use a clean area of the wipe or clean wipe for each stroke. See the bed bath procedure in Chapter 6 for a reminder on how to give perineal care.
   Improper cleaning can infect urinary tract and contaminate the sample.
8. Ask the resident to urinate a small amount into the bedpan, urinal, or toilet, and to stop before urination is complete.
9. Place the container under the urine stream. Have the resident start urinating again. Fill the container at least half full. Ask the resident to stop urinating and remove the container. Have the resident finish urinating in bedpan, urinal, or toilet.
10. After urination, provide a plastic bag so the resident can discard toilet paper. Give perineal care if help is needed. Ask the resident to clean his hands with a wipe if he is able.
11. Cover the urine container with its lid. Do not touch the inside of the container. Wipe off the outside with a paper towel. Discard the paper towel.
12. Apply label. Place the container in a clean specimen bag. Seal the bag.
    Provides for safe transport.
13. Discard extra urine in the toilet. Turn the faucet on with a paper towel. Rinse the bedpan or urinal with cold water and empty it into the toilet. Flush the toilet. Place equipment in proper area for cleaning or clean it according to facility policy.
14. Remove and discard gloves.
15. Wash your hands.
    Promotes infection prevention.
16. Place call light within resident's reach.
    Allows resident to communicate with staff as necessary.
17. Report any changes in resident to the nurse.
    Provides nurse with information to assess resident.
18. Take specimen and lab slip to proper area. Document procedure using facility guidelines. Note amount and characteristics of urine.
    If you do not document the care, legally it did not happen.

The NA should ask the resident to let her know when he can have a bowel movement. She should be ready to collect the specimen.

Collecting a stool specimen

Equipment: specimen container and lid, completed label (labeled with resident's name, date of birth, room number, date, and time), specimen bag, 2 pairs of gloves, 2 tongue blades, bedpan (if resident cannot use portable commode or toilet), hat for toilet (if resident uses portable commode or toilet), plastic bag, toilet paper, disposable wipes, paper towels, supplies for perineal care, lab slip

1. Identify yourself by name. Identify the resident by name.
   Resident has right to know identity of his or her caregiver. Addressing resident by name shows respect and establishes correct identification.
2. Wash your hands.
   Provides for infection prevention.
3. Explain procedure to resident. Speak clearly, slowly, and directly. Maintain face-to-face contact whenever possible.
   Promotes understanding and independence.
4. Provide for resident's privacy with curtain, screen, or door.
   Maintains resident's right to privacy and dignity.
5. Put on gloves.
   Prevents you from coming into contact with body fluids.
6. Ask the resident not to urinate when he is ready to move his bowels. Ask him not to put toilet paper in with the sample. Provide a plastic bag to discard toilet paper separately.
   Urine and paper ruin the sample.
7. Fit hat to toilet or commode, or provide resident with bedpan.
8. Make sure bed is in its lowest position. Place toilet paper and disposable wipes within resident's reach. Ask the resident to clean his hands with a wipe when finished if he is able.
9. Remove and discard gloves. Wash your hands.
   Promotes infection prevention.
10. Place the call light within resident's reach. Ask the resident to signal when done. Leave the room and close the door.
    Promotes resident's privacy and dignity.
11. When called by the resident, return and wash your hands. Put on clean gloves. Give perineal care if help is needed.
12. Using the two tongue blades, take about two tablespoons of stool and put it in the container. Without touching the inside of the container, cover it tightly. Apply the label and place the container in a clean specimen bag. Seal the bag.
    Prevents contamination.
13. Wrap the tongue blades in toilet paper. Put them in the plastic bag with the used toilet paper. Discard bag in proper container.
14. Empty the bedpan or container into the toilet. Turn the faucet on with a paper towel. Rinse the bedpan with cold water and empty it into the toilet. Flush the toilet. Place equipment in the proper area for cleaning or clean it according to facility policy.
15. Remove and discard gloves.
16. Wash your hands.
    Provides for infection prevention.
17. Place call light within resident's reach.
    Allows resident to communicate with staff as necessary.
18. Report any changes in resident to the nurse.
    Provides nurse with information to assess resident.
19. Take specimen and lab slip to proper area. Document procedure using facility guidelines. Note amount and characteristics of stool.
    If you do not document the care, legally it did not happen.

Sputum specimens are collected to check for respiratory problems or illness. Early morning is the best time to collect sputum. The resident should cough up the sputum and spit it directly into the specimen container. Proper personal protective equipment (PPE) must be worn when collecting sputum. The required PPE are gloves and a special mask.

6. Explain care guidelines for urinary catheters, oxygen therapy, and IV therapy

A **catheter** is a thin tube inserted into the body that is used to drain fluids or inject fluids. A **urinary catheter** is used to drain urine from the bladder. A **straight catheter** is a type of catheter that is inserted to drain urine from the bladder. It is removed immediately after urine is drained. It does not remain inside the person. An **indwelling catheter** (also called a *Foley catheter*) remains inside the bladder for a period of time (Fig. 7-35). The urine drains into a bag.

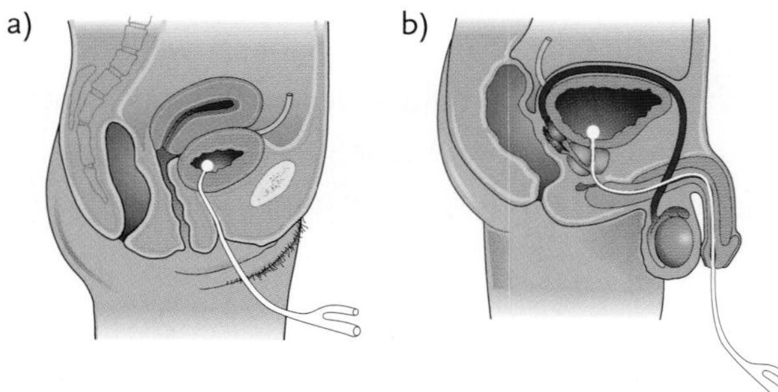

Fig. 7-35. *An illustration of a) an indwelling catheter (female) and b) an indwelling catheter (male).*

Another catheter that is used for males is an external, or **condom catheter** (also called a *Texas catheter*). It has an attachment on the end that fits onto the penis and is fastened with special tape. Urine drains through the catheter into the tubing, then into the drainage bag. A smaller bag, called a *leg bag*, attaches to the leg and collects the urine. The condom catheter is changed daily or as needed.

Nursing assistants do not insert, remove, or irrigate catheters. NAs may be asked to give daily catheter care, clean the area around the urethral opening, and empty the drainage bag.

Guidelines: Urinary Catheters

G Thoroughly wash your hands before giving catheter care.

G Keep the genital area clean to prevent infection. Because the catheter goes all the way into the bladder, bacteria can enter the bladder more easily. Daily care of the genital area (perineal care) is especially important.

G Make sure that the drainage bag always hangs lower than the hips or bladder. Urine must never flow from the bag or tubing back into the bladder. This can cause infection.

G Keep the drainage bag off the floor. Make sure the catheter tubing does not touch the floor.

G Keep the tubing as straight as possible. It should not be kinked.

Observing and Reporting: Urinary Catheters

Report any of these to the nurse:

O/R Blood in the urine or urine that looks unusual in any way

O/R Catheter bag does not fill after several hours

O/R Catheter bag fills suddenly

O/R Catheter is not in place

O/R Urine leaks from the catheter

O/R Resident reports pain or pressure

O/R Odor is present

Providing catheter care 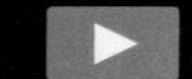

Equipment: bath blanket, disposable bed protector, bath basin with warm water, soap, bath thermometer, 2–4 washcloths or disposable wipes, towel, gloves

1. Identify yourself by name. Identify the resident by name.
   Resident has right to know identity of his or her caregiver. Addressing resident by name shows respect and establishes correct identification.

2. Wash your hands.
   Provides for infection prevention.

3. Explain procedure to resident. Speak clearly, slowly, and directly. Maintain face-to-face contact whenever possible.
   Promotes understanding and independence.

4. Provide for resident's privacy with curtain, screen, or door.
   Maintains resident's right to privacy and dignity.

5. Adjust bed to a safe level, usually waist high. Lock bed wheels.
   Prevents injury to you and to resident.

6. Lower the head of the bed. Position the resident lying flat on her back.

7. Remove or fold back top bedding. Keep the resident covered with the bath blanket.
   Promotes resident's privacy.

8. Test water temperature with a thermometer or against the inside of your wrist. Water temperature should be no higher than 105°F. Have resident check water temperature. Adjust if necessary.
   Resident's sense of touch may be different than yours; therefore, resident is best able to identify a comfortable water temperature.

9. Put on gloves.
   Prevents you from coming into contact with body fluids.

10. Ask the resident to flex her knees and raise her buttocks off the bed by pushing against the mattress with her feet. Place a clean bed protector under her perineal area, including her buttocks.
    Keeps linen from getting wet.

11. Expose only the area necessary to clean the catheter. Avoid overexposing the resident.
    Promotes resident's privacy.

12. Place a towel under the catheter tubing before washing.
    Helps keep linen from getting wet.

13. Wet a washcloth in the basin. Apply soap to the washcloth. Clean the area around the meatus. Use a clean area of the washcloth for each stroke.

14. Hold the catheter near the meatus. Avoid tugging the catheter.

15. Clean at least four inches of catheter nearest meatus. Move in only one direction, away from the meatus. Use a clean area of the washcloth for each stroke.
    Prevents infection.

16. Dip a clean washcloth in the water. Rinse area around the meatus, using a clean area of the washcloth for each stroke. With a clean, dry towel, dry the area around the meatus.

17. Dip a clean washcloth in the water. Rinse at least four inches of the catheter nearest the meatus. Move in only one direction, away from the meatus (Fig. 7-36). Use a clean area of the washcloth for each stroke.

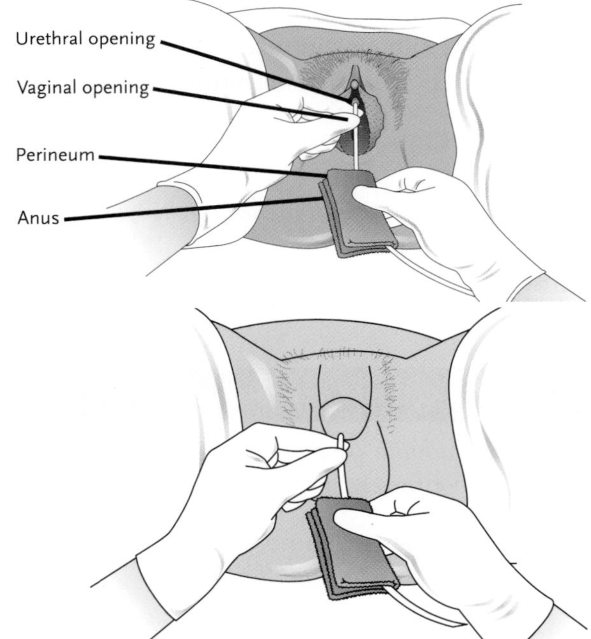

Fig. 7-36. *Hold the catheter near the meatus to avoid tugging the catheter. Moving in only one direction, away from meatus, helps prevent infection. Use a clean area of the washcloth for each stroke.*

18. With a clean, dry towel, dry at least four inches of catheter nearest the meatus. Move in only one direction, away from the meatus. Do not tug the catheter.
19. Remove bed protector from under resident and discard. Remove towel from under the catheter tubing and place in proper container. Replace top covers. Remove bath blanket and place in proper container.
20. Place used washcloths in proper container.
21. Empty the basin into the toilet and flush the toilet. Place basin in proper area for cleaning or clean and store it according to facility policy.
22. Remove and discard gloves.
23. Wash your hands.
Provides for infection prevention.
24. Return bed to lowest position.
Lowering the bed provides for safety.
25. Place call light within resident's reach.
Allows resident to communicate with staff as needed.
26. Report any changes in resident to the nurse.
Provides nurse with information to assess resident.
27. Document procedure using facility guidelines.
If you do not document the care, legally it did not happen.

Emptying the catheter drainage bag

Equipment: graduate (measuring container), alcohol wipes, paper towels, gloves

1. Identify yourself by name. Identify the resident by name.
Resident has right to know identity of his or her caregiver. Addressing resident by name shows respect and establishes correct identification.
2. Wash your hands.
Provides for infection prevention.
3. Explain procedure to resident. Speak clearly, slowly, and directly. Maintain face-to-face contact whenever possible.
Promotes understanding and independence.
4. Provide for resident's privacy with curtain, screen, or door.
Maintains resident's right to privacy and dignity.
5. Put on gloves.
6. Place a paper towel on the floor under the drainage bag. Place the graduate on the paper towel.
7. Open the clamp on the bag so that the urine flows out of the bag and into the graduate (Fig. 7-37). Do not let the spout or clamp touch the graduate.

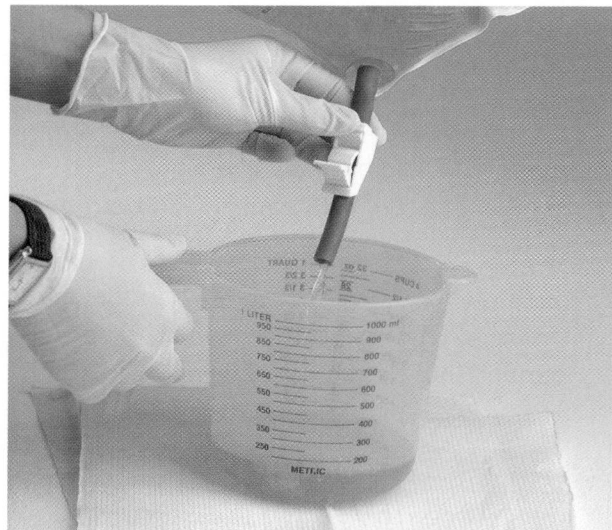

Fig. 7-37. *Keep the spout and clamp from touching the graduate while draining urine.*

8. When the urine has drained from the bag, close the clamp. Using alcohol wipes, clean the drain spout. Place the drain spout back in its holder on the bag.
9. Go into the bathroom. Place graduate on a flat surface and measure at eye level. Note the amount and characteristics of urine. Empty into the toilet and flush the toilet.
10. Clean and store graduate. Discard paper towels.

11. Remove and discard gloves.

12. Wash your hands.
    Provides for infection prevention.

13. Document procedure using facility guidelines. Note amount and characteristics of urine.
    If you do not document the care, legally it did not happen.

Oxygen therapy is the administration of oxygen to increase the supply of oxygen to the lungs. This increases oxygen to the body tissues. Oxygen therapy is used to treat breathing problems. It is prescribed by a doctor. Nursing assistants never stop, adjust, or administer oxygen.

Oxygen may be piped into a resident's room through a central system. It may be in tanks or produced by an oxygen concentrator. An oxygen concentrator is a box-like device that changes air in the room into air with more oxygen.

Some residents receive oxygen through a nasal cannula. A nasal cannula is a piece of plastic tubing that fits around the face and is secured by a strap that goes over the ears and around the back of the head. The face piece has two short prongs made of tubing. These prongs fit inside the nose, and oxygen is delivered through them (Fig. 7-38). A nurse or respiratory therapist fits the cannula. The resident can talk and eat while wearing the cannula.

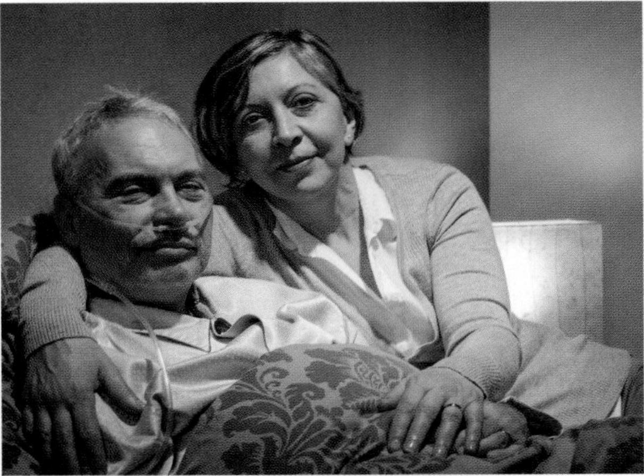

Fig. 7-38. *This man is using a nasal cannula.*

Residents who do not need concentrated oxygen all the time may use a face mask when they need oxygen (Fig. 7-39). The face mask fits over the nose and mouth. It is secured by a strap that goes over the ears and around the back of the head. Plastic tubing connects the mask to the oxygen source. It is difficult for a resident to talk while wearing the face mask. It must be removed for the resident to eat or drink anything.

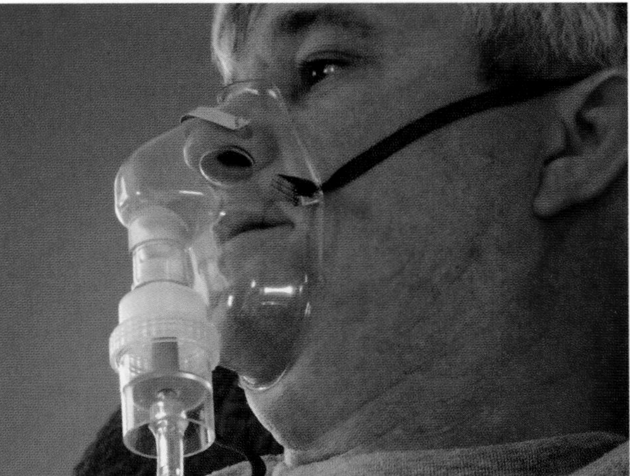

Fig. 7-39. *Residents who need oxygen only occasionally may use a face mask.*

Combustion means the process of burning. Oxygen is a very dangerous fire hazard because it supports combustion (makes other things burn). Working around oxygen requires special safety precautions.

Guidelines: Working Safely Around Oxygen

G Post *No Smoking* and *Oxygen in Use* signs. Never allow smoking where oxygen is used or stored.

G Remove all fire hazards from the room or area. Fire hazards include electrical equipment, such as electric razors and hair dryers. Other fire hazards are cigarettes, matches, and flammable liquids. **Flammable** means easily ignited and capable of burning quickly. Alcohol and nail polish remover are examples of flammable liquids. Notify the nurse if a resident does not want a fire hazard removed.

- **G** Do not burn candles, light matches, or use lighters around oxygen. Any type of open flame that is present around oxygen is a dangerous fire hazard.
- **G** Do not use an extension cord with an oxygen concentrator.
- **G** Do not place electrical cords or oxygen tubing under rugs or furniture.
- **G** Avoid using fabrics such as nylon and wool that can cause static electricity discharges.
- **G** Report if the nasal cannula or face mask causes skin irritation. Check the nasal area and behind the ears for signs of irritation.
- **G** Do not use any petroleum-based products, such as Vaseline or Chapstick, on the resident or on any part of the cannula or mask. Oil-based lubricants can be a fire hazard.
- **G** Learn how to turn off oxygen in case of fire. Never adjust the oxygen setting or dose.

Intravenous therapy, often called *IV therapy*, is the delivery of medication, nutrition, or fluids through a vein. When a doctor prescribes IV therapy, a nurse inserts a needle or tube into a vein. This gives direct access to the bloodstream. Medication, nutrition, or fluids either drip from a bag suspended on a pole or are pumped by a portable pump through a tube and into the vein. Some residents with chronic conditions may have a permanent opening for IV lines, called a *port*. It has been surgically created to allow easy access for IV fluids. Nursing assistants never insert or remove IV lines. They are not responsible for care of the IV site. Their only responsibility for IV care is to report and document any observations of changes or problems with the IV line.

Observing and Reporting: IV Therapy

Report any of the following to the nurse:

- O/R The tube/needle falls out or is removed
- O/R The tubing disconnects
- O/R The dressing around the IV site is loose or not intact
- O/R Blood is in the tubing or around the IV site
- O/R The site is swollen or discolored
- O/R The bag is broken or the level of fluid does not seem to decrease
- O/R The IV fluid is not dripping or is leaking
- O/R The IV fluid is nearly gone
- O/R The pump beeps, indicating a problem
- O/R The pump is dropped
- O/R The resident complains of pain or has trouble breathing

The NA should document her observations and the care given. The NA should not do any of the following:

- Measure blood pressure on an arm with an IV line
- Get the IV site wet
- Pull or catch the tubing on anything, such as clothing (special gowns with sleeves that snap and unsnap are available to lessen the risk of pulling out IV lines)
- Leave the tubing kinked
- Lower the IV bag below the IV site
- Touch the clamp
- Disconnect the IV from the pump or turn off the alarm

7. Discuss a resident's unit and related care

A resident's unit is the room or area where the resident lives. It contains furniture and personal items. The unit is the resident's home. It must be treated with respect. NAs must always knock and wait for permission before entering. Residents' units must be kept neat and clean. Providing a clean, safe, and orderly environment is an essential part of the NA's job.

Standard equipment often found in each resident's unit includes the following:

- Electric or manual bed
- Bedside stand
- Urinal/bedpan and covers
- Wash basin
- Emesis basin
- Soap dish and soap
- Bath blanket
- Toilet paper
- Personal hygiene items
- Overbed table
- Chair
- Call light
- Privacy curtain or screen

Small items are usually stored in bedside stands. The water pitcher and cup are often placed on top of the bedside stand. A telephone, radio, and other items, such as photos, may also be placed there.

The overbed table may be used for meals or personal care. It is a clean area. It must be kept clean and free of clutter. Bedpans, urinals, soiled linen, and other contaminated items should not be placed on overbed tables.

The intercom system is the most common call system. When the resident presses the button, a light will be seen and/or a bell will be heard at the nurses' station. The call light allows the resident to contact staff when necessary. NAs must always place the call light within the resident's reach and answer all call lights immediately.

Residents' Rights

Privacy Curtains

All residents in a facility have the legal right to personal privacy. This means that they must always be protected from public view when receiving care. Each bed usually has a privacy curtain that extends all the way around the bed. Curtains keep others from seeing a resident undressed or while having care procedures done. To protect the resident's privacy, NAs must keep this curtain closed when giving care (Fig. 7-40). Although curtains and screens block vision, they do not block sound. NAs should keep their voices low. They should not discuss a resident's care near others. Closing the door, when possible, gives more complete privacy.

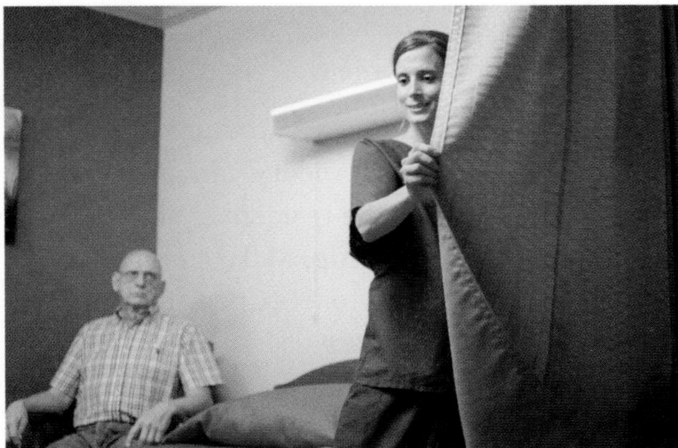

Fig. 7-40. *Nursing assistants should pull the privacy curtain around the bed before giving care.*

There are many types of equipment in a care facility. NAs must know how to use and care for all equipment properly. This helps prevent infection and injury. An NA should ask for help when needed. She should not try to use equipment that she does not know how to use.

Guidelines: Resident's Unit

- **G** Clean the overbed table after use. Place it within the resident's reach before leaving.
- **G** Keep the call light within the resident's reach. Check to see that it is within reach of the resident's stronger/unaffected hand before you leave the room.
- **G** Keep equipment clean and in good condition. If any equipment appears damaged, report it

to the nurse and/or file the proper paperwork to get it repaired. Do not use broken or damaged equipment.

- **G** OBRA requires that long-term care facilities have comfortable and safe environments by maintaining a temperature range of 71–81°F. Older people may feel cold often. Layer clothing and bed covers for warmth. Keep residents away from drafty areas. If residents control the heat and air conditioning in their rooms, do not change it for your comfort.
- **G** Remove meal trays right after meals. Check to make sure that there are no crumbs in the bed. Straighten bed linens as needed. Change linens if they become wet, soiled, or wrinkled.
- **G** Restock supplies. Make sure the resident has fresh drinking water and a clean cup within reach. Check that the resident is able to lift the pitcher and the cup. Make sure that tissues, paper towels, toilet paper, soap, and other supplies that are used daily are stocked before you leave.
- **G** If trash needs to be emptied or the bathroom needs to be cleaned, notify the housekeeping department. Trash should be emptied at least daily. Remove the trash when you leave the room if housekeeping staff is not available.
- **G** Report signs of insects or pests right away.
- **G** Do not move a resident's belongings. Do not discard any personal items. Respect the resident's things.
- **G** Clean equipment and return it to storage or take it to the proper area for cleaning. Tidy the area.

8. Explain the importance of sleep and perform proper bedmaking

Sleep is a natural period of rest for the mind and body. As a person sleeps, the mind and body's energy is restored. During sleep, vital functions are performed. These include repairing and renewing cells, processing information, and organizing memory. Sleep is essential to a person's health and well-being.

A lack of sleep causes many problems. These include decreased mental function, reduced reaction time, and irritability. Sleep deprivation also decreases immune system function.

Many elderly persons, especially those who are living away from their homes, have sleep problems. Many things can affect sleep, such as fear, anxiety, stress, noise, diet, medications, and illness. Sharing a room with another person can disturb sleep.

Observing and Reporting: Sleep Issues

When a resident complains that he or she is not sleeping well, observe and report the following:

- O/R Sleeping too much during the day
- O/R Eating or drinking items that contain caffeine late in the day
- O/R Wearing nightclothes during the day
- O/R Eating heavy meals late at night
- O/R Refusing to take medication ordered for sleep
- O/R Taking new medications
- O/R Having the TV, radio, computer, phone, or light on late at night
- O/R Having pain

Some residents spend much or all of their time in bed. Careful bedmaking is essential for comfort, cleanliness, and health. Linens should always be changed after personal care, such as bed baths. They should also be changed any time bedding or sheets are damp, soiled, or in need of straightening. Bed linens should be changed often for these reasons:

- Sheets that are damp, wrinkled, or bunched up are uncomfortable. They may keep the resident from sleeping well.

- Microorganisms thrive in moist, warm places. Bedding that is damp or unclean may cause infection and disease.
- Residents who spend long hours in bed are at risk for pressure injuries. Sheets that do not lie flat increase this risk by cutting off circulation.

Guidelines: Bedmaking

G Keep linens wrinkle-free and tidy. Change linen whenever it is wet, damp, wrinkled, or dirty.

G Wash your hands before handling clean linen (Fig. 7-41).

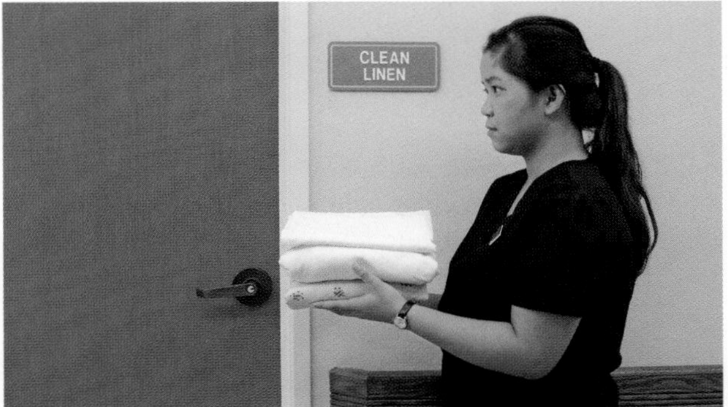

Fig. 7-41. *Make sure you have washed your hands before gathering clean linen.*

G Place clean linen on a clean surface within reach, such as a bedside stand, overbed table, or chair. Do not place clean linen on the floor or on a contaminated area.

G Don (put on) gloves before removing bed linen from the bed.

G Look for personal items, such as dentures, hearing aids, jewelry, and glasses, before removing linen.

G When removing linen, fold or roll linen so that the dirtiest area is inside. Rolling puts the dirtiest surface of the linen inward. This lessens contamination.

G Do not shake linen or clothes. It may spread airborne contaminants.

G Bag soiled linen at the point of origin. Do not take it to other residents' rooms.

G Sort soiled linen away from resident care areas.

G Place wet linen in leakproof bags.

G Wear gloves when handling soiled linen. Hold soiled linen away from your body. Place it in the proper container or area immediately. If dirty linen touches your uniform, your uniform becomes contaminated.

G Change disposable bed protectors whenever they become soiled or wet. Discard them in the proper container. Put a clean bed protector on the bed when you change linen.

If a resident cannot get out of bed, an NA must change the linens with the resident in bed. An **occupied bed** is a bed made while the resident is still in the bed. When making the bed, the NA should use a wide stance and bend her knees. Bending from the waist should be avoided, especially when tucking sheets under the mattress. The height of the bed should be raised to make the job easier and safer.

Making an occupied bed 

Equipment: clean linen—mattress pad, fitted or flat bottom sheet, disposable bed protector (if needed), cotton draw sheet, flat top sheet, blanket(s), bedspread (if used), bath blanket, pillowcase(s), gloves

1. Identify yourself by name. Identify the resident by name.
   Resident has right to know identity of his or her caregiver. Addressing resident by name shows respect and establishes correct identification.
2. Wash your hands.
   Provides for infection prevention.
3. Explain procedure to resident. Speak clearly, slowly, and directly. Maintain face-to-face contact whenever possible.
   Promotes understanding and independence.
4. Provide for resident's privacy with curtain, screen, or door.
   Maintains resident's right to privacy and dignity.

5. Place clean linen on clean surface within reach (e.g., bedside stand, overbed table, or chair).
   Prevents contamination of linen.

6. Adjust bed to a safe level, usually waist high. Lower the head of the bed. Lock bed wheels.
   When bed is flat, resident can be moved without working against gravity. Adjusting bed level and locking wheels prevents injury to you and resident.

7. Put on gloves.
   Prevents you from coming into contact with body fluids.

8. Loosen top linen from the end of the bed on the working side.

9. Unfold the bath blanket over the top sheet to cover the resident. Remove the top sheet. Keep the resident covered at all times with the bath blanket.

10. You will make the bed one side at a time. Raise the far side rail (if used). Then go to the other side of the bed. Help the resident to turn onto her side, toward the raised side rail.

11. Loosen the bottom soiled linen, mattress pad, and protector, if present, on the working side.

12. Roll the bottom soiled linen toward the resident, soiled side inside. Tuck it snugly against the resident's back.
    Rolling puts dirtiest surface of linen inward, lessening contamination. The closer the linen is rolled to resident, the easier it is to remove from the other side.

13. Place the mattress pad (if used) on the bed, attaching elastic at corners on the working side.

14. Place and tuck in the clean bottom linen. Make hospital corners to keep the bottom sheet wrinkle-free (Fig. 7-42). Finish with the bottom sheet free of wrinkles.
    Hospital corners prevent a resident's feet from being restricted by or tangled in linen when getting in and out of bed.

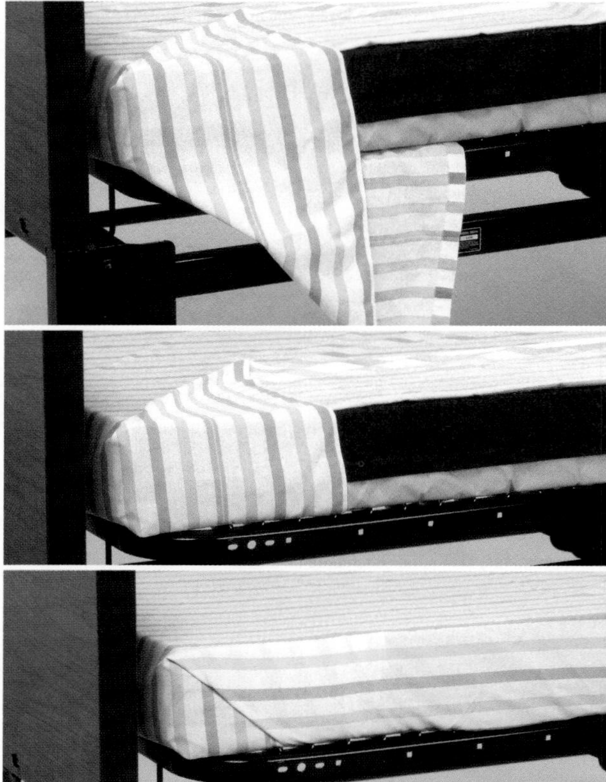

Fig. 7-42. *Hospital corners help keep the flat sheet smooth under the resident.*

15. Smooth the bottom sheet out toward the resident. Be sure there are no wrinkles in the mattress pad. Roll the extra material toward the resident. Tuck it under the resident's body (Fig. 7-43).

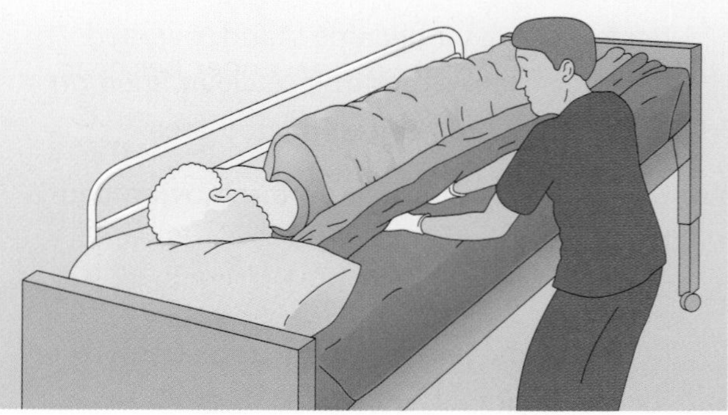

Fig. 7-43. *Tuck extra material under the resident's body.*

16. If using a disposable bed protector, unfold it and center it on the bed. Tuck the side near you under the mattress. Smooth it out toward the resident. Tuck as you did with the sheet.

17. If using a draw sheet, place it on the bed. Tuck in on your side, smooth, and tuck as you did with the other bedding.

18. Raise the side rail (if used) nearest you. Go to the other side of the bed and lower that side rail. Help the resident roll or turn onto clean bottom sheet, toward you. Protect the resident from any soiled matter on the old linens.

19. Loosen the soiled linen. Check for any personal items. Roll the linen from the head to the foot of the bed. Avoid contact with your skin or clothes. Place it in a hamper or bag. Do not put it on the floor or furniture. Do not shake it. Soiled linens are full of microorganisms that should not be spread to other parts of the room.
Always work from cleanest (head of bed) to dirtiest (foot of bed) area to prevent spread of infection. Rolling puts dirtiest surface of linen inward, lessening contamination.

20. Pull the clean linen through as quickly as possible. Start with the mattress pad and wrap around corners. Pull and tuck in the clean bottom linen just like the other side. Pull and tuck in the bed protector and draw sheet (if used). Make hospital corners with the bottom sheet. Finish with bottom sheet free of wrinkles.

21. Ask the resident to turn onto her back. Help as needed. Keep the resident covered and comfortable, with a pillow under her head. Raise the side rail.

22. Unfold the top sheet. Place it over the resident and center it. Ask the resident to hold the top sheet. Slip the bath blanket out from underneath (Fig. 7-44). Put it in the hamper or bag.

23. Place a blanket over the top sheet. Match the top edges. Place the bedspread over the blanket (if used), matching the top edges. Tuck the bottom edges of the top sheet, blanket, and bedspread under the foot of the bed. Make hospital corners on each side. Loosen the top linens over the resident's feet. At the head of the bed, fold the top sheet over the blanket about six inches.
Loosening the top linens over the feet prevents pressure on the feet, which can cause pressure injuries.

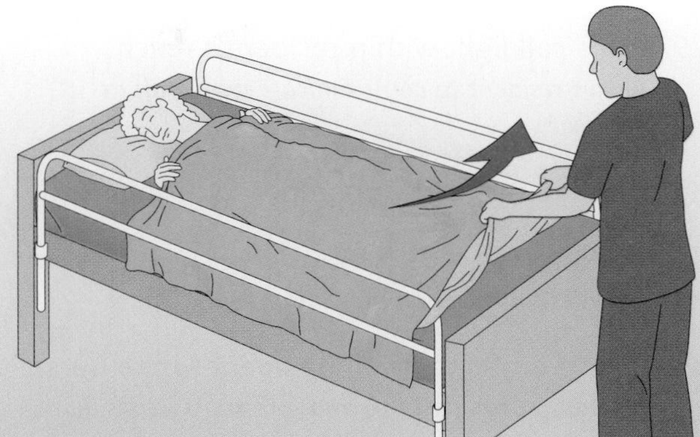

Fig. 7-44. *With the resident holding on to the top sheet, pull the bath blanket out.*

24. Remove the pillow. Do not hold it near your face. Remove the soiled pillowcase by turning it inside out. Place it in the hamper or bag.

25. Remove and discard gloves. Wash your hands.
Provides for infection prevention.

26. With one hand, grasp the clean pillowcase at the closed end. Turn it inside out over your arm. Next, using the same hand that has the pillowcase over it, grasp the center of the end of the pillow. Pull the pillowcase over it with your free hand (Fig. 7-45). Do the same for any other pillows. Place them under resident's head with open end away from door.

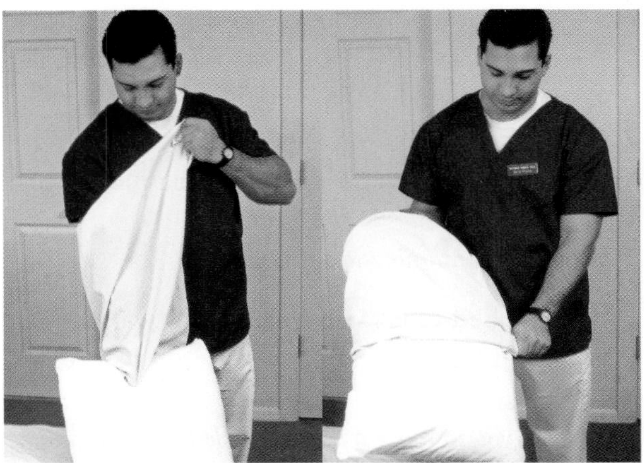

Fig. 7-45. *After the pillowcase is turned inside out over your arm, grasp the center of the end of the pillow. Pull the pillowcase over the pillow.*

27. Make resident comfortable.

28. Return bed to lowest position. Leave side rails in the ordered position.
 Lowering the bed provides for safety.

29. Place call light within resident's reach.
 Allows resident to communicate with staff as necessary.

30. Take laundry bag or hamper to proper area.

31. Wash your hands.
 Provides for infection prevention.

32. Report any changes in resident to the nurse.
 Provides nurse with information to assess resident.

33. Document procedure using facility guidelines.
 If you do not document the care, legally it did not happen.

Mattresses can be heavy. It is easier to make an empty bed than one with a resident in it. An **unoccupied bed** is a bed made while no resident is in the bed. If the resident can be moved, the NA's job will be easier.

Making an unoccupied bed 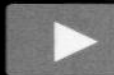

Equipment: clean linen—mattress pad, fitted or flat bottom sheet, disposable bed protector if needed, blanket(s), cotton draw sheet, flat top sheet, bedspread (if used), pillowcase(s), gloves

1. Wash your hands.
 Provides for infection prevention.

2. Place clean linen on clean surface within reach (e.g., bedside stand, overbed table, or chair).
 Prevents contamination of linen.

3. Adjust bed to a safe level, usually waist high. Put bed in flattest position. Lock bed wheels.
 Allows you to make a neat, wrinkle-free bed.

4. Put on gloves.
 Prevents you from coming into contact with body fluids.

5. Loosen soiled linen. Roll soiled linen (soiled side inside) from the head to the foot of the bed. Avoid contact with your skin or clothes. Place it in a hamper or bag. Do not put it on the floor or furniture. Do not shake it. Remove pillows and pillowcases and place pillowcases in hamper or bag.
 Always work from cleanest (head of bed) to dirtiest (foot of bed) area to prevent spread of infection. Rolling puts dirtiest surface of linen inward, lessening risk of contamination.

6. Remove and discard gloves. Wash your hands.
 Provides for infection prevention.

7. Remake the bed. Start with the mattress pad and wrap around corners. Place and tuck in the clean bottom linen. Make hospital corners to keep the bottom sheet wrinkle-free. Put on the disposable bed protector and draw sheet (if used), smooth, and tuck under sides of the bed.

8. Place top sheet, blanket, and bedspread (if used) over bed. Center these, tuck under the end of the bed, and make hospital corners. Fold down the top sheet over the blanket about six inches. Fold both the top sheet and blanket down so the resident can easily get into bed. If the resident will not be returning to bed immediately, leave bedding up.

9. Put on clean pillowcases. Replace pillows.

10. Return bed to lowest position.

11. Take laundry bag or hamper to proper area.

12. Wash your hands.
 Provides for infection prevention.

13. Document procedure using facility guidelines.
 If you do not document the care, legally it did not happen.

A **closed bed** is a bed completely made with the bedspread and blankets in place. It is made for residents who will be out of bed most of the day. It is also made when a resident is discharged. A closed bed is turned into an **open bed** by folding the linen down to the foot of the bed. An open bed is a bed that is ready to receive a resident who has been out of bed all day or who is being admitted to the facility.

9. Discuss dressings and bandages

Sterile dressings cover new, open, or draining wounds. A nurse changes these dressings. Non-sterile dressings are applied to dry, closed wounds that have less chance of infection. Nursing assistants may change non-sterile dressings. State regulations vary, so NAs should follow state and facility policies.

Changing a dry dressing using non-sterile technique

Equipment: package of square gauze dressings, adhesive tape, scissors, 2 pairs of gloves, plastic bag

1. Identify yourself by name. Identify the resident by name.
   Resident has right to know identity of his or her caregiver. Addressing resident by name shows respect and establishes correct identification.

2. Wash your hands.
   Provides for infection prevention.

3. Explain procedure to resident. Speak clearly, slowly, and directly. Maintain face-to-face contact whenever possible.
   Promotes understanding and independence.

4. Provide for resident's privacy with curtain, screen, or door.
   Maintains resident's right to privacy and dignity.

5. Cut pieces of tape long enough to secure the dressing. Hang tape on the edge of a table within reach. Open the four-inch gauze square package without touching the gauze. Place the opened package on a flat surface.

6. Put on gloves.
   Protects you from coming into contact with body fluids.

7. Remove soiled dressing by gently peeling the tape toward the wound. Lift the dressing off the wound. Do not drag it over the wound. Observe dressing for any odor or drainage. Notice the color and size of the wound. Discard used dressing in plastic bag.
   Avoids disturbing wound healing. Reduces risk of contamination.

8. Remove and discard gloves in plastic bag. Wash your hands.
   Provides for infection prevention.

9. Put on clean gloves. Touching only the outer edges of the new gauze, remove it from package. Apply it to the wound. Tape gauze in place. Secure it firmly (Fig. 7-46).
   Keeps gauze as clean as possible.

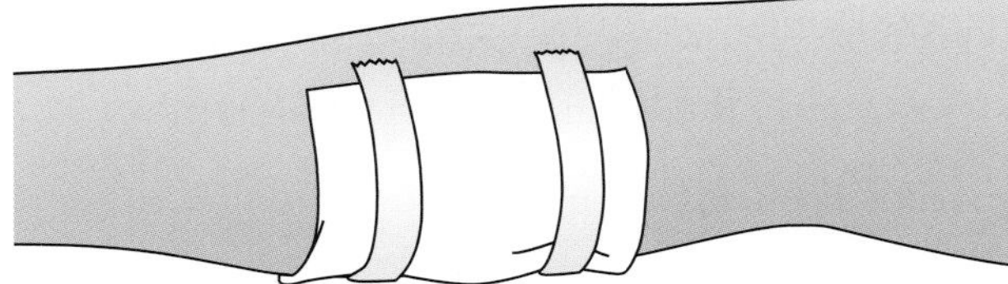

Fig. 7-46. *Tape gauze in place to secure the dressing. Do not completely cover all areas of the dressing with tape.*

10. Discard supplies in proper container.

11. Remove and discard gloves.

12. Wash your hands.
    Provides for infection prevention.

13. Place call light within resident's reach.
    Allows resident to communicate with staff as necessary.

14. Report any changes in resident to the nurse.
    Provides nurse with information to assess resident.

15. Document procedure according to facility guidelines.
    If you do not document the care, legally it did not happen.

Elastic bandages (also called *non-sterile bandages, ACE bandages,* or *ACE wraps*) are used to hold dressings in place, secure splints, and support and protect body parts. In addition, these bandages may decrease swelling that occurs from an injury (Fig. 7-47).

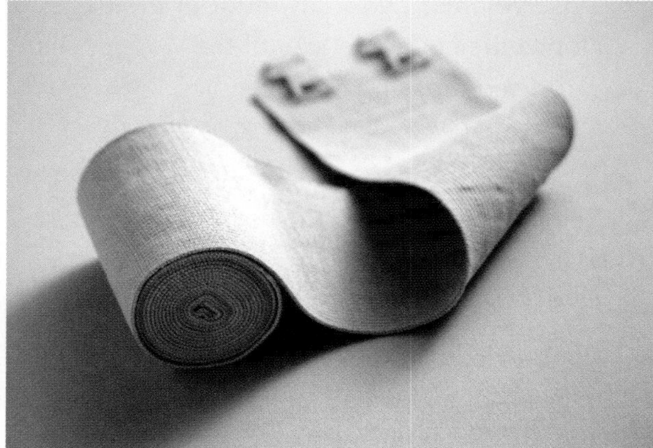

Fig. 7-47. *This is one type of elastic bandage.*

NAs may be required to help with elastic bandages. Duties may include the following:

- Bringing the bandage to the resident
- Positioning the resident to apply the bandage
- Washing and storing the bandage
- Documenting observations about the bandage

Some states allow NAs to apply and remove elastic bandages. They should follow their facility's policies and the care plan regarding elastic bandages.

Guidelines: Elastic Bandages

G Keep the area to be wrapped clean and dry.

G Apply bandage snugly enough to control bleeding and prevent movement of dressings. Make sure that the body part is not wrapped too tightly, which can decrease circulation.

G Wrap the bandage evenly, in a figure-eight pattern, so that no part of the wrapped area is pinched.

G Do not tie the bandage, because this cuts off circulation to the body part; the end is held in place with special clips or tape.

G Remove the bandage as often as indicated in the care plan.

G Check the bandage often. It can become wrinkled or loose, which causes it to lose effectiveness. It can also become bunched up, which causes pressure and possible discomfort.

G Check on the resident 10 to 15 minutes after the bandage is applied to check for signs of poor circulation. Signs and symptoms of poor circulation include the following:

- Swelling
- Pale, gray, cyanotic (bluish), or white skin
- Shiny, tight skin
- Skin that is cold to the touch
- Sores
- Numbness
- Tingling
- Pain or discomfort

Loosen the bandage if you note any signs of poor circulation, and notify the nurse immediately.

8 Nutrition and Hydration

1. Identify the six basic nutrients and explain MyPlate

Proper nutrition is very important. **Nutrition** is how the body uses food to maintain health. Bodies need a well-balanced diet with nutrients and plenty of fluids. This helps the body grow new cells, maintain normal body function, and have energy. Proper nutrition in early life helps ensure health later in life. For the ill or elderly, a well-balanced diet helps maintain muscle and skin tissues and prevent pressure injuries. A healthy diet promotes the healing of wounds. It also helps a person cope with stress.

A **nutrient** is a necessary substance that provides energy, promotes growth and health, and helps regulate metabolism. Metabolism is the process by which nutrients are broken down to be used by the body for energy, growth, and maintenance. The body needs the following six nutrients for growth and development:

1. **Water**: Water is the most essential nutrient for life. It is needed by every cell in the body. Without it, a person can only live for a few days. Water assists in the digestion and absorption of food. It helps with waste elimination. Through perspiration, water also helps maintain normal body temperature. Keeping enough fluid in the body is necessary for health.

The fluids a person drinks—water, juice, soda, coffee, tea, and milk—provide most of the water the body uses. Some foods are also sources of water, including soup, celery, lettuce, and apples.

2. **Carbohydrates**: Carbohydrates supply the body with energy and extra protein. They help the body use fat efficiently. Carbohydrates also provide fiber, which is necessary for bowel elimination. Carbohydrates can be divided into two basic types: complex and simple. Complex carbohydrates are found in bread, cereal, potatoes, rice, pasta, vegetables, and fruits (Fig. 8-1). Simple carbohydrates are found in sugars, sweets, syrups, and jellies. Simple carbohydrates do not have the same nutritional value that complex carbohydrates have.

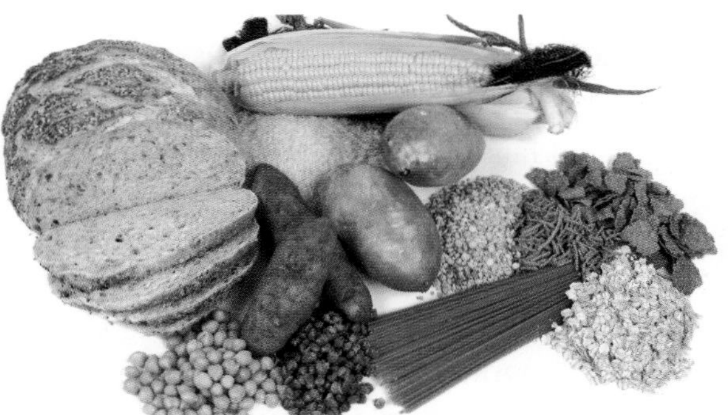

Fig. 8-1. *Some sources of complex carbohydrates.*

3. **Protein**: Proteins are part of every body cell. They are needed for tissue growth and repair. Proteins also supply energy for the body. Excess proteins are excreted by the kidneys or stored as body fat. Sources of protein include seafood, poultry, meat, eggs, milk, cheese, nuts, nut butters, peas, beans or legumes, and vegetarian meat substitutes from a variety of food sources (Fig. 8-2). Whole-grain cereals, pastas, rice, and breads contain some proteins, too.

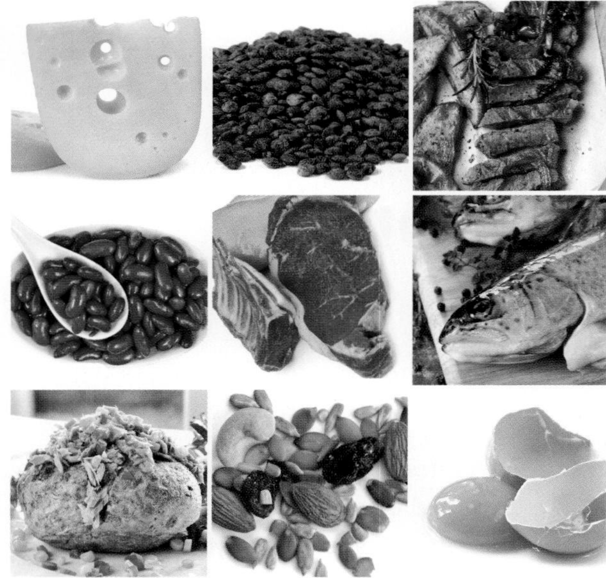

Fig. 8-2. Some sources of protein.

4. **Fats**: Fat helps the body store energy. Fats add flavor to food and are important for the absorption of certain vitamins. Excess fat in the diet is stored as fat in the body.

Fat falls into four categories: saturated, trans, monounsaturated, and polyunsaturated. Saturated and trans fats can increase cholesterol levels and the risk of some diseases, such as cardiovascular disease. Monounsaturated and polyunsaturated fats can be helpful in the diet, and can decrease the risk of cardiovascular disease and type 2 diabetes.

Some fats come from animal sources, such as butter, beef, pork, fowl, fish, and dairy products. Some fats come from plant sources, such as olives, nuts, and seeds (Fig. 8-3).

5. **Vitamins**: Vitamins are substances needed by the body to function. The body cannot make most vitamins. They can only be obtained from certain foods. Vitamins A, D, E, and K are fat-soluble vitamins. This means they are carried and stored in body fat. Vitamins B and C are water-soluble vitamins. They are broken down by water in the body and cannot be stored. Excess vitamins B and C are eliminated in urine and feces.

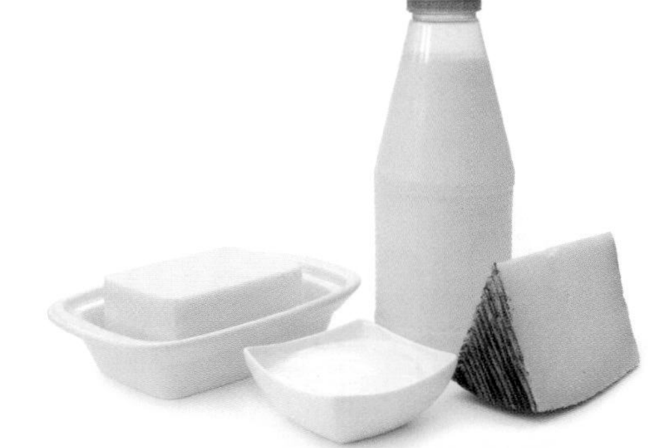

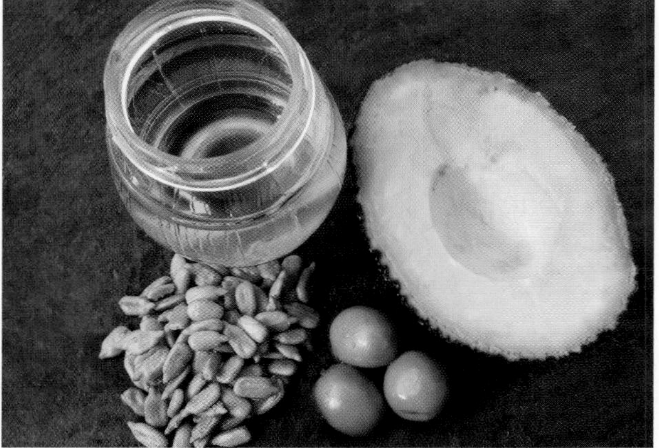

Fig. 8-3. Some animal sources of fat are in the top photo and plant sources are in the bottom photo.

6. **Minerals**: Minerals maintain body functions. Minerals help build bones, make hormones, and help in blood formation. They provide energy and control body processes. Zinc, iron, calcium, and magnesium are examples of minerals. Minerals are found in many foods.

Most foods have several nutrients. However, no one food has all the nutrients needed for a healthy body. This is why it is important to eat a daily diet that is well balanced. There is not one single dietary plan that is right for everyone. People have different nutritional needs depending upon their age, gender, and activity level.

In 2011, in response to increasing rates of obesity, the United States Department of Agriculture (USDA, usda.gov) developed MyPlate to help people build a healthy plate at mealtimes (Fig. 8-4). The MyPlate icon emphasizes vegetables, fruits, grains, protein, and low-fat dairy products.

MyPlate gives suggestions and tools for making healthy choices. It does not provide specific messages about what a person should eat. The MyPlate icon includes the following food groups:

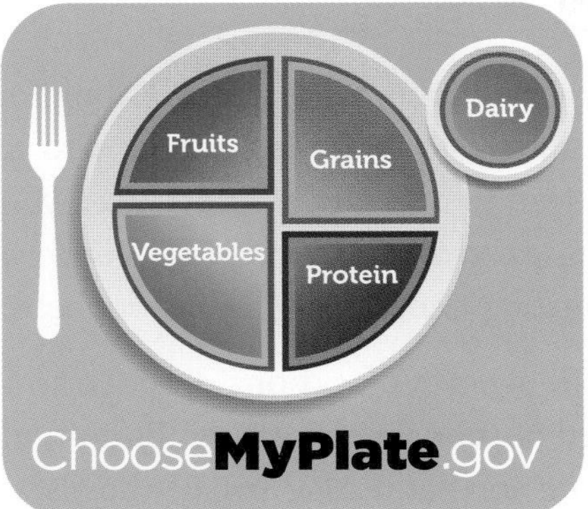

Fig. 8-4. The U.S. Department of Agriculture developed the MyPlate icon and website (ChooseMyPlate.gov) to help promote healthy eating practices.

Vegetables and fruits: Vegetables and fruits should make up half of a person's plate. Vegetables include all fresh, frozen, canned, and dried vegetables, and vegetable juices. There are five subgroups within the vegetable group, organized by their nutritional content. These are dark green vegetables, red and orange vegetables, beans and peas, starchy vegetables, and other vegetables. A variety of vegetables from these subgroups should be eaten every day. Dark green, red, and orange vegetables have the best nutritional content (Fig. 8-5).

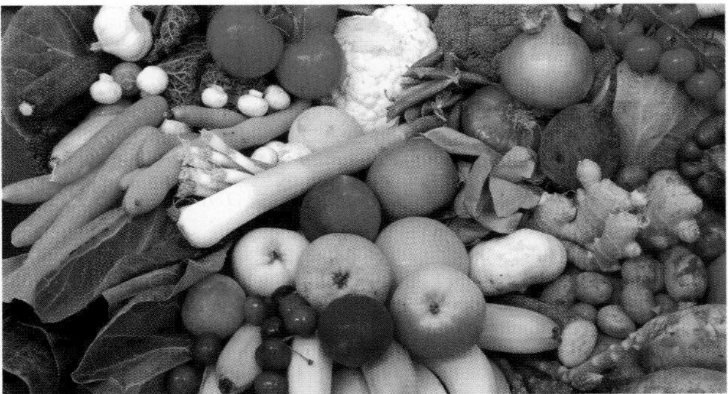

Fig. 8-5. Eating a variety of vegetables every day, especially dark green, red, and orange vegetables, helps promote health.

Vegetables are low in fat and calories and have no cholesterol (although sauces and seasonings may add fat, calories, and cholesterol). They are good sources of dietary fiber, potassium, vitamin A, vitamin E, and vitamin C.

Fruits include all fresh, frozen, canned, and dried fruits, and 100% fruit juices. Most choices should be whole, cut-up, or pureed fruit, rather than juice, for the additional dietary fiber provided. Fruit can be added as a main dish, side dish, or dessert.

Fruits, like vegetables, are naturally low in fat, sodium, and calories and have no cholesterol. They are important sources of dietary fiber and many nutrients, including folic acid, potassium, and vitamin C. Foods containing dietary fiber help provide a feeling of fullness with fewer calories. Folic acid helps the body form red blood cells. Vitamin C is important for growth and repair of body tissues.

Grains: A person should make half his grain intake whole grains. There are many different grains. Some common ones are wheat, rice, oats, cornmeal, and barley. Foods made from grains include bread, pasta, oatmeal, breakfast cereals, tortillas, and grits. Grains can be divided into two groups: whole grains and refined grains. Whole grains contain bran and germ, as well as the endosperm. Refined grains retain only the endosperm. The endosperm is the tissue within flowering plants. It surrounds and nourishes the plant embryo. Examples of whole grains include brown rice, wild rice, bulgur, oatmeal, whole-grain corn, whole oats, whole wheat, and whole rye. Foods rich in fiber reduce the risk of heart disease and other diseases and may reduce constipation.

Protein: MyPlate guidelines emphasize the importance of eating a variety of protein foods every week. Meat, poultry, seafood, and eggs are animal sources of proteins. Beans, peas, soy products, vegetarian meat substitutes, nuts, and seeds are plant sources of proteins. Seafood should be eaten twice a week in place of meat or poultry. Seafood that is higher in oils and low in mercury, such as salmon or trout, is a better choice (Fig. 8-6). Lean meats and poultry, as well as eggs and egg whites, can be eaten on a regular basis. A person should eat plant-based protein foods more often. Beans and peas, soy products (tofu, tempeh, many vegetarian products), vegetarian meat substitutes, nuts, and seeds are low in saturated fat and high in fiber. Some nuts and seeds (flax, walnuts) are excellent sources of essential fatty acids. These acids may reduce the risk of heart disease. Sunflower seeds and almonds are good sources of vitamin E.

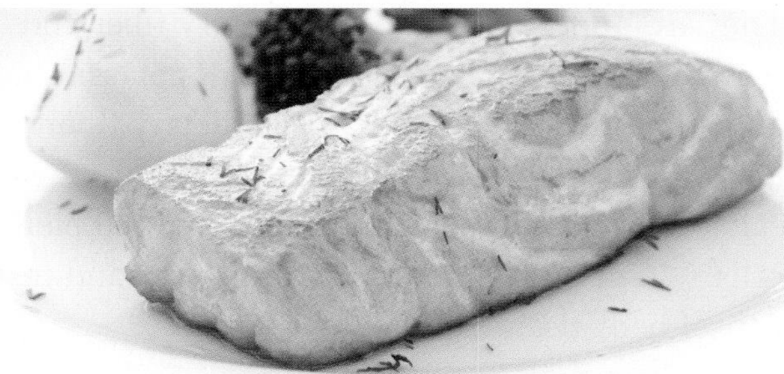

Fig. 8-6. *Fish, like this salmon, contains healthy oils and is a good source of protein.*

Dairy: All milk products and foods made from milk that retain their calcium content, such as yogurt and cheese, are part of the dairy category. Most dairy group choices should be fat-free (0%) or low-fat (1%). Fat-free or low-fat milk or yogurt should be chosen more often than cheese. Milk and yogurt contain less sodium than most cheeses.

Milk provides nutrients that are vital for the health and maintenance of the body. These nutrients include calcium, potassium, vitamin D, and protein. Fat-free or low-fat milk provides these nutrients without the extra calories and saturated fat. Soy products enriched with calcium are an alternative to dairy foods.

The following guidelines provide additional tips for making healthy food choices:

Guidelines: Healthy Food Choices

- G Balance calories. Calorie balance is the relationship between the calories obtained from food and fluids consumed and the calories used during normal body functions and physical activity. Proper calorie intake varies from person to person. To find the proper calorie intake, the USDA suggests visiting ChooseMyPlate.gov.
- G Enjoy your food, but eat less. Eating too fast or eating without paying attention to your food can lead to overeating. Know when you feel hungry and when you are full. Notice what you are eating. Stop eating when you feel satisfied.
- G Avoid oversized portions. Choose smaller-sized portions when eating. Portion out food before you eat it. Use smaller bowls and plates for meals. When eating out, split food with others or take part of your meal home.
- G Eat these foods more often: vegetables, fruits, whole grains, and fat-free or 1% milk and low-fat dairy products. These foods have better nutrients for health.
- G Eat these foods less often: foods high in solid fats, added sugars, and salt. These foods include fatty meats like bacon and hot dogs, cheese, fried foods, ice cream, and cookies.
- G Check sodium content in foods. Read product labels to determine if they contain salt or sodium. Foods high in sodium include the following:
  - Cured meats, including ham, bacon, lunch meat, sausage, and hot dogs
  - Salty or smoked fish, including herring, sardines, anchovies, and smoked salmon
  - Processed cheese and some other cheeses
  - Salted foods, including nuts, pretzels, potato chips, and dips
  - Vegetables preserved in brine, such as pickles, sauerkraut, and olives
  - Sauces with high concentrations of salt, including steak and soy sauces, ketchup, mustard, and mayonnaise
  - Commercially-prepared foods such as breads, canned soups and vegetables, and certain breakfast cereals

Select canned foods that are labeled *sodium-free, very low sodium, low sodium,* or *reduced sodium.*

G Drink water instead of sugary drinks. Drinking water or unsweetened beverages reduces sugar and calorie intake. Sweetened beverages, such as soda, fruit punch, and sports drinks, are a major source of sugar and calories in diets.

2. Describe factors that influence food preferences

Culture, ethnicity, income, education, religion, and geography all affect ideas about nutrition. Food preferences may be formed by what a person ate as a child, by what tastes good, or by personal beliefs about what should be eaten (Fig. 8-7). Some people choose not to eat any animals or animal products, such as steak, chicken, butter, or eggs. These people are *vegetarians* or *vegans,* depending on what they eat.

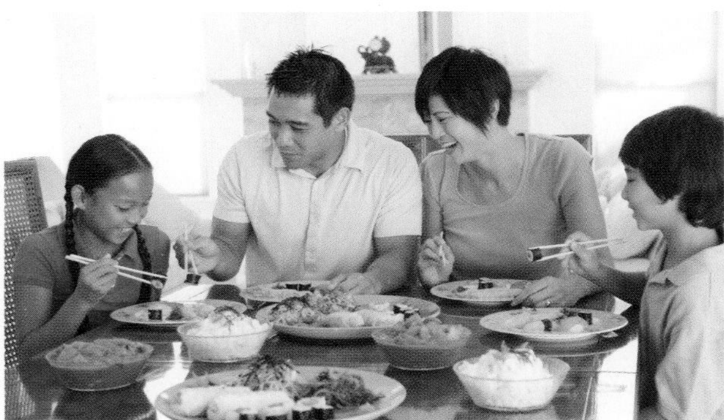

Fig. 8-7. *Food likes and dislikes are influenced by what a person ate as a child.*

The region or culture a person grows up in often affects his food preferences. People from the southwestern United States may like spicy foods. Southern cooking may include fried foods, such as fried chicken or fried okra. Ethnic groups often share common foods. These may be eaten at certain times of the year or all the time. Religious beliefs affect diet, too. Some Muslims and Jewish people do not eat any pork. Mormons may not drink alcohol, coffee, or tea.

Food preferences may change while a resident is living at a facility. Just as anyone may decide that he likes some foods for a time and then change his mind, so may a resident. Providing person-centered care means respecting each resident's preferences. It is never appropriate to make fun of personal preferences. If an NA notices that certain food is not being eaten—no matter how small the amount—she should report it to the nurse.

Residents' Rights

Food Choices

Residents have the legal right to make choices about their food. They can choose what kind of food they want to eat. They can refuse the food and drink being offered. NAs must honor a resident's personal beliefs and preferences about selecting and avoiding specific foods. Although residents have the right to refuse, it is best to ask questions when they do. For example, if a resident refuses dinner, the NA can ask if there is something wrong with the food. The resident may say he is Jewish and cannot eat a pork chop because it is not kosher. NAs should respond to requests for different food in a pleasant way. The NA can explain that she will report to the nurse and will get him another meal as quickly as possible. She can take the tray to the dietitian or dietary department so that an alternative may be offered.

3. Explain special diets

Residents who do not have any health problems that require a change in diet often eat a *regular* diet. However, residents who are ill may be placed on **therapeutic**, **modified**, or **special diets**. With special diets, certain nutrients or fluids may need to be restricted or removed. Some medications may also interact with certain foods, which then must be eliminated. Residents who do not eat enough may be placed on supplementary diets. Diets are also used for weight control and food allergies.

Several types of diets are available for different illnesses. Some residents may be on a combination of special diets. The care plan should specify any special diet the resident needs. NAs must never modify a resident's diet. Special diets can only be prescribed by doctors and planned by dietitians, along with residents.

Low-Sodium Diet: People are most familiar with sodium as one of the two components of salt. Salt is restricted first in a low-sodium diet because it is high in sodium. Residents who have high blood pressure, heart disease, or kidney disease may be placed on a low-sodium diet. A modified fluid intake may also be required for people with these conditions. For residents on a low-sodium diet, salt will not be used. Salt shakers or packets will not be on the diet tray. Common abbreviations for this diet are *Low Na*, which means low sodium, or *NAS*, which stands for *No Added Salt*.

Fluid-Restricted Diet: The fluid taken into the body through food and fluids must equal the fluid that leaves the body through perspiration, stool, urine, and expiration. This is fluid balance. When fluid intake is greater than fluid output, body tissue becomes swollen with fluid. People with severe heart disease or kidney disease may have trouble processing fluid. To prevent further damage, doctors may restrict fluid intake. For residents on fluid restriction, the NA will measure and document exact amounts of fluid intake and report excesses to the nurse. Additional fluids or foods that count as fluids, such as ice cream, puddings, gelatin, etc., should not be offered. If the resident complains of thirst or requests fluids, the NA should tell the nurse. A common abbreviation for this diet is *RF*, which stands for *Restrict Fluids*.

Low-Protein Diet: People who have kidney disease may be on low-protein diets. Protein is restricted because it breaks down into compounds that may lead to further kidney damage. The extent of the restrictions depends on the stage of the disease and if the resident is on dialysis. Vegetables and starches, such as breads and pasta, are encouraged.

Low-Fat Diet: Eating a diet high in saturated fats may put a person at risk for heart disease. Choosing to eat unsaturated fat can reduce the risk of heart disease and improve HDL (good) cholesterol levels. People who have heart disease or who have had heart attacks are often prescribed a diet that is low in saturated fat. People with gallbladder disease, diseases that interfere with fat digestion, and liver disease are also placed on a low-fat diet. This diet limits the intake of saturated fat (trans fat should be avoided). Foods high in saturated fat include fatty meats, high-fat dairy products (especially cheese), hydrogenated oils, and desserts and baked goods. Foods that contain healthier fats include olive oil, nuts, avocado, and fatty fish like salmon (Fig. 8-8). People who have gallbladder disease or other digestive problems may be placed on a diet that restricts all fats. *Low-Fat* may be listed on the diet card for this diet. Sometimes *Cardiac Diet* may be listed on the diet card, which means a diet that is low in sodium, fat, and cholesterol, as well as in excess sugar.

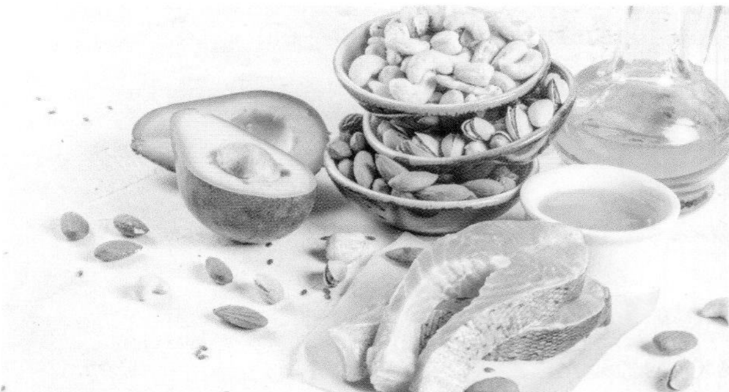

Fig. 8-8. *Healthier fats come from olives, nuts, avocados, and fatty fish.*

Modified Calorie Diet: Some residents may need to reduce calories to lose weight or prevent weight gain. Other residents may need to gain weight or increase calories because of malnutrition, surgery, illness, or fever. Common abbreviations for this diet are *Low-Cal* or *High-Cal*.

Diabetic Diet: Calories and carbohydrates are carefully controlled in the diets of residents who have diabetes. Protein and fats are also regulated. The types and amounts of food are determined by nutritional and energy needs. A dietitian and the resident will make up a meal plan. It will include all the right types and amounts of food for each day. The meal plan may use a carbohydrate-counting approach (often called *carb counting*). After the proper amount of carbohydrates is determined by the dietitian, they need to be counted in each meal or snack. Nutrition labels need to be read, paying attention to serving size and carbohydrate content. Food portions may need to be measured.

To keep their blood glucose levels near normal, residents who have diabetes must eat the right amount of the right type of food at the right time. They must eat all that is served. NAs should encourage them to do so. Other foods should not be offered without the nurse's approval. If a resident will not eat what is recommended, does not finish meals, or is not following the diet, the NA should tell the nurse.

People who have diabetes should avoid foods that are high in sugar. Sugary foods can cause problems with insulin balance. A meal tray for a resident with diabetes may have artificial sweetener, low-calorie jelly, and/or low-calorie maple syrup. Artificial sweeteners, rather than sugar, may be used in coffee or tea. The American Diabetes Association's (ADA) website, diabetes.org, has more information.

Vegetarian Diet: Health issues, such as diabetes or obesity, may cause a person to require a vegetarian diet. A person may also choose to eat a vegetarian diet for religious reasons, or due to a dislike of meat, a compassion for animals, a belief in nonviolence, or financial issues. There are different types of vegetarian diets:

- A lacto-ovo vegetarian diet excludes all meats, fish, and poultry, but allows eggs and dairy products.
- A lacto-vegetarian diet eliminates poultry, meats, fish, and eggs, but allows dairy products.
- An ovo-vegetarian diet omits all meats, fish, poultry, and dairy products, but allows eggs.
- A vegan diet eliminates poultry, meats, fish, eggs, and dairy products, along with all foods that are derived from animals.

A person might choose to limit his intake of animal-based foods by being a pescatarian. A pescatarian diet eliminates all meats and poultry, but allows fish and other seafood. Eggs and dairy products may be consumed.

Liquid Diet: A liquid diet is usually ordered for a short time due to a medical condition or before or after a test or surgery. It is ordered when a resident needs to keep the intestinal tract free of food. A liquid diet consists of foods that are in a liquid state at body temperature. Liquid diets are usually ordered as *clear* or *full*. A clear liquid diet includes clear juices, broth, gelatin, and popsicles. A full liquid diet includes all the liquids served on a clear liquid diet, with the addition of cream soups, milk, and ice cream.

Soft Diet and Mechanical Soft Diet: The soft diet is soft in texture and consists of soft or chopped foods that are easier to chew and swallow. Foods that are hard to chew and swallow, such as raw fruits and vegetables and some meats, will be restricted. High-fiber foods, fried foods, and spicy foods may also be limited. Doctors order this diet for residents who have trouble chewing and swallowing due to dental problems or other medical conditions. It is also ordered for people who are going from a liquid diet to a regular diet.

The mechanical soft diet consists of chopped or blended foods that are easier to chew and swallow. Foods are prepared with blenders, food processors, or cutting utensils. Unlike the soft diet, the mechanical soft diet does not limit spices, fat, and fiber. Only the texture of foods is changed. This diet is used for people recovering from surgery or who have trouble chewing and swallowing.

Pureed Diet: To **puree** a food means to blend or grind it into a thick paste of baby food consistency. The food should be thick enough to hold its form in the mouth. This diet does not require a person to chew his food. A pureed diet is often used for people who have trouble chewing and/or swallowing more textured foods.

Nutritional Supplements

Illness and injury may call for nutritional supplements to be added to the resident's diet. Certain medications also change the need for nutrients. For example, some medication prescribed for high blood pressure increases the need for potassium.

Nutritional supplements may come in a powdered or liquid form. Some supplements may be premixed and ready to drink. Powdered supplements need to be mixed with a liquid before being taken. NAs may not be allowed to prepare supplements and/or hand them to residents. They should follow facility policy.

The NA may need to make sure the resident takes the supplement at the ordered time. A resident who is ill, tired, or in pain may not have much of an appetite. It may take a long time for him to drink a large glass of a thick liquid. The NA should be patient and encouraging. If a resident does not want to drink the supplement, the NA should not insist that he do so. However, she should report this to the nurse.

4. Describe how to assist residents in maintaining fluid balance

Water is an essential nutrient for life. Proper fluid intake is important. Drinking enough water or other fluids per day can help prevent constipation and urinary incontinence. Without enough fluid, urine becomes concentrated. More concentrated urine creates a higher risk for infection. Proper fluid intake also helps to dilute wastes and flush out the urinary system. It may even help prevent confusion.

The sense of thirst can lessen as people age. Infection, fever, diarrhea, and some medications will also increase the need for fluid intake. NAs should remind residents to drink fluids often (Fig. 8-9). Some residents will drink more fluids if they are offered them in smaller amounts, rather than in one large glassful. Some residents will have an order to encourage or restrict fluids because of medical conditions. When a resident has a restrict fluids (RF) order, the NA should not give the resident any extra fluids or a water pitcher unless the nurse approves it.

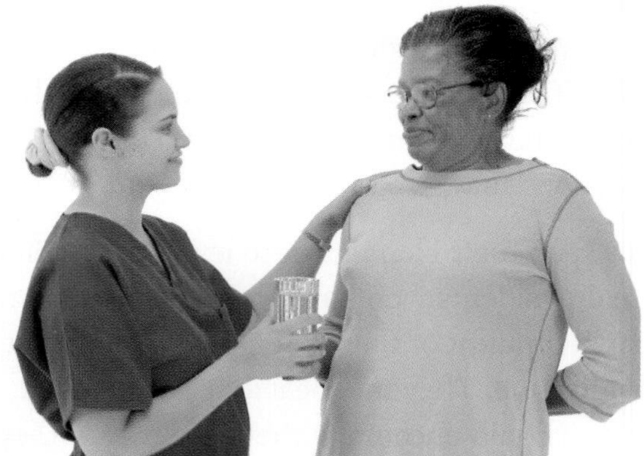

Fig. 8-9. *Drinking enough water and other fluids promotes health. NAs should encourage residents to drink fluids often.*

The abbreviation **NPO** means *nothing by mouth*. This means that a resident is not allowed to have anything to eat or drink. Some residents have such a severe problem with swallowing that it is unsafe to give them anything by mouth. These residents will receive nutrition through a feeding tube or intravenously. Some residents may not be able to eat and drink for a short time before a medical test or surgery. NAs need to know this abbreviation. They should never offer any food or drink, even water, to a resident with this order.

Dehydration occurs when a person does not have enough fluid in the body. Dehydration is a serious condition. It is a major problem among the elderly. People can become dehydrated if they do not drink enough or if they have diarrhea or are vomiting. Preventing dehydration is very important.

Guidelines: Preventing Dehydration

G Report observations and warning signs to the nurse immediately.

G Encourage residents to drink every time you see them.

G Offer fresh water or other fluids often. Offer drinks that the resident enjoys. Some residents may prefer water or sparkling water (seltzer water). Some may not like water and prefer other types of beverages, such as juice, soda, tea, or milk. Some residents do not want ice in their drinks. As always, it is important to provide person-centered care. Honor personal preferences. Report to the nurse if the resident tells you she does not like the fluids being served.

G Ice chips, frozen flavored ice sticks, and gelatin are also forms of liquids. Offer them often. Do not offer ice chips or sticks if a resident has a swallowing problem.

G If appropriate, offer sips of liquid between bites of food at meals and snacks.

G Make sure the pitcher and cup are nearby and are light enough for the resident to lift.

G Offer assistance if the resident cannot drink without help. Use adaptive cups as needed.

G Record fluid intake and output.

Observing and Reporting: Dehydration

Report any of these to the nurse:

O/R Resident drinks fewer than six 8-ounce glasses of liquid per day

O/R Resident drinks little or no fluids at meals

O/R Resident needs help drinking from a cup or glass

O/R Resident has trouble swallowing liquids

O/R Resident has frequent vomiting, diarrhea, or fever

O/R Resident is easily confused or tired

Report any of these signs and symptoms:

O/R Dry mouth

O/R Cracked lips

O/R Sunken eyes

O/R Dark urine

O/R Strong-smelling urine

O/R Weight loss

O/R Complaints of abdominal pain

Serving fresh water

Equipment: water pitcher, ice scoop, cup, straw, gloves

1. Identify yourself by name. Identify the resident by name.
   Resident has right to know identity of his or her caregiver. Addressing resident by name shows respect and establishes correct identification.
2. Wash your hands.
   Provides for infection prevention.
3. Put on gloves.
   Promotes infection prevention.
4. Scoop ice into the water pitcher without touching the ice scoop to the pitcher. Add fresh water. Do not touch the pitcher to the spout or faucet.
5. Use and store the ice scoop properly. Do not allow ice to touch your gloved hand and fall back into the container. Place the scoop in the proper receptacle after each use.
   Avoids contamination of ice.
6. Take the pitcher to the resident.
7. Pour water into the resident's cup. Offer the resident a drink of water. Leave the pitcher and cup at the bedside.
   Encourages resident to maintain hydration.
8. Make sure that the pitcher and cup are light enough for the resident to lift. Leave a straw if the resident desires and does not have swallowing problems.
   Demonstrates understanding of resident's abilities and/or limitations. Prevents dehydration.
9. Place call light within resident's reach.
   Allows resident to communicate with staff as necessary.
10. Remove and discard gloves.

11. Wash your hands.
    Provides for infection prevention.

Fluid overload occurs when the body cannot handle the fluid consumed. This often affects people with heart or kidney disease.

Observing and Reporting: Fluid Overload

Report any of these to the nurse:

- O/R Swelling/edema of extremities (ankles, feet, fingers, hands); **edema** is swelling caused by excess fluid in body tissues.
- O/R Weight gain (daily weight gain of one to two pounds)
- O/R Decreased urine output
- O/R Shortness of breath
- O/R Increased heart rate
- O/R Anxiety
- O/R Skin that appears tight, smooth, or shiny

5. List ways to identify and prevent unintended weight loss

Unintended weight loss is a serious problem for the elderly. Weight loss can mean that the resident has a serious medical condition. It can lead to skin breakdown. This leads to pressure injuries. It is very important for NAs to report any weight loss, no matter how small. If a resident has diabetes, COPD, cancer, HIV, or other diseases, he is at a greater risk for malnutrition. (Chapter 4 has more information.)

Guidelines: Preventing Unintended Weight Loss

- G Report observations and warning signs to the nurse.
- G Food should look, taste, and smell good. The resident may have a poor sense of taste and smell.
- G Encourage residents to eat. Talk about food being served in a positive tone of voice. Use positive words (Fig. 8-10).

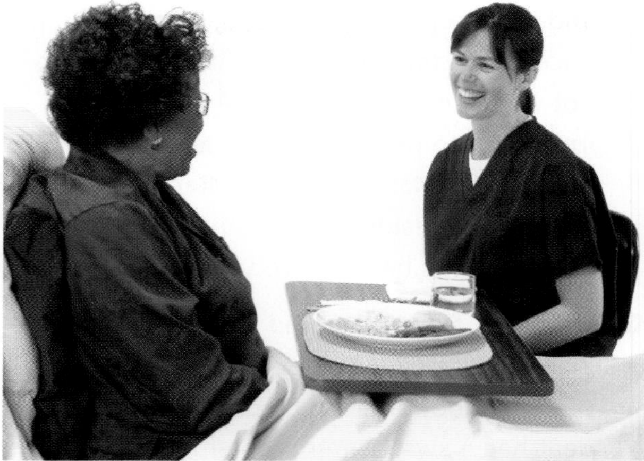

Fig. 8-10. *Be friendly and positive while helping residents with eating. This helps promote appetite and may prevent weight loss.*

- G Honor residents' food likes and dislikes.
- G Offer different kinds of foods and beverages.
- G Help residents who have trouble feeding themselves.
- G Season foods to residents' preferences.
- G Allow time for residents to finish eating.
- G Tell the nurse if residents have trouble using utensils.
- G Record meal/snack intake.
- G Give oral care before and after meals if the resident requests it.
- G Position residents sitting upright for eating.
- G If resident has had a loss of appetite and/or seems sad, ask about it.

Observing and Reporting: Unintended Weight Loss

Report any of these to the nurse:

- O/R Resident needs help eating or drinking
- O/R Resident eats less than 75% of meals served

O/R Resident has mouth pain

O/R Resident has dentures that do not fit

O/R Resident has difficulty chewing or swallowing

O/R Resident coughs or chokes while eating

O/R Resident is sad, has crying spells, or withdraws from others

O/R Resident is confused, wanders, or paces

6. Identify ways to promote appetites at mealtime

Mealtime is often one of the most anticipated times of a resident's day. Mealtime is important for getting proper nourishment. It is also a time for socializing, which has a positive effect on eating. Socializing can help prevent weight loss, dehydration, and malnutrition. It can also prevent loneliness and boredom. Promoting healthy eating is an important part of a nursing assistant's job. Mealtime should be pleasant and enjoyable.

Guidelines: Promoting Appetites

G Assist residents with grooming and hygiene tasks before dining as needed.

G Give oral care before eating if requested.

G Offer a trip to the bathroom or help with elimination needs before eating.

G Help residents wash hands before eating.

G Encourage the use of dentures, eyeglasses, and hearing aids. If these are damaged, notify the nurse.

G Check the environment. The temperature should be comfortable. Address any odors. Keep the noise level low. Televisions should be off. Do not shout or raise your voice. Do not bang plates or cups.

G Seat residents next to their friends or people with like interests. Encourage conversation.

G Properly position residents for eating. Usually the proper position is upright, at a 90-degree angle. This helps prevent swallowing problems. If residents use a wheelchair, make sure they are sitting at a table that is the right height. Most facilities have adjustable tables for wheelchairs. Residents who use geri-chairs—reclining chairs on wheels—should be upright, not reclined, while eating.

G Serve food promptly to maintain the correct temperature. Keep food covered until ready to serve.

G Plates and trays should look appetizing. If they do not, inform your supervisor.

G Give the resident the proper eating tools. Use assistive utensils if needed (Fig. 8-11).

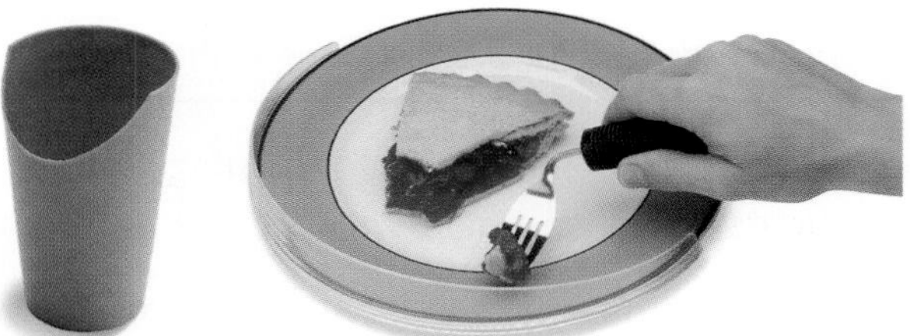

Fig. 8-11. *Special cups, plates with guards on them, and utensils with thick handles that are easier to hold are examples of assistive devices that can help with eating.* (PHOTOS COURTESY OF NORTH COAST MEDICAL, INC., WWW.NCMEDICAL.COM, 800-821-9319)

G Be cheerful, positive, and helpful. Make conversation if the resident wishes to talk.

G Honor requests regarding food. Residents have the legal right to ask for and receive different food. They can also ask for additional food.

7. Demonstrate how to assist with eating

Residents will need different levels of help with eating. Some residents will not need any help. Other residents will only need help setting up. They may only need someone to open cartons and cut and season their food. Once that is done, they can feed themselves. The NA should check with these residents from time to time to see if they need anything else.

Other residents will be completely unable to feed themselves. It will be the NA's job to feed them. Residents who must be fed are often embarrassed and depressed about their dependence on another person. NAs should be sensitive to this and give privacy while residents are eating. Residents should not be rushed through their meals.

NAs should only give assistance as specified, when necessary, or when residents request it. They should encourage residents to do what they can. For example, if a resident can hold and use a napkin, she should. If she can hold and eat finger foods, the NA should offer them. There are devices that help residents eat more independently (Fig. 8-11 on previous page). More adaptive devices are shown in Chapter 9.

Guidelines: Assisting a Resident with Eating

G Before you begin serving or helping residents, wash your hands.

G It is very important to identify residents before serving a meal tray. Feeding a resident the wrong food can cause serious problems, even death. Verify that you have the right resident. Check the diet card against the name listed outside the door (if available). Ask the resident to state his name. Check that the diet on the tray is correct and matches the diet card.

G Sit at a resident's eye level. The resident should be sitting upright, at a 90-degree angle. Make eye contact with the resident.

G If the resident wishes, allow time for prayer.

G Never treat the resident like a child. This is embarrassing and disrespectful. It is hard for many people to accept help with eating. Be supportive and encouraging.

G Test the temperature of the food by putting your hand over the dish to sense the heat. Do not touch food to test its temperature. If you think the food is too hot, do not blow on it to cool it. Offer other food to give it time to cool.

G Cut foods and pour liquids as needed. Season foods to the resident's preference.

G Identify the foods and fluids that are in front of the resident. Call pureed foods by the correct name. For example, ask, "Would you like green beans?" rather than referring to it as "some green stuff."

G Ask the resident which food he wants to eat first. Allow him to make the choice, even if he wants to eat dessert first.

G Do not mix foods unless the resident requests it.

G Do not rush the meal. Allow time for the resident to chew and swallow each bite. Be relaxed.

G Be social and friendly. Make simple conversation if the resident wishes to do so. Use appropriate topics, such as the news, weather, the resident's life, things the resident enjoys, and food preferences. Say positive things about the food being served, such as, "This smells really good," and, "This looks really fresh."

G Give the resident your full attention while she is eating. Do not talk to other staff members while helping a resident eat.

G Alternate food and drink. Alternating cold and hot foods or bland foods and sweets can help increase appetite.

G If the resident wants a different food from what is being served, inform the dietitian so that an alternative may be offered.

Residents' Rights

Clothing Protectors

Residents have the right to refuse to wear a clothing protector. An NA can offer a clothing protector but should not insist that a resident wear one. The resident's wishes should be respected. A clothing protector should not be referred to as a *bib*. Residents are not children, and this is disrespectful.

Feeding a resident 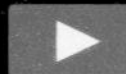

Equipment: meal and beverage; eating utensils; clothing protector; washcloths, wipes, or towel

1. Identify yourself by name. Identify the resident by name.
   Resident has right to know identity of his or her caregiver. Addressing resident by name shows respect and establishes correct identification.
2. Wash your hands.
   Provides for infection prevention.
3. Explain procedure to resident. Speak clearly, slowly, and directly. Maintain face-to-face contact whenever possible.
   Promotes understanding and independence.
4. Provide for resident's privacy with curtain, screen, or door.
   Maintains resident's right to privacy and dignity.
5. Look at the diet card or menu. Ask the resident to state her name. If the resident is unable to state her name, check identification another way, such as looking at a photo ID or an armband. Verify that the resident has received the right tray.
   Tray should only contain foods, fluids, and condiments permitted on the diet.
6. Raise the head of the bed. Make sure the resident is in an upright sitting position (at a 90-degree angle).
   Promotes ease of swallowing. Prevents aspiration of food and beverage.
7. Adjust bed height to where you will be able to sit at the resident's eye level. Lock bed wheels.
8. Place the tray where it can be easily seen by the resident, such as on the overbed table.
9. Help the resident to clean her hands if she cannot do it herself.
   Promotes good hygiene and infection prevention.
10. Help the resident put on clothing protector if desired.
    Protects resident's clothing from food and beverage spills.
11. Sit in a chair facing the resident at the resident's eye level (Fig. 8-12). Sit on the stronger side if the resident has one-sided weakness.
    Promotes good communication. Lets resident know that he or she will not be rushed while eating.

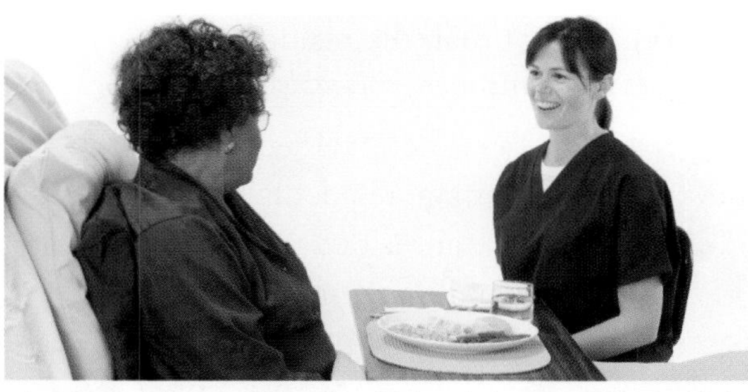

Fig. 8-12. *The resident should be sitting upright, and the NA should be sitting at her eye level.*

12. Tell the resident what foods and beverage are on the tray. Offer a drink of beverage. Ask what the resident would like to eat first.
    Resident has legal right to make decisions.
13. Check the temperature of the food. Using utensils, offer the food in bite-sized pieces. Tell the resident the content of each bite of food offered (Fig. 8-13). Alternate types of food, allowing for the resident's preferences. Do not feed all of one type before offering another type. Make sure the resident's mouth is empty before the next bite or sip. Report any swallowing problems to the nurse immediately.
    Small pieces are easier to chew and lessen the risk of choking. If the mouth is empty before offering more food, it lessens the risk of choking.

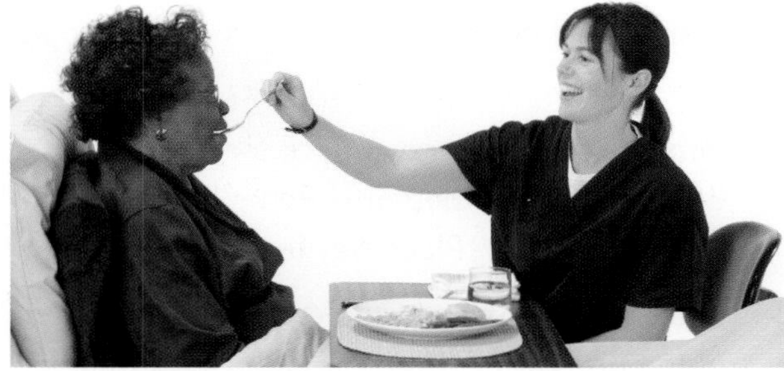

Fig. 8-13. *Offer the food in bite-sized pieces. Tell the resident the content of each bite of food.*

14. Offer sips of beverage throughout the meal. If you are holding the cup, touch it to the resident's lips before you tip it. Give small, frequent sips.
Promotes ease of swallowing.

15. Talk with the resident during the meal (Fig. 8-14). Do not rush the resident.
Makes mealtime more enjoyable.

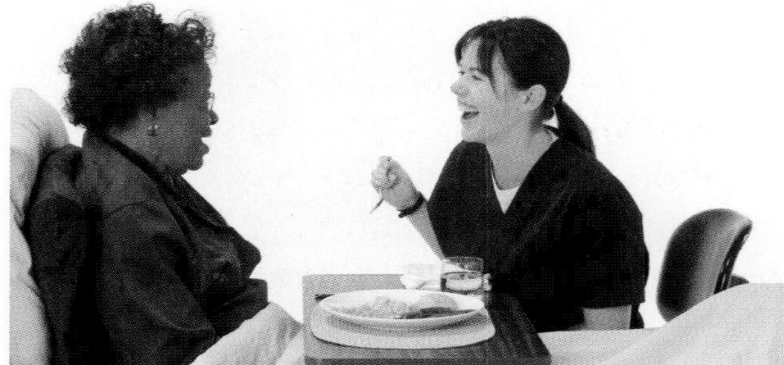

Fig. 8-14. *Socializing during mealtime makes eating more enjoyable. It may help promote a healthy appetite.*

16. Wipe food from the resident's mouth and hands as needed during the meal (Fig. 8-15). Wipe again at the end of the meal.
Maintains resident's dignity.

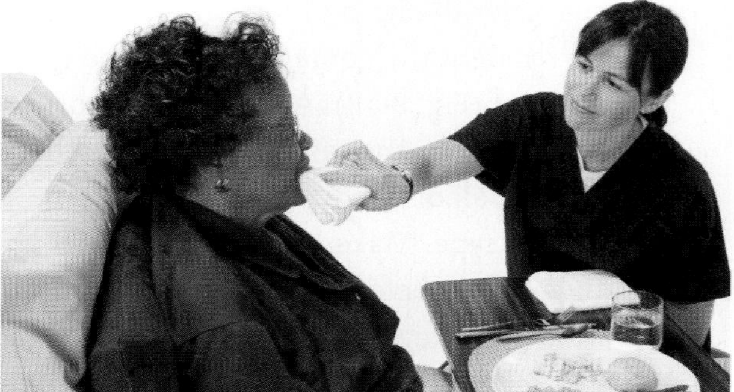

Fig. 8-15. *Wiping food from the mouth during the meal helps to maintain the resident's dignity.*

17. Remove the clothing protector if used. Place it and used washcloths or wipes in the proper containers.

18. Remove the food tray. Check for eyeglasses, dentures, or any personal items before removing the tray. Place tray in the proper area.

19. Make resident comfortable. Keep the resident in the upright position for at least 30 minutes. Make sure the bed is free of crumbs.
Food left on sheets can cause skin breakdown.

20. Return bed to lowest position. Remove privacy measures.
Provides for safety.

21. Place call light within resident's reach.
Allows resident to communicate with staff as necessary.

22. Wash your hands.
Provides for infection prevention.

23. Report any changes in resident to the nurse.
Provides nurse with information to assess resident.

24. Document procedure using facility guidelines.
If you do not document the care, legally it did not happen.

Food trays and plates should also be observed after the meal. This helps to identify residents with poor appetites. It may also signal illness, a problem such as dentures that do not fit properly, or a change in food preferences.

All facilities keep track of how much food and fluid a resident consumes. Percentages are often used to document food intake, but the method can vary. The dietitian calculates the percentages for meals. The NA may be asked to document how much of the entire meal a resident ate. For example, if the resident ate the entire meal served, the NA would document that 100% was eaten. If the resident ate about half of the meal, the NA would document 50% eaten, and so on. NAs must document food intake accurately. They should follow their facility's policies.

8. Identify signs and symptoms of swallowing problems

Residents may have conditions that make eating or swallowing difficult. **Dysphagia** means difficulty in swallowing. A stroke, or CVA, can cause weakness and paralysis on one side of the body. Nerve and muscle damage from head and neck cancer, multiple sclerosis, Parkinson's disease, or Alzheimer's disease may also be present. If a resident has trouble swallowing, soft foods and thickened liquids will be served. A special cup will help make swallowing easier.

NAs need to be able to recognize and report signs that a resident has a swallowing problem. Signs and symptoms of swallowing problems include the following:

- Coughing during or after meals
- Choking during meals
- Dribbling saliva, food, or fluid from the mouth
- Having food residue inside the mouth or cheeks during or after meals
- Gurgling during or after meals or losing one's voice
- Eating slowly
- Avoiding eating
- Spitting out pieces of food
- Swallowing several times per mouthful
- Clearing the throat frequently during and after meals
- Watering eyes when eating or drinking
- Food or fluid coming up into the nose
- Making a visible effort to swallow
- Breathing rapidly or with shorter breaths while eating or drinking
- Difficulty chewing food
- Difficulty swallowing medications

Residents with swallowing problems may be restricted to consuming only thickened liquids. Thickened liquids have a thickening powder or agent added to them. This improves the ability to control fluid in the mouth and throat. A doctor orders the necessary thickness after the resident has been evaluated by a speech-language pathologist.

Some beverages arrive already thickened and ready to drink. Other beverages must have the thickening agent added before serving. If thickening is ordered, it must be used with all liquids. This means that regular liquids, such as water or other beverages, should not be offered to residents who must have thickened liquids. There are three basic thickened consistencies:

1. **Nectar Thick**: This consistency is thicker than water. It is the thickness of a thick juice, such as a pear nectar or tomato juice. A resident can drink this from a cup.
2. **Honey Thick**: This consistency has the thickness of honey. It will pour very slowly. A resident will usually use a spoon to consume it.
3. **Pudding Thick**: With this consistency, the liquids have become semi-solid, much like pudding. A spoon should stand up straight in the glass when put into the middle of the drink. A resident must consume these liquids with a spoon.

Swallowing problems put residents at high risk for choking on food or drink. Inhaling food, fluid, or foreign material into the lungs is called **aspiration**. Aspiration can cause pneumonia or death. An NA should alert the nurse immediately if any problems occur while eating.

Guidelines: Preventing Aspiration

- **G** Position residents in an upright position (90-degree angle) for eating and drinking. Do not feed residents in a reclined position.
- **G** Offer small pieces of food or small spoonfuls of pureed food.
- **G** Feed residents slowly. Do not rush them.
- **G** Place food in the unaffected, or stronger, side of the mouth.
- **G** Make sure the mouth is empty before offering another bite of food or sip of drink.
- **G** Keep residents in the upright position for at least 30 minutes after eating and drinking.

When the digestive system does not function properly, **parenteral nutrition** (**PN**) (sometimes referred to as *total parenteral nutrition*) may be needed. With parenteral nutrition, a solution of nutrients goes directly into the bloodstream. It bypasses the digestive system. NAs are not responsible for parenteral nutrition. They may be assigned to measure the resident's temperature or assemble supplies. In addition, duties include observing, reporting, and documenting any changes in the resident or problems with the feeding.

When a person is unable to swallow, he may be fed through a tube. A **nasogastric tube** is inserted into the nose and goes to the stomach. A tube can also be placed into the stomach through the abdominal wall. This is called a **percutaneous endoscopic gastrostomy** (**PEG**) **tube**. The surgically-created opening into the stomach that allows the insertion of a tube is called a **gastrostomy** (Fig. 8-16). Tube feedings are used when residents cannot swallow but can digest food. Conditions that may prevent swallowing include coma, cancer, stroke, refusal to eat, and extreme weakness. It is important to remember that residents have the legal right to refuse treatment. This includes the insertion of tubes.

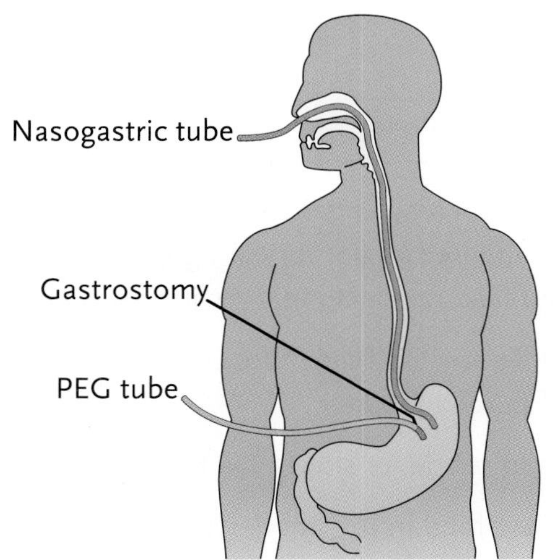

Fig. 8-16. *Nasogastric tubes are inserted through the nose. PEG tubes are inserted through the abdominal wall into the stomach.*

NAs never insert or remove tubes, do the feeding, or irrigate (clean) the tubes. They may assemble equipment and supplies and hand them to the nurse. NAs may position residents in a sitting position for feeding. They may also discard or clean and store used equipment and supplies. In addition, NAs may observe, report, and document any changes in the resident or problems with the feeding.

Guidelines: Tube Feedings

- **G** Wash your hands before assisting with any aspect of tube feedings.
- **G** Make sure the tubing is not coiled, kinked, or resting underneath the resident.
- **G** Be aware if resident has an order for *nothing by mouth* or *NPO*.
- **G** The tube is only inserted and removed by a doctor or nurse. If it comes out, report it immediately.
- **G** A doctor will prescribe the type and amount of feeding. The feedings should be at room temperature and in liquid form.
- **G** A resident with a feeding tube should always have the head of the bed elevated 30 degrees. However, during a feeding, the resident should remain in a sitting position with the head of the bed elevated at least 45 degrees. This helps prevent serious problems, such as aspiration. The elderly can develop pneumonia or even die from improper positioning during tube feedings. After the feeding, keep the resident upright for as long as ordered, at least 30 minutes.
- **G** If the resident must remain in bed for long periods during feedings, give careful skin care. This helps to prevent pressure injuries on the hips and sacral area.

Observing and Reporting: Tube Feedings

Report any of these to the nurse immediately:

- O/R Redness or drainage around the opening
- O/R Skin sores or bruises

- O/R Cyanotic skin
- O/R Resident complaints of pain or nausea
- O/R Choking or coughing
- O/R Vomiting
- O/R Diarrhea
- O/R Swollen abdomen
- O/R Fever
- O/R Tube falls out
- O/R Problems with equipment
- O/R Sound of feeding pump alarm
- O/R Change of resident's inclined position

9. Describe how to assist residents with special needs

Residents with specific diseases or conditions, such as stroke, Parkinson's disease, Alzheimer's disease or other dementias, head trauma, blindness, confusion, or those recovering from a stroke, may need special assistance when eating.

Guidelines: Dining Techniques

- G Use assistive devices such as utensils with built-up handle grips and plate guards. Assistive devices for eating help people feed themselves. These devices should be included on the meal tray.
- G Residents may benefit from physical and verbal cues. These promote independence. A cue is something that signals that a person should do something. The hand-over-hand approach is an example of a physical cue. The resident lifts a utensil if he is able. You put your hand over his to help with eating. With your hand placed over the resident's hand, help him get food on the utensil. Steer the utensil from the plate to the mouth and back. Repeat this until the resident is finished.
- G Verbal cues must be short and clear. The cues should prompt the resident to do something. Give verbal cues one at a time. Wait until the resident has finished one task before asking him to do another. Repeat the cues until the resident is done eating. Examples of verbal cues include the following:
  - "Pick up your spoon."
  - "Put some carrots on your spoon."
  - "Raise the spoon to your lips."
  - "Open your mouth."
  - "Place the spoon in your mouth."
  - "Close your mouth."
  - "Take the spoon out of your mouth."
  - "Chew."
  - "Swallow."
  - "Drink some water."
- G For residents who have a visual impairment, read menus to them if needed. When helping with eating, place the tray directly in front of residents. Use the face of an imaginary clock to explain the position of what is in front of them (Fig. 8-17).

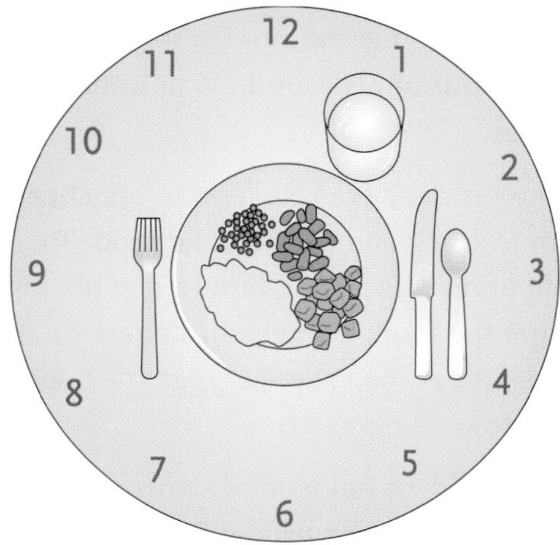

Fig. 8-17. *Use the face of an imaginary clock to explain the position of food to residents who have a visual impairment.*

- **G** For residents who have had a stroke and have a paralyzed or weaker side, place food in the stronger side of the mouth. Make sure food is swallowed before offering another bite.
- **G** Place food in the resident's field of vision. The nurse will determine a resident's field of vision.
- **G** For residents who have Parkinson's disease, tremors or shaking can make it difficult to eat. Help by using physical cues. Place food and drinks close so that the resident can easily reach them. Use assistive devices as needed.
- **G** If a resident has poor sitting balance, seat him in a regular dining room chair with armrests, rather than in a wheelchair. Proper position in a chair means hips are at a 90-degree angle, knees are flexed, and feet and arms are fully supported. Push the chair under the table. Place forearms on the table. If a resident tends to lean to one side, ask him to keep his elbows on the table.
- **G** If a resident has poor neck control, a neck brace may be used to stabilize the head. Use assistive devices as needed. If resident is in a geri-chair, a wedge cushion behind the head and shoulders may be used.
- **G** If the resident bites down on utensils, ask him to open his mouth. Do not pull the utensil out of his mouth. Wait until his jaw relaxes.
- **G** If the resident pockets food in his cheeks, ask him to chew and swallow the food. Touch the side of his cheek. Ask him to use his tongue to get the food. Using your fingers on the cheek (near the lower jaw), gently push the food toward his teeth.
- **G** If the resident holds food in his mouth, ask him to chew and swallow the food. You may need to trigger swallowing. To do this, gently press down on the tongue when taking the spoon out of his mouth. You can also try to gently press down on the top of his head with your hand. Make sure the resident has swallowed the food before offering more.

Residents' Rights

Residents with Special Needs

Residents have the right to be treated with dignity and as adults. They have the right to self-determination. This means, in part, that they should be given the opportunity to choose and state their preferences for care and services. For example, a resident who is blind may want to feed herself without using utensils. This may not look dignified to others, but it is the resident's choice.

9 Rehabilitation and Restorative Care

1. Discuss rehabilitation and restorative care

When a resident loses some ability to function due to illness or injury, rehabilitation may be ordered. **Rehabilitation** is care that is managed by professionals. It helps to restore a person to his highest possible level of functioning. It involves helping residents move from illness, disability, and dependence toward health, ability, and independence. Rehabilitation involves all parts of the person's disability. This includes physical (e.g., eating, elimination) and psychosocial (e.g., independence, self-esteem) needs. Goals of a rehabilitation program include the following:

- To help a resident regain function or recover from illness
- To develop and promote a resident's independence
- To help a resident to feel in control of his life
- To help a resident accept or adapt to the limitations of a disability

Rehabilitation will be used for many residents, particularly those who have suffered a stroke, accident, joint replacement, or trauma. **Restorative care** usually follows rehabilitation. The goal of restorative care is to keep the resident at the level achieved by rehabilitative services. Restorative care works to maintain a resident's functioning, to improve his quality of life, and to increase independence. Both rehabilitation and restorative care take a person-centered, team approach (Fig. 9-1).

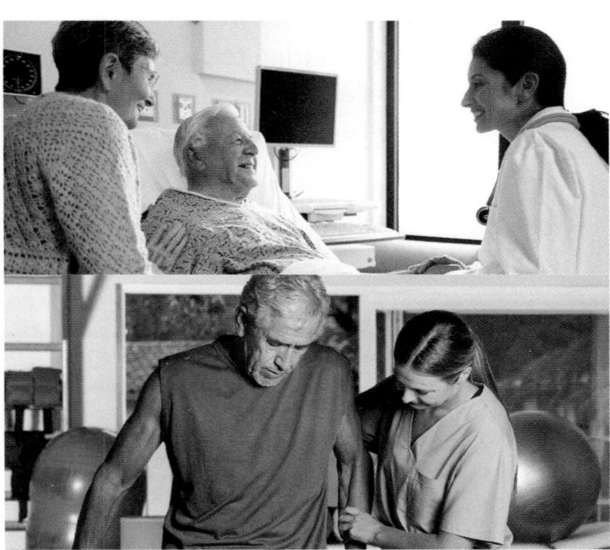

Fig. 9-1. *A team of specialists, including doctors, nurses, physical therapists, and other kinds of therapists, helps residents with rehabilitation.*

Because nursing assistants spend many hours with these residents, they are a very important part of the team. NAs play a critical role in helping residents recover and regain independence.

Guidelines: Restorative Care

G Be patient. Progress may be slow. The more patient you are, the easier it will be for them to regain abilities and confidence.

G Be positive and supportive.

- G Focus on small tasks and small accomplishments. Break tasks down into small steps. Take everything one step at a time.
- G Recognize that setbacks occur. Progress occurs at different rates. Reassure residents that setbacks are normal.
- G Be sensitive to the resident's needs. Some residents may need more encouragement than others. Some may be embarrassed by encouragement. Understand what motivates your residents.
- G Encourage independence. Independence improves self-image and attitude. It also helps speed recovery.
- G Provide privacy. Ensuring privacy while residents try to do skills promotes dignity and maintains their legal rights.
- G Involve residents in their care. Residents who feel involved and valued may be more motivated to work hard in rehabilitation.

Observing and Reporting: Restorative Care

- O/R Any increase or decrease in abilities
- O/R Any change in attitude or motivation, positive or negative
- O/R Any change in general health, such as changes in skin condition, appetite, energy level, or general appearance
- O/R Signs of depression or mood changes

Residents' Rights

Call Lights

Residents may need help often while going through rehabilitation. No matter how often a resident uses his call light or how demanding he is, it is never acceptable for an NA to unplug a resident's call light. Call lights should always be left within reach of the resident's unaffected/stronger hand. Staff must respond kindly and promptly to call lights every time they are used.

2. Describe the importance of promoting independence and list ways exercise improves health

Maintaining independence is vital during and after rehabilitation and restorative services. When an active and independent person is dependent, physical and mental problems may result. The body becomes less mobile. The mind is less focused. Studies show that the more active a person is, the better the mind and body work.

Inactivity and immobility can result in many problems, including the following:

- Loss of self-esteem
- Depression
- Anxiety
- Boredom
- Pneumonia
- Urinary tract infection
- Skin breakdown and pressure injuries
- Constipation
- Blood clots
- Dulling of the senses
- Muscle atrophy
- Contractures
- Problems with independence and self-esteem

The staff's job is to keep residents as active as possible—whether they are bedbound or are able to walk (ambulate). Regular ambulation and exercise help improve these things:

- Quality and health of the skin
- Circulation
- Strength
- Sleep and relaxation
- Mood
- Self-esteem
- Appetite

- Elimination
- Blood flow
- Oxygen level

Promoting social interaction and thinking abilities is important too. Most facilities have activities geared to residents' ages and abilities. Social involvement should be encouraged. When possible, NAs should join in activities with residents. This promotes independence. It also gives NAs a chance to observe residents' abilities.

3. Discuss ambulation and describe assistive devices and equipment

Ambulation is walking. A resident who is **ambulatory** is one who can get out of bed and walk. Many older residents are ambulatory, but need help to walk safely. Several tools, including gait belts, canes, walkers, and crutches, help with ambulation. The NA should check the care plan before helping a resident ambulate. It is important to know the resident's abilities, limitations, and disabilities. The NA should communicate what she would like to do and allow the resident to do what he can.

Assisting a resident to ambulate 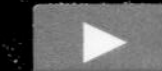

Equipment: gait belt, nonskid shoes for resident

1. Identify yourself by name. Identify the resident by name.
   Resident has right to know identity of his or her caregiver. Addressing resident by name shows respect and establishes correct identification.
2. Wash your hands.
   Provides for infection prevention.
3. Explain procedure to resident. Speak clearly, slowly, and directly. Maintain face-to-face contact whenever possible.
   Promotes understanding and independence.
4. Provide for resident's privacy with curtain, screen, or door.
   Maintains resident's right to privacy and dignity.
5. Adjust the bed to its lowest position. Lock bed wheels. Assist the resident into a sitting position. Make sure his feet are flat on the floor. Adjust the bed height if needed.
   Prevents injury and promotes stability.
6. Before ambulating, put nonskid footwear on the resident and fasten securely.
   Promotes resident's safety. Prevents falls.
7. Stand in front of and face the resident. Place your feet about shoulder-width apart.
   Promotes proper body mechanics.
8. Place the gait belt around the resident's waist over his clothing (not on bare skin). Grasp the belt securely on both sides, with hands in an upward position.
9. If the resident is unable to stand without help, brace (support) the resident's lower extremities. This can be done by placing one or both of your knees against the resident's knees (Fig. 9-2). Or you can stand toe to toe with the resident. Bend your knees. Keep your back straight.

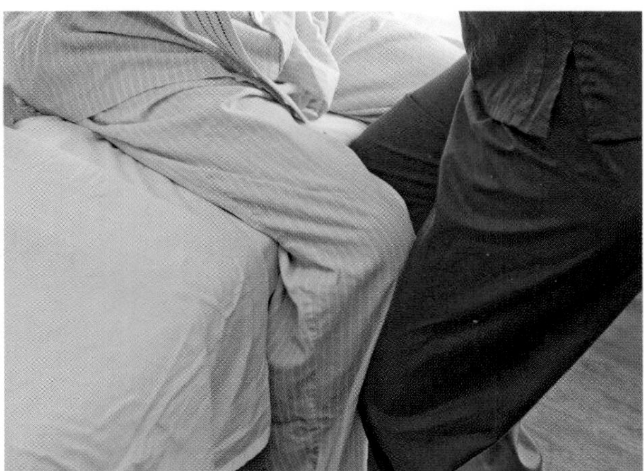

Fig. 9-2. *If the resident has a weak knee, brace it against your knee.*

10. Hold the resident close to your center of gravity. Provide instructions to allow the resident to help with standing. Tell the resident to lean forward, push down on the bed with his hands, and stand on the count of three. When you start to count, begin to rock. On

three, with hands still grasping the gait belt on both sides and moving upward, rock your weight onto your back foot. Slowly help the resident to stand.

11. Walk slightly behind and to one side of the resident for the full distance, while holding onto the gait belt (Fig. 9-3). If the resident has a weaker side, stand on the weaker side. Use the hand that is not holding the belt to offer support on the weak side. Ask the resident to look forward, not down at the floor, during ambulation.
Promotes resident's safety. Prevents injury.

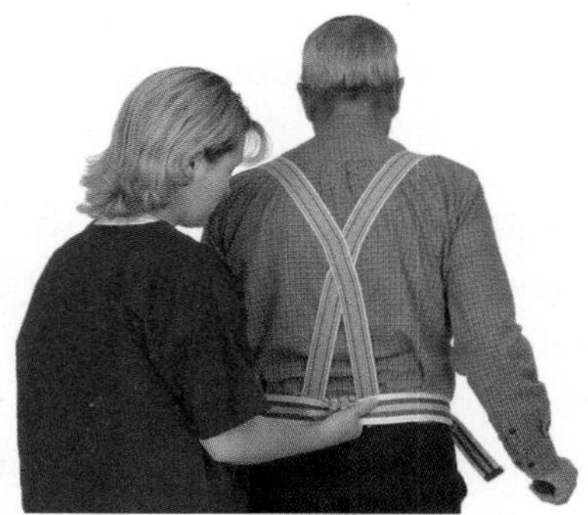

Fig. 9-3. *Standing on the weaker side, walk behind the resident while holding onto the gait belt.*

12. After ambulation, remove the gait belt. Help the resident to the bed or chair. Check that the resident is in proper alignment.
13. Leave bed in its lowest position.
Provides for safety.
14. Place call light within resident's reach.
Allows resident to communicate with staff as necessary.
15. Wash your hands.
Provides for infection prevention.
16. Report any changes in resident to nurse.
Provides nurse with information to assess resident.
17. Document procedure using facility guidelines.
If you do not document the care, legally it did not happen.

When helping a resident who has a visual impairment walk, the NA should be beside and slightly ahead of the resident. The resident should be able to place his hand on the NA's elbow. The NA should walk at a normal pace. She should let the resident know when they are about to turn a corner or when a step is approaching. The NA should state whether they will be stepping up or down.

Residents who have trouble walking may use canes, walkers, or crutches to help themselves. Canes help with balance. Residents using canes should be able to bear weight on both legs. If one leg is weaker, the cane should be held in the hand on the stronger side.

Types of canes are the C cane, the functional grip cane, and the quad cane. The C cane is a straight cane with a curved handle at the top. It has a rubber-tipped bottom to prevent slipping. A C cane is used to improve balance. A functional grip cane is similar to the C cane, except that it has a straight grip handle rather than a curved handle. The grip handle helps improve grip control. It provides more support than the C cane. A quad cane has four rubber-tipped feet and a rectangular base. It is designed to bear more weight than the other canes (Fig. 9-4).

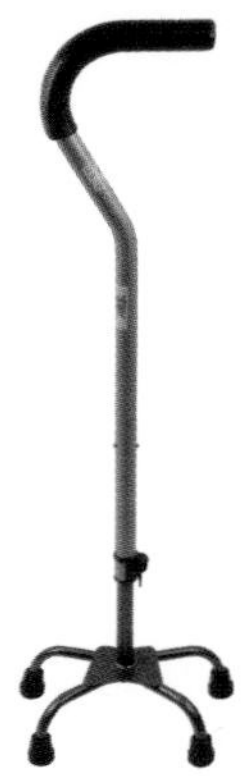

Fig. 9-4. *A quad cane has four rubber-tipped feet and can bear more weight than other canes.*

A walker is used when the resident can bear some weight on both legs. The walker gives stability for residents who are unsteady or lack balance. The metal frame may have rubber-tipped feet and/or wheels (Fig. 9-5). Crutches are used for residents who can bear no weight or limited weight on one leg. Crutches have rubber-tipped feet to prevent sliding. Some people use one crutch. Some use two.

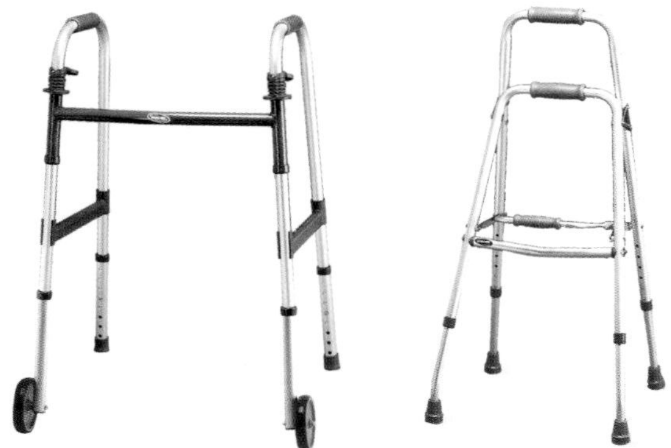

Fig. 9-5. The photo on the left shows a standard walker and the photo on the right shows a Hemi Walker, which is a walker that is designed for people who have difficulty using an arm or a hand. (© INVACARE CORPORATION. USED WITH PERMISSION. WWW.INVACARE.COM)

Guidelines: Cane or Walker Use

- G Be sure the walker or cane is in good condition. It must have rubber tips on the bottom. The tips should not be cracked. Walkers may have wheels. If so, roll the walker to make sure the wheels are moving properly.
- G Be sure the resident is wearing securely fastened, nonskid shoes before ambulating.
- G When using a cane, the resident should place it on his stronger side.
- G When using a walker, have the resident place both hands on the walker. The walker should not be overextended. It should be placed no more than six inches in front of the resident.
- G Stay near the resident on the weaker side.
- G Do not hang purses or clothing on the walker.
- G If height of the cane or walker does not appear to be correct (too short, too tall, etc.), tell the nurse.

Assisting with ambulation for a resident using a cane, walker, or crutches

Equipment: gait belt, nonskid shoes for the resident, cane, walker, or crutches

1. Identify yourself by name. Identify the resident by name.
   Resident has right to know identity of his or her caregiver. Addressing resident by name shows respect and establishes correct identification.
2. Wash your hands.
   Provides for infection prevention.
3. Explain procedure to resident. Speak clearly, slowly, and directly. Maintain face-to-face contact whenever possible.
   Promotes understanding and independence.
4. Provide for resident's privacy with curtain, screen, or door.
   Maintains resident's right to privacy and dignity.
5. Adjust the bed to its lowest position so that the feet are flat on the floor. Lock bed wheels.
   Prevents injury and promotes stability.
6. Before ambulating, put nonskid footwear on the resident and securely fasten.
   Promotes resident's safety. Prevents falls.
7. Stand in front of and face the resident. Place your feet about shoulder-width apart.
   Promotes proper body mechanics.
8. Place the gait belt around the resident's waist over his clothing (not on bare skin). Grasp the belt securely on both sides, with hands in an upward position.
9. If the resident is unable to stand without help, brace (support) resident's lower extremities (see previous procedure). Bend your knees. Keep your back straight. Help the resident to stand as described in the previous procedure.
10. Help as needed with ambulation.

a. **Cane**: Resident places cane about six inches, or a comfortable distance, in front of his stronger leg. He brings his weaker leg even with the cane. He then brings his stronger leg forward slightly ahead of the cane. Repeat.

b. **Walker**: Resident picks up or rolls the walker. He places it about six inches, or a comfortable distance, in front of him. All four feet or wheels of the walker should be on the ground before the resident steps forward to the walker. The walker should not be moved again until the resident has moved both feet forward and is steady. The resident should never put his feet ahead of the walker.
Promotes stability and prevents falls.

c. **Crutches**: Resident should be fitted for crutches and taught to use them correctly by a physical therapist or a nurse. The resident may use the crutches several different ways. It depends on his weakness. No matter how they are used, the resident's weight should be on his hands and arms. Weight should not be on the underarm area.

11. Walk slightly behind and to one side of the resident for the full distance, while holding onto the gait belt. If the resident has a weaker side, stand on the weaker side.
Provides security.

12. Watch for obstacles in the resident's path. Ask the resident to look forward, not down at the floor, during ambulation.
Promotes resident's safety. Prevents injury.

13. Encourage resident to rest if he is tired. When a person is tired, it increases the chance of a fall. Let the resident set the pace. Discuss how far he plans to go based on the care plan.

14. After ambulation, remove the gait belt. Help the resident to the bed or chair. Check that the resident is in proper alignment.

15. Leave bed in its lowest position.
Provides for safety.

16. Place call light within resident's reach.
Allows resident to communicate with staff as necessary.

17. Wash your hands.
Provides for infection prevention.

18. Report any changes in resident to nurse.
Provides nurse with information to assess resident.

19. Document procedure using facility guidelines.
If you do not document the care, legally it did not happen.

Many devices are available to help people who are recovering from or adapting to a physical condition. **Assistive** or **adaptive devices** help residents perform their activities of daily living (ADLs). Each device is made to support a particular disability. Raised seating, for example, makes it easier for a resident with weak legs to stand.

Personal care equipment includes long-handled brushes and combs. Plate guards prevent food from being pushed off the plate. They make it easier to scoop food onto utensils. Reachers can help put on underwear or pants. A sock aid can pull on socks. A long-handled shoehorn assists in putting shoes on without bending. Long-handled sponges help with bathing.

Supportive devices, such as canes, walkers, and crutches, are used to assist residents with ambulation. Safety devices, such as shower chairs and gait or transfer belts, help prevent accidents. Safety bars/grab bars are often installed in and near the tub and toilet to give the resident something to hold on to while changing position. More examples of assistive devices are shown in Figure 9-6.

4. Explain guidelines for maintaining proper body alignment

Residents who are confined to bed need proper body alignment. This aids recovery and prevents injury to muscles and joints. By following these guidelines, NAs can help residents maintain proper alignment:

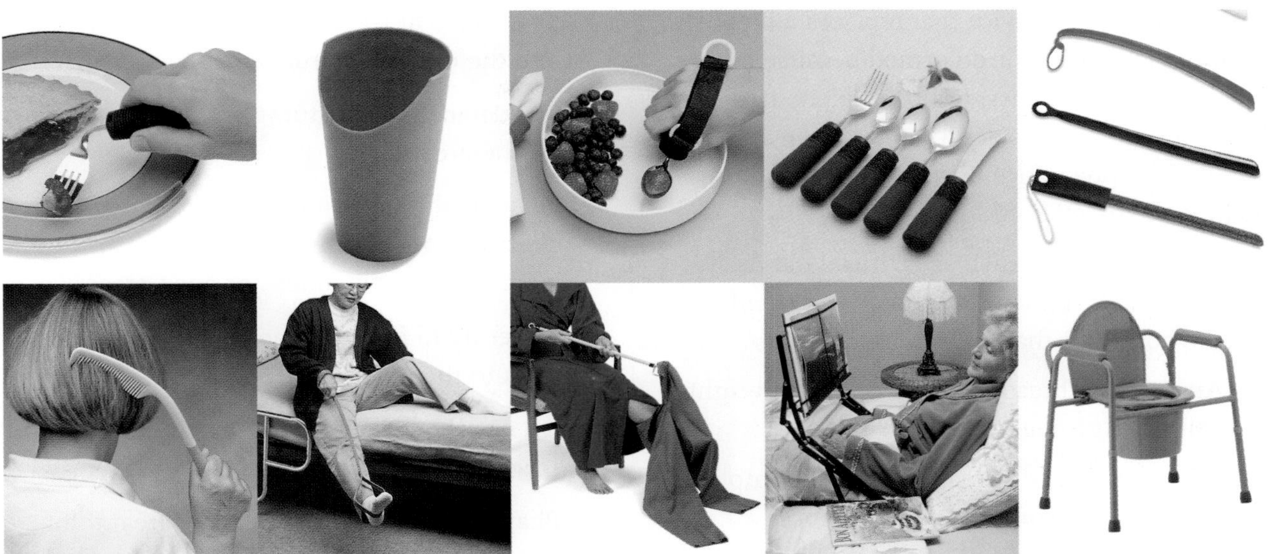

Fig. 9-6. Many assistive items are available to help residents adapt to physical changes. (PHOTOS COURTESY OF NORTH COAST MEDICAL, INC. WWW.NCMEDICAL.COM, 800-821-9319)

Guidelines: Alignment and Positioning

- **G** Observe principles of alignment. Proper alignment is based on straight lines. The spine should lie in a straight line. Pillows or rolled or folded blankets can support the small of the back and raise the knees or head in the supine position. They can support the head and one leg in the lateral position (Fig. 9-7).

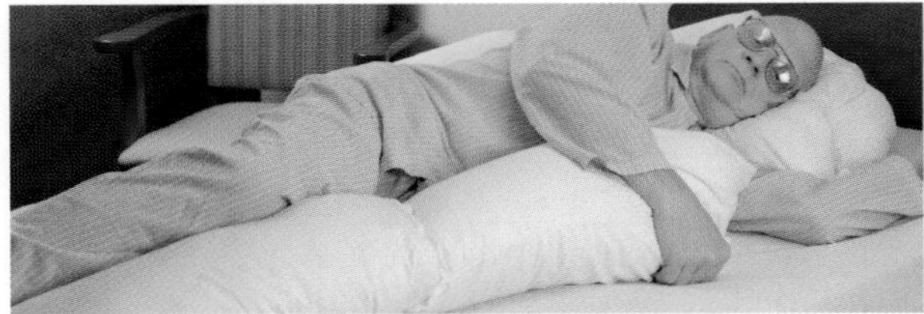

Fig. 9-7. Pillows or rolled or folded blankets help provide extra support.

- **G** Keep body parts in natural positions. In a natural hand position, the fingers are slightly curled. Use a rolled washcloth, gauze bandage, or a rubber ball inside the palm to support the fingers in this position. Use bed cradles to keep covers from resting on feet in the supine position.
- **G** Prevent external rotation of hips. When legs and hips turn outward during bedrest, hip contractures can result. A rolled blanket or towel tucked alongside the hip and thigh can keep the leg from turning outward.
- **G** Change positions often to prevent muscle stiffness and pressure injuries. This should be done at least every two hours. The position used will depend on the resident's condition and preference. Check the resident's skin every time you reposition him.
- **G** Give back rubs as ordered for comfort and relaxation.

5. Describe care guidelines for prosthetic devices

Amputation is the surgical removal of some or all of a body part, usually an arm, hand, leg, or foot. Amputation may be the result of an injury or disease. After amputation, some people feel that the limb is still there. They may feel pain in the part that has been amputated. **Phantom sensation** is the term used when a person feels that the body part is still there. **Phantom limb pain** occurs when the person feels pain in a limb (or extremity) that has been amputated. It may last for a short time or for years. The pain or sensation is real. It should not be ignored. Medication or physical therapy may be used to treat these conditions.

A **prosthesis** is a device that replaces a body part that is missing or deformed because of an accident, injury, illness, or birth defect. It is used to improve a person's ability to function and/or to improve appearance. Examples of prostheses include the following:

- Artificial limbs, such as artificial hands, arms, feet, and legs, are made to resemble the body part that they are replacing.
- An artificial breast is made of a lightweight, soft, spongy material.
- A hearing aid is a small device that amplifies sound for persons with hearing loss.
- An artificial eye, or ocular prosthetic, replaces an eye that has been lost to disease or injury. An ocular prosthetic does not provide vision. It can, however, improve appearance.
- Dentures are artificial teeth. They may be necessary when a tooth or teeth have been damaged, lost, or must be removed.

Guidelines: Amputation and Prosthesis Care

G Residents who have had a body part amputated must make many physical, psychological, social, and occupational adjustments due to disability. Be supportive.

G Help residents with their ADLs.

G Prostheses are specially fitted, expensive pieces of equipment (some cost tens of thousands of dollars). Care for them as assigned. Handle them carefully.

G A therapist or nurse will demonstrate application of a prosthesis. Follow instructions to apply and remove the prosthesis. Follow the manufacturer's care directions.

G Respect a resident's decision not to wear a prosthetic limb. Some residents may find the limb uncomfortable and only wish to wear it for special occasions.

G Keep a prosthesis and the skin under it dry and clean. The socket of the prosthesis must be cleaned at least daily. Follow the care plan and the nurse's instructions.

G If ordered, apply a stump sock before putting on the prosthesis.

G Observe the skin on the stump. Watch for skin breakdown caused by pressure and abrasion. Report any redness or open areas.

G Never try to fix a prosthesis. Report any problems to the nurse.

G Do not show negative feelings about the stump during care.

G Phantom limb pain is real pain. Treat it that way. Report complaints of pain to the nurse.

G If the resident has an artificial eye, review the care plan with the nurse. Always wash your hands and don gloves before handling an artificial eye. Provide privacy for the resident. Never clean or soak the eye in rubbing alcohol. It will crack the plastic and destroy it. If the eye is to be removed and not reinserted, store it in water or saline solution. Make sure the container is labeled with the resident's name and room number. The resident may be able to remove, clean, and insert the eye himself. Know any needed instructions for care.

Information on care of hearing aids is in Chapter 2. Denture care is located in Chapter 6.

6. Describe how to assist with range of motion exercises

Range of motion (**ROM**) exercises put a joint through its full arc of motion. The goals of these exercises are to decrease or prevent contractures or atrophy, improve strength, and increase circulation. Active range of motion (AROM) exercises are done by a resident himself, without help. The NA's role is to encourage the resident. Active assisted range of motion (AAROM) exercises are done by the resident with some help and support from the NA. Passive range of motion (PROM) exercises are used when residents are not able to move on their own. These exercises are done by a staff member, without the resident's help.

ROM exercises are specific for each body area. They include these movements (Fig. 9-8):

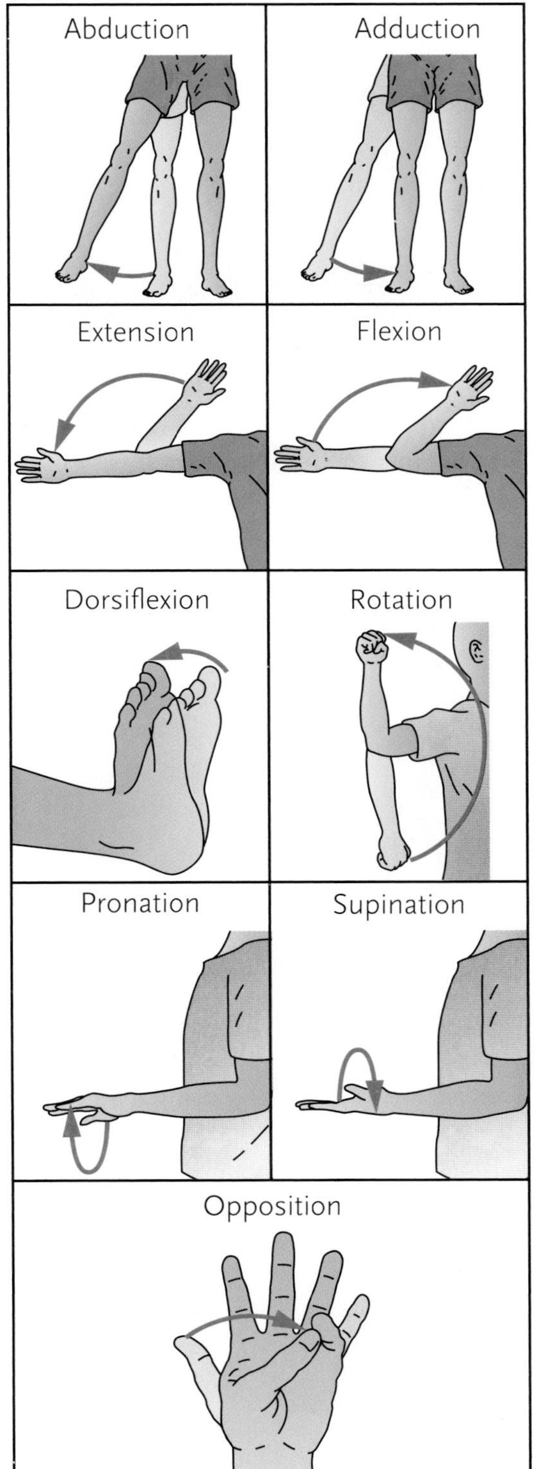

Fig. 9-8. *The different range of motion body movements.*

- **Abduction**: moving a body part away from the midline of the body
- **Adduction**: moving a body part toward the midline of the body
- **Extension**: straightening a body part
- **Flexion**: bending a body part
- **Dorsiflexion**: bending backward
- **Rotation**: turning a joint
- **Pronation**: turning downward
- **Supination**: turning upward
- **Opposition**: touching the thumb to any other finger

Range of motion exercises are not done without an order from a doctor, nurse, or physical therapist. The NA will repeat each exercise three to five times, once or twice a day, working on both sides of the body. When doing ROM exercises, the NA should begin at the resident's shoulders and work down the body. The upper extremities (arms) should be exercised before the lower extremities (legs). The NA should give support above and below the joint. The joints should be moved gently, slowly, and smoothly. It is important to ask if the exercises are causing pain. The NA should stop the exercises if the resident complains of pain and report the pain to the nurse.

Assisting with passive range of motion exercises

1. Identify yourself by name. Identify the resident by name.
   Resident has right to know identity of his or her caregiver. Addressing resident by name shows respect and establishes correct identification.

2. Wash your hands.
   Provides for infection prevention.

3. Explain procedure to resident. Speak clearly, slowly, and directly. Maintain face-to-face contact whenever possible.
   Promotes understanding and independence.

4. Provide for resident's privacy with curtain, screen, or door.
   Maintains resident's right to privacy and dignity.

5. Adjust bed to a safe level, usually waist high. Lock bed wheels.
   Prevents injury to you and to resident.

6. Position the resident lying supine—flat on her back—on the bed. Use proper alignment. Ask the resident to let you know if she has any pain during the procedure.
   Reduces stress to joints. Pain is a warning sign for injury.

7. While supporting the limbs, move all joints gently, slowly, and smoothly through the range of motion to the point of resistance. Repeat each exercise at least three times. Ask the resident if an exercise is causing pain. Watch for signs of pain. Stop if resident appears to be in pain or reports pain.
   Rapid movement may cause injury. Pain is a warning sign for injury.

8. **Shoulder**: Support the resident's arm at the elbow and wrist while performing ROM for the shoulder. Place one hand under the elbow and the other hand under the wrist. Raise the straightened arm from the side position upward toward the head to ear level. Return the arm down to the side of the body (extension/flexion) (Fig. 9-9).

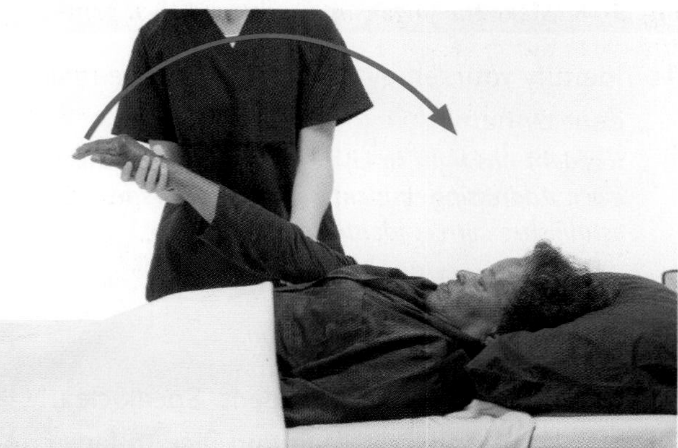

Fig. 9-9. *Raise the straightened arm upward toward head to ear level and return it to the side of the body.*

   Keep one hand under the elbow and one hand under the wrist. Move the straightened arm away from the side of the body to shoulder level. Return the arm to the side of the body (abduction/adduction) (Fig. 9-10).

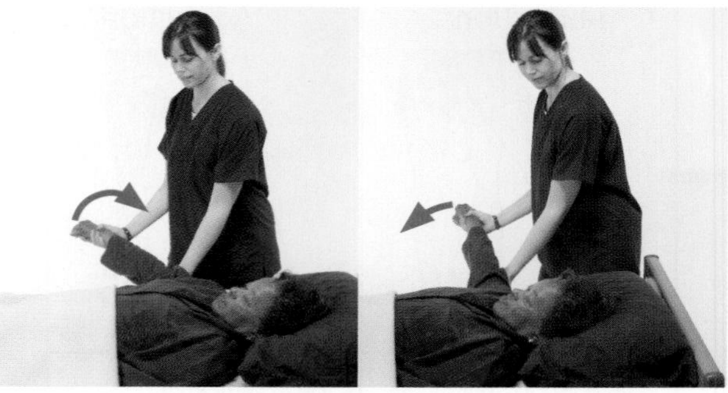

Fig. 9-10. *Move the straightened arm away from the side of the body to shoulder level and return the arm to side.*

9. **Elbow**: Hold the resident's wrist with one hand and the elbow with the other hand. Bend the elbow so that the hand touches the shoulder on that same side (flexion). Straighten the arm (extension) (Fig. 9-11).

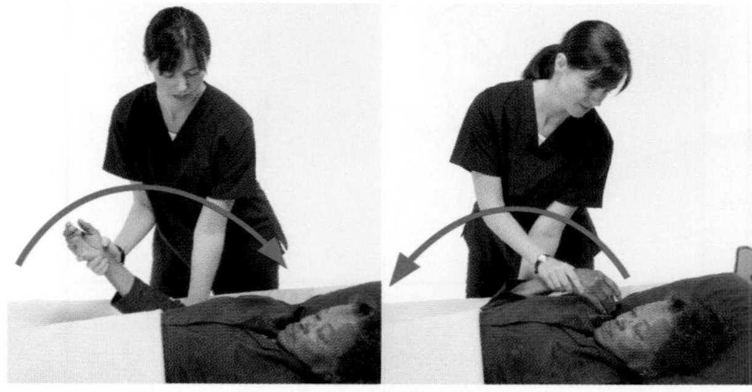

Fig. 9-11. *Bend the elbow so that the hand touches the shoulder on the same side. Then straighten the arm.*

   Exercise the forearm by moving it so the palm is facing downward (pronation) and then the palm is facing upward (supination) (Fig. 9-12).

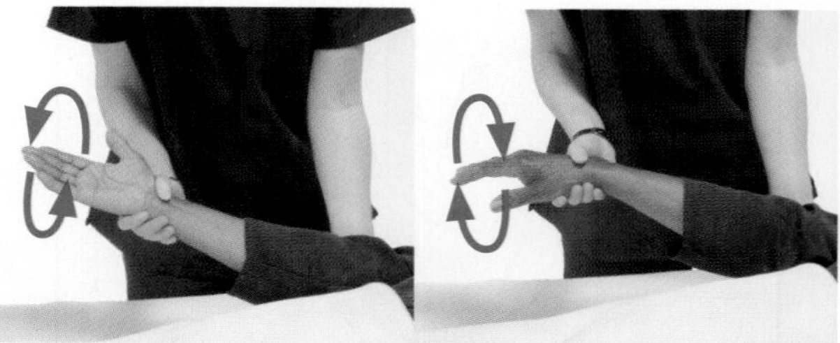

Fig. 9-12. *Exercise the forearm so that the palm is facing downward and then upward.*

10. **Wrist**: Hold the wrist with one hand. Use the fingers of the other hand to help move the joint through the motions. Bend the hand down (flexion). Bend the hand backward (dorsiflexion) (Fig. 9-13).

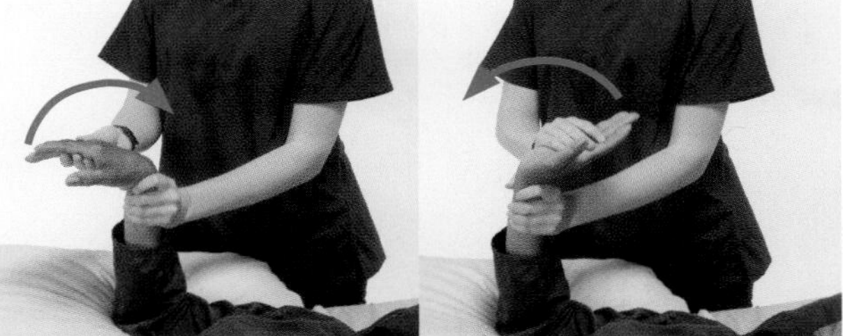

Fig. 9-13. *While supporting the wrist, gently bend the hand down and then backward.*

Turn the hand in the direction of the thumb (radial flexion). Then turn the hand in the direction of the little finger (ulnar flexion) (Fig. 9-14).

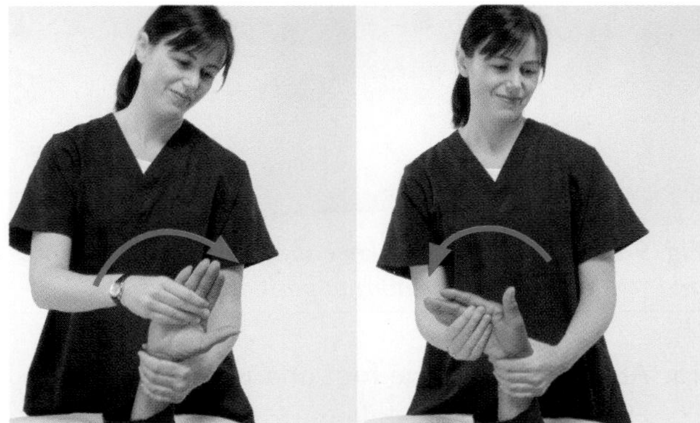

Fig. 9-14. *Turn the hand in the direction of the thumb, then turn it in the direction of the little finger.*

11. **Thumb**: Move the thumb away from the index finger (abduction). Move the thumb back next to the index finger (adduction) (Fig. 9-15).

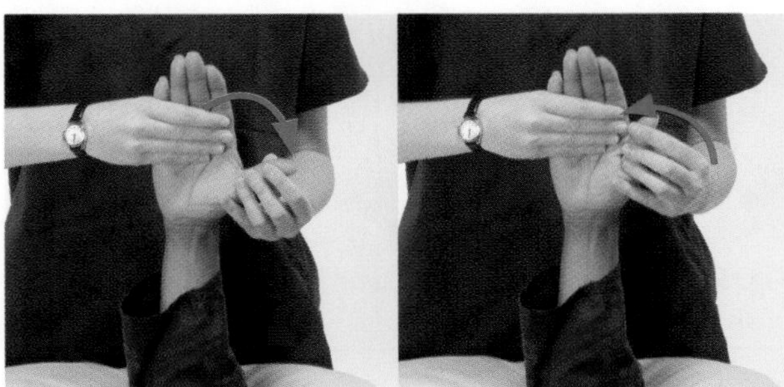

Fig. 9-15. *Move the thumb away from the index finger and then back to the index finger.*

Touch each fingertip with the thumb (opposition) (Fig. 9-16).

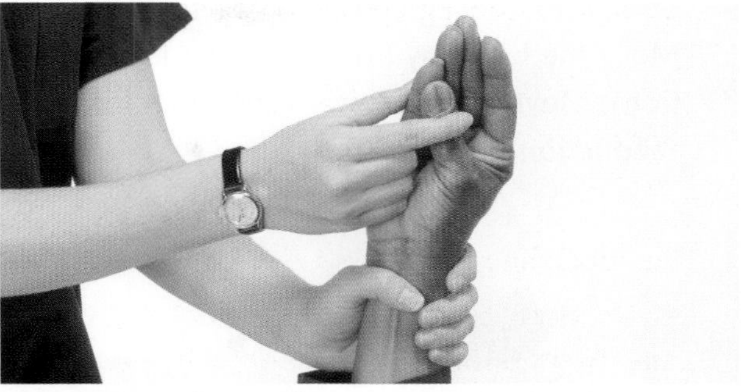

Fig. 9-16. *Touch each fingertip with the thumb.*

Bend the thumb into the palm (flexion) and out to the side (extension) (Fig. 9-17).

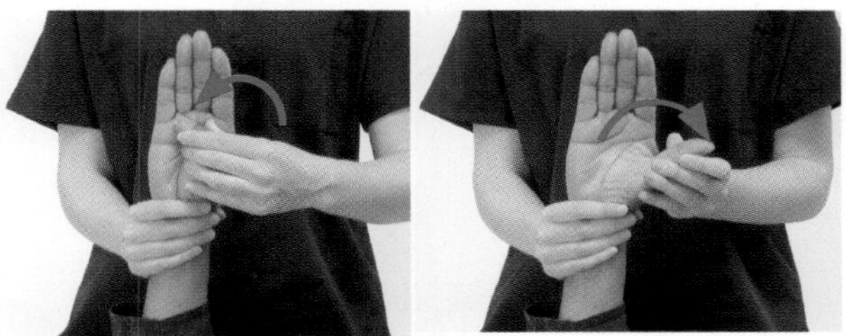

Fig. 9-17. *Bend the thumb into the palm and then out to the side.*

12. **Fingers**: Make the hand into a fist (flexion). Gently straighten out the fist (extension) (Fig. 9-18).

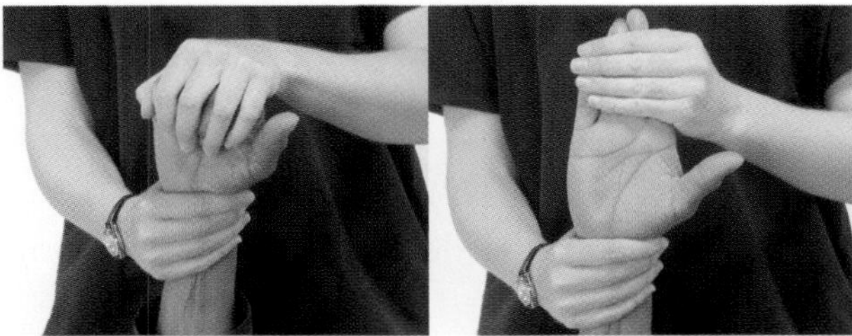

Fig. 9-18. *Make the fingers into a fist and then gently straighten out the fist.*

Spread the fingers and the thumb far apart from each other (abduction). Bring the fingers back next to each other (adduction) (Fig. 9-19).

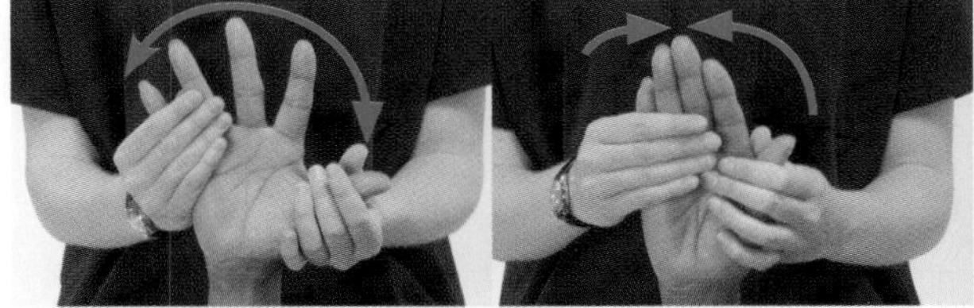

Fig. 9-19. *Spread the fingers and thumb far apart from each other and then bring them back next to each other.*

13. **Hip**: Support the leg by placing one hand under the knee and one under the ankle. Straighten the leg and gently raise it upward. Move the leg away from the other leg (abduction). Move the leg toward the other leg (adduction) (Fig. 9-20).

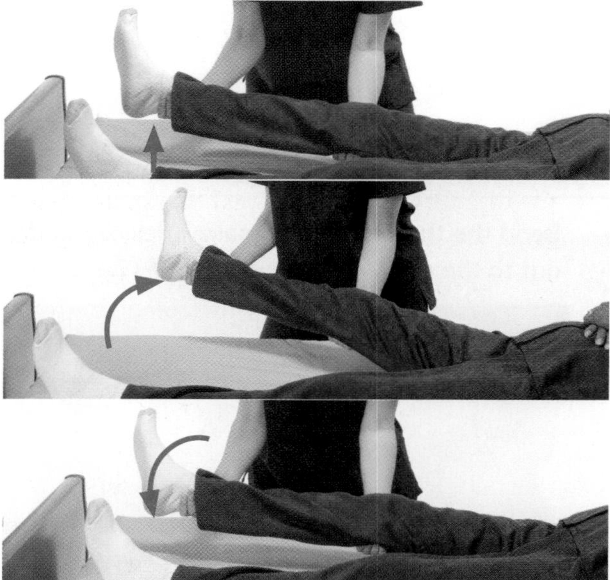

Fig. 9-20. *Straighten the leg and gently raise it. Move the leg away from the other leg and then back toward the other leg.*

Gently turn the leg inward (internal rotation), then turn the leg outward (external rotation) (Fig. 9-21).

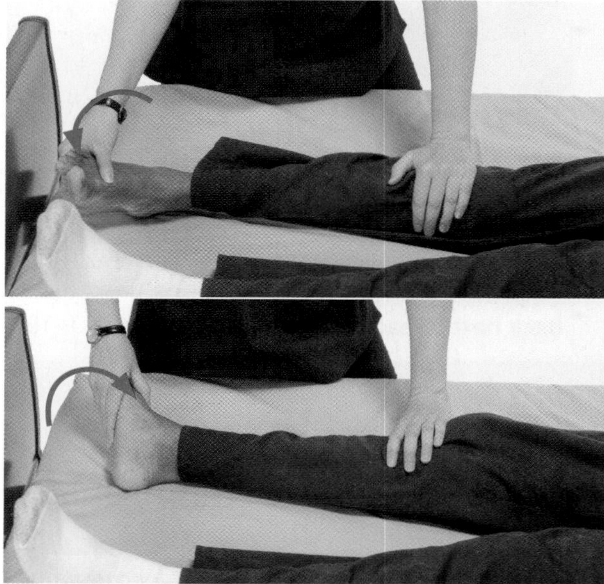

Fig. 9-21. *Gently turn the leg inward and then outward.*

14. **Knee**: Support the leg under the knee and under the ankle while performing ROM for the knee. Bend the knee to the point of resistance (flexion). Return the leg to resident's normal position (extension) (Fig. 9-22).

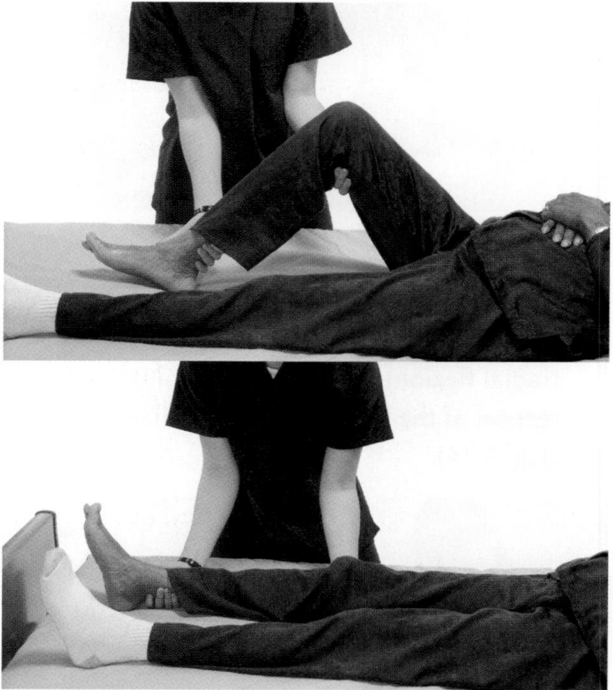

Fig. 9-22. *Gently bend the knee to the point of resistance and return the leg to its normal position.*

15. **Ankle**: Support the foot and under the ankle close to the bed while performing ROM for the ankle. Push/pull foot up toward the head (dorsiflexion). Push/pull foot down, with the toes pointed down (plantar flexion) (Fig. 9-23).

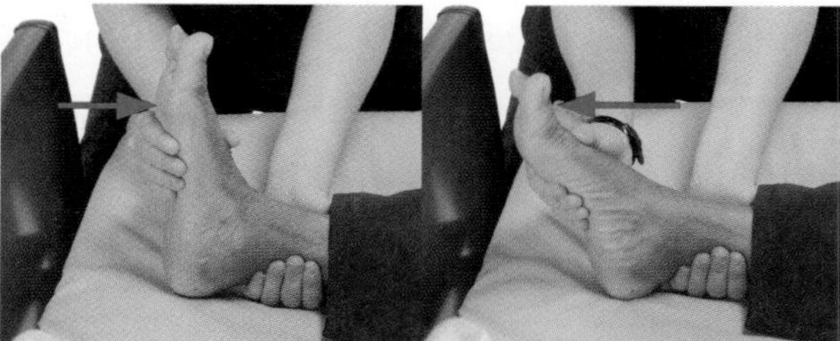

Fig. 9-23. *Push the foot up toward the head and then push it back down.*

Turn the inside of the foot inward toward the body (supination). Bend the sole of the foot so that it faces away from the body (pronation) (Fig. 9-24).

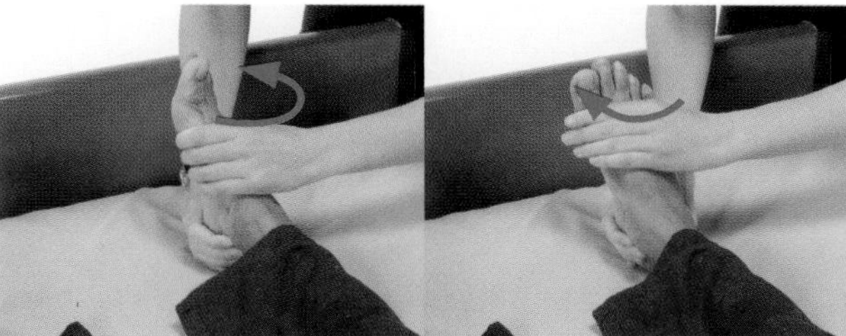

Fig. 9-24. *Turn the inside of the foot inward, toward the body, and then bend it to face away from the body.*

16. **Toes**: Curl and straighten the toes (flexion and extension) (Fig. 9-25).

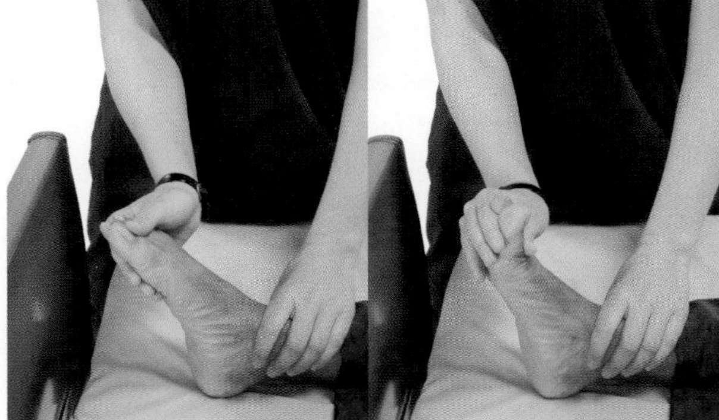

Fig. 9-25. *Curl and straighten the toes.*

Gently spread the toes apart (abduction) (Fig. 9-26).

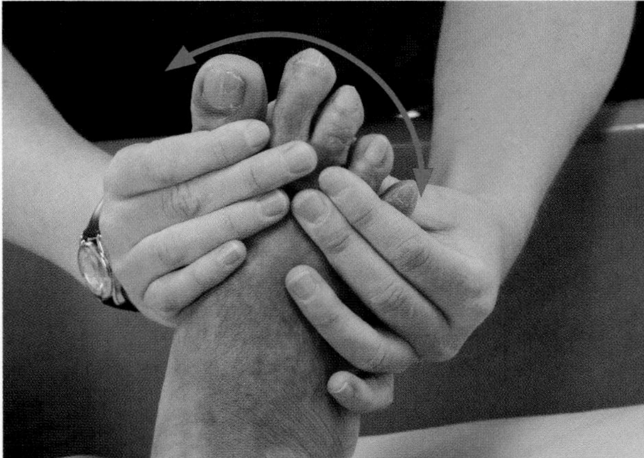

Fig. 9-26. *Gently spread the toes apart.*

17. Return resident to a comfortable position. Return bed to lowest position.
Promotes resident's safety.

18. Place call light within resident's reach.
Allows resident to communicate with staff as necessary.

19. Wash your hands.
Provides for infection prevention.

20. Report any changes in resident to nurse.
Provides nurse with information to assess resident.

21. Document procedure using facility guidelines. Note any decrease in range of motion or any pain experienced by the resident. Notify the nurse or the physical therapist if you find increased stiffness or physical resistance. Resistance may be a sign that a contracture is developing.
If you do not document the care, legally it did not happen.

7. List guidelines for assisting with bladder and bowel retraining

Injury, illness, or inactivity may cause a loss of normal bladder or bowel function. Residents may need help to reestablish a regular routine and normal function. Problems with elimination can be embarrassing or difficult to discuss. NAs should be sensitive to this. They should be professional when handling incontinence or working to reestablish routines.

Guidelines: Bladder or Bowel Retraining

G Follow Standard Precautions. Wear gloves when handling body wastes.

G Explain the training schedule to the resident. Follow the schedule carefully.

G Keep a record of the resident's bladder and bowel habits. When you see a pattern of elimination, you can predict when the resident will need a bedpan or a trip to the bathroom.

G Offer a bedpan or a trip to the bathroom before beginning long procedures.

- **G** Encourage the resident to drink plenty of fluids. Do this even if urinary incontinence is a problem. About 30 minutes after fluids are taken, offer a trip to the bathroom or a bedpan or urinal.
- **G** Encourage the resident to eat foods that are high in fiber. Encourage residents to follow special diets as ordered.
- **G** Answer call lights promptly. Residents cannot wait long when the urge to go to the bathroom occurs. Leave call lights within reach.
- **G** Provide privacy for elimination—both in the bed and in the bathroom.
- **G** If a resident has trouble urinating, try running water in the sink. Have her lean forward slightly. This puts pressure on the bladder.
- **G** Do not rush the resident.
- **G** Help the resident with careful perineal care. This helps prevent skin breakdown and promotes proper hygiene. Observe for skin changes.
- **G** Discard wastes according to facility policy.
- **G** Discard clothing protectors and incontinence briefs properly (Fig. 9-27). Double-bag these items if ordered. This stops odors from collecting.

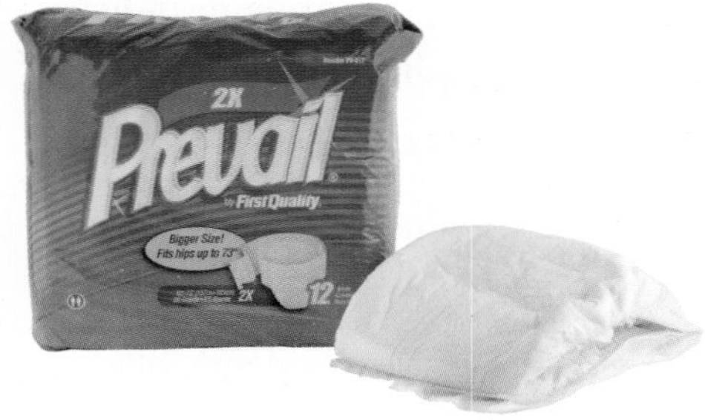

Fig. 9-27. *A type of incontinence pad.*

- **G** Some facilities use washable bed pads or briefs. Follow Standard Precautions when handling these items.
- **G** Keep an accurate record of urination and bowel movements. This includes episodes of incontinence.
- **G** Praise successes or even attempts to control the bladder and bowels. However, do not talk to residents as if they are children. Keep your voice low. Do not draw attention to any aspect of retraining. Do not discuss accidents or retraining in public areas.
- **G** Never show frustration or anger toward residents who are incontinent. The problem is out of their control. Negative reactions will only make things worse. Be kind, supportive, and professional.
- **G** When the resident is incontinent or cannot use the toilet when asked, be positive. Never make the resident feel like a failure. Praise and encouragement are essential for a successful program. Each resident has different needs and may respond to different types of encouragement. Finding out each resident's needs and preferences is part of giving person-centered care.
- **G** Some residents will always be incontinent. Be patient. Offer these residents extra care and attention. Skin breakdown may lead to pressure injuries without proper care. Always report changes in skin.

Changing Incontinence Briefs

When changing an incontinence brief, the NA should assemble all needed items beforehand, including a protective pad, perineal care supplies, disposable wipes, gloves, and a clean brief. She should don gloves before handling the brief. When removing the soiled brief, the NA should roll it inward, soiled side inside, without spilling its contents. Working from front to back, she should carefully remove all urine and/or feces from the skin. After cleaning the area thoroughly, she should blot it dry and put on the clean brief.

10 Caring for Yourself

The first nine chapters of this book introduce readers to the long-term care setting. They cover the knowledge, skills, and qualities a person needs to work as a nursing assistant. This final chapter is more personal. It addresses the reader directly. This chapter has to do with finding and keeping a job, as well as advice about building good working relationships. It also includes helpful tips for managing stress and staying healthy.

1. Describe how to find a job

Once your training is complete, you may soon be looking for a job. Nursing assistants may be able to work in long-term care facilities, in assisted living facilities, in hospitals, in the home, and in other places. To find a job, you must first find potential employers. Then you must contact them to find out about job opportunities. To find employers, use the internet, a newspaper, or personal contacts (Fig. 10-1). You can also ask your instructor about potential employers.

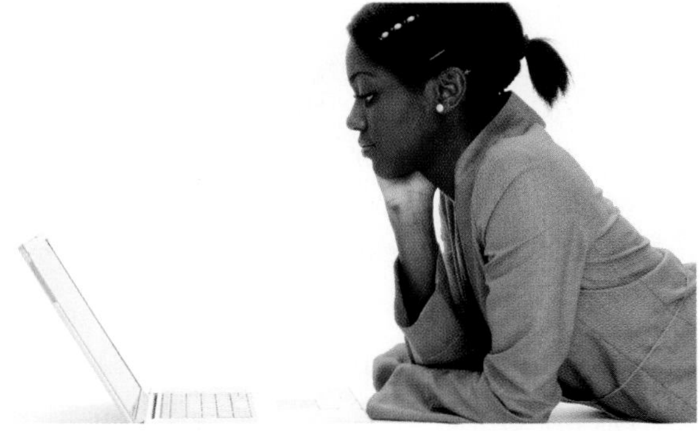

Fig. 10-1. *Using the internet is a good way to find a job.*

Once you have a list of potential employers, you need to contact them. Emailing or phoning first, unless they mention not to do so, is a good way to find out what jobs are available. Ask how to apply for a job with each potential employer.

When making an appointment, ask what information to bring with you. Make sure you have this information with you when you go. Some of these documents may be required:

- Identification, including driver's license, social security card, birth certificate, passport, or other official form of identification
- Proof of your legal status in this country and proof that you are legally able to work, even if you are a US citizen. All employers must have files showing that all employees are legally allowed to work in this country. Do not be offended by this request.
- High school diploma or equivalency, school transcripts, and diploma or certificate from your nursing assistant training course. Take your instructor's name, phone number, and email address with you as well.
- References are people who can be contacted to recommend you as an employee. They include former employers and/or former teachers. Do not use relatives or friends as references. You can ask references beforehand to write general letters for you. They can be addressed "To Whom It May Concern" and should explain how they know you

and describe your skills, qualities, and work habits. Take copies of these with you.

Some potential employers will ask you for a résumé. A *résumé* is a summary or listing of relevant job experience and education. When creating your résumé, keep it brief (one page is best) and clear. Include this information:

- Your contact details: name, address, phone number, and email address
- Your educational experience, starting with the most current first
- Your work experience, starting with the most current first
- Any special skills, such as knowledge of computer software, typing skills, or speaking other languages
- Any memberships in professional organizations
- Volunteer work

A job application may need to be completed. Write down the general information you will need. Take this information with you, along with your résumé if you have one. This will save time and avoid mistakes. Include this information:

- Your address, phone number, and email address
- Your birth date
- Your social security number
- Name and address of the school or program where you were trained, and the date you completed your training, as well as your certification number and information about other certifications such as CPR and first aid
- Names, titles, addresses, phone numbers, and email addresses of former employers, and the dates you worked there
- Salary information from your former jobs
- Reasons why you left each of your former jobs
- Names, addresses, phone numbers, and email addresses of your references
- Days and hours you can work
- A brief statement about why you are changing jobs or why you want to work as a nursing assistant

Fill out the application carefully and neatly. Never lie. Before you write anything, read it all the way through once. If you are not sure what is being asked, find out before filling in that space. Fill in all of the blanks. Write *N/A* (not applicable) if the question does not apply to you.

Your employer may require that a criminal background check be done on new employees. You may be asked to sign a form granting permission to do this. Do not take it personally. It is a law intended to protect patients and residents.

To make the best impression at a job interview, be professional. Do the following:

- Shower or bathe. Use deodorant.
- Brush your teeth.
- Wash your hands and clean and file your nails. Nails should be medium length or shorter. Do not wear artificial nails.
- Wear only simple makeup and jewelry or none at all.
- Your hair should be clean and out of your eyes. Wear it in a simple style.
- Shave or trim facial hair before the interview.
- Dress neatly and appropriately. Make sure clothing is clean, ironed, and has no holes in it. Do not wear jeans, shorts, or short dresses or skirts (no shorter than knee-length). Do not wear t-shirts or anything with a logo or writing on it. Shoes should be clean and polished. Do not wear sneakers or flip-flops.
- Do not wear perfume or cologne. Many people dislike or are allergic to scents.
- Do not smoke beforehand. You will smell like smoke during the interview.

- Arrive 10 or 15 minutes early.
- Do not bring friends or children with you.
- Turn off your phone.
- Introduce yourself. Smile and shake hands (Fig. 10-2). Your handshake should be firm and confident.

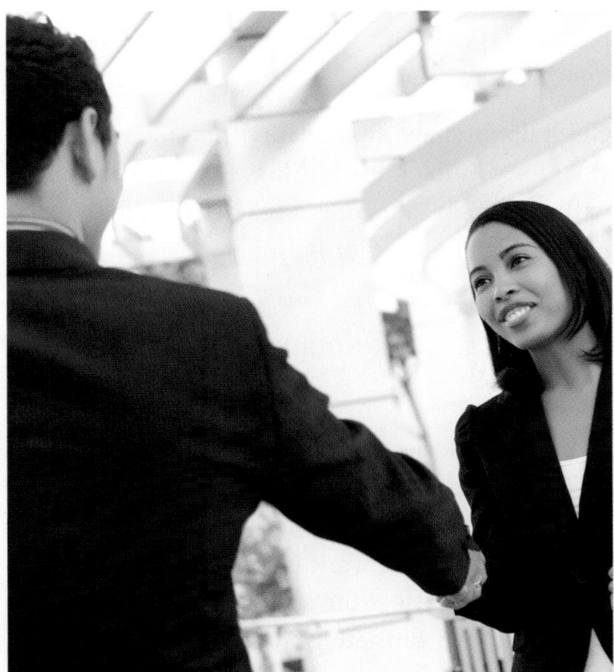

Fig. 10-2. *Smile and shake hands confidently when you arrive at a job interview.*

- Answer questions clearly and completely.
- Make eye contact to show you are sincere.
- Avoid slang words or expressions.
- Do not eat, drink, chew gum, or smoke in an interview.
- Sit up or stand up straight. Look happy to be there.
- Relax and be confident. You have worked hard to get this far.

Be positive when answering questions. Emphasize what you enjoy or think you will enjoy about the job. Do not complain about any previous jobs you have had. Make it clear that you are hardworking and willing to work with all kinds of residents.

Usually interviewers will ask if you have any questions. Have some prepared. Write them down so you do not forget things you really want to know. Questions you may want to ask include

- What hours would I work? Is there any mandatory overtime I would need to work?
- What benefits does the job include? Is health insurance available? Would I get paid sick days or holidays?
- What is the average caseload for nursing assistants?
- What orientation or training is provided?
- How will I contact my supervisor when I need to do so?
- Are there any policies regarding ongoing education or advancement?
- How soon will you be making a decision about this position?

Later in the interview, you may want to ask about salary or wages if you have not already been given this information. Listen carefully to the answers to your questions. Take notes if needed. You will probably be told when you can expect to hear from the employer about the job. Do not expect to be offered a job at the interview. When the interview is over, stand up and shake hands again. Thank the employer for meeting with you.

Send an email or letter after the interview to say thank you. Express your continued interest in the job. If you have not heard back from the employer within the time frame you discussed with your interviewer, call and politely ask if the job has been filled.

2. Describe a standard job description and explain how to manage time and assignments

A job description is an agreement between the employer and the employee. When you start a new job, you will receive a job description. It states the responsibilities and tasks of the job. It also describes the skills required for the job, to whom you must report, and the salary range.

The job description provides protection for you and your employer. It protects you, the employee, from the facility changing duties without notifying you. It protects you from being fired based on something not related to your job description. The employer is protected if you ever were to claim you did not know certain duties were part of the job. The job description reduces misunderstandings. It can be used to document what was agreed upon if legal issues occur.

When taking care of residents, you must be able to manage your time well. There are many tasks that must be done during your shift. Managing time properly helps you complete these tasks. Many of the following ideas for managing time on the job can be used to manage personal time as well:

Plan ahead. Planning is the single best way to manage time better. Sometimes it is hard even to find time to plan, but it is important to sit down and list everything that has to be done. It is helpful to take time to check to see if you have all the supplies needed for a procedure before you begin. Often just making the list and taking time to recheck will help you focus and feel better.

The nurse creates nursing assistants' work assignments based on the needs of residents and availability of staff. The assignments allow staff to work as a team. Your responsibilities in completing assignments include the following:

- Helping others when needed
- Never ignoring a resident who needs help
- Answering all call lights even when not assigned to a particular resident
- Notifying the nurse if you cannot complete an assignment

Prioritize. Identify the most important things to get done and do them first.

Make a schedule. Write out the hours of the day and fill in what needs to be done and when. This allows for a realistic schedule.

Combine activities. You can visit with residents while providing care, which combines two important tasks. Work more efficiently whenever possible.

Get help. It is a simple reality that it is not possible for you to do everything. Sometimes you will need help to ensure a resident's safety. Do not be afraid to ask for help.

3. Discuss how to manage and resolve conflict

Everyone experiences conflict at some point in his life. For example, families may argue at home, coworkers may disagree on the job, and so on. If conflict at work is not managed or resolved, it may affect the ability to function well. The work environment may suffer. When conflict occurs, there is a proper time and place to address it. You may need to talk to your supervisor for help. In general, follow these guidelines:

Guidelines: Resolving Conflict

G Plan to discuss the issue at the right time. Do not start a conversation while you are helping residents. Wait until the supervisor has decided on the right time and place. Privacy is important. Shut the door. Limit distractions, such as TV and conversations.

G Agree not to interrupt the person. Do not be rude or sarcastic, or name-call. Use active listening. Take turns speaking.

G Do not get emotional. Some situations may be upsetting. However, you will be more effective in communicating if you can keep your emotions out of it.

- **G** Check your body language. Make sure it is not tense, unwelcoming, or threatening. Maintain eye contact. Use a posture that says you are listening and interested. Lean forward slightly. Do not slouch.
- **G** Keep the focus on the issue at hand. When discussing conflict, state how you feel when a behavior occurs. Use "I" statements. First describe the actual behavior. Then use "feeling" words to describe how you feel. Let the person know how the problem is affecting you. For example, "When you are late to work, I feel upset because I end up doing your work along with my own."
- **G** People involved in the conflict may need to come up with possible solutions. Think of ways that the conflict can be resolved. A solution may be chosen by a supervisor that does not satisfy everyone. You may have to compromise. Be prepared to do this.

4. Describe employee evaluations and discuss appropriate responses to feedback

From time to time you will get evaluations from your employer. They contain ideas to help you improve your job performance, which is often referred to as *constructive feedback*. Constructive feedback involves giving opinions about a person's work and making helpful suggestions for change. The feedback may be positive or negative, but it is given in a nonaggressive way. Here are some ideas for handling feedback and using it to your benefit:

- Listen to the message that is being sent. Try not to get upset so you can understand the message.
- Hostile criticism is not the same as constructive feedback. Hostile criticism is angry and negative. Examples are, "You are useless!" or, "You are lazy and slow." Hostile criticism should not come from your employer or supervisor. You may hear hostile criticism from residents, family members, or others. The best response is something like, "I'm sorry you are so disappointed," and nothing more. Give the person a chance to calm down before trying to discuss their comments.
- Constructive feedback may come from your employer, supervisor, or others. Constructive feedback is meant to help you improve. Examples are, "You really need to be more accurate in your charting," or, "You are late too often. You'll have to make more of an effort to be on time." Listening to, accepting, and acting on constructive feedback can help you be more successful in your job. Pay attention to it.
- If you are not sure how to avoid a mistake you have made, always ask for suggestions on improving your performance (Fig. 10-3).

I think you are having a problem organizing your time.
RN

Yes, I have felt rushed lately. Do you have any suggestions on how I can prioritize my time?

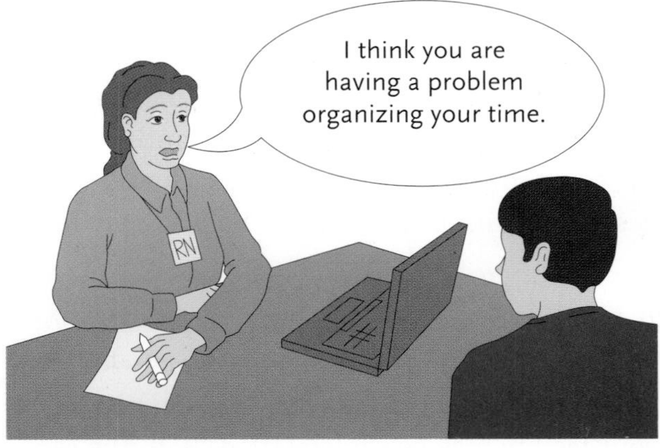

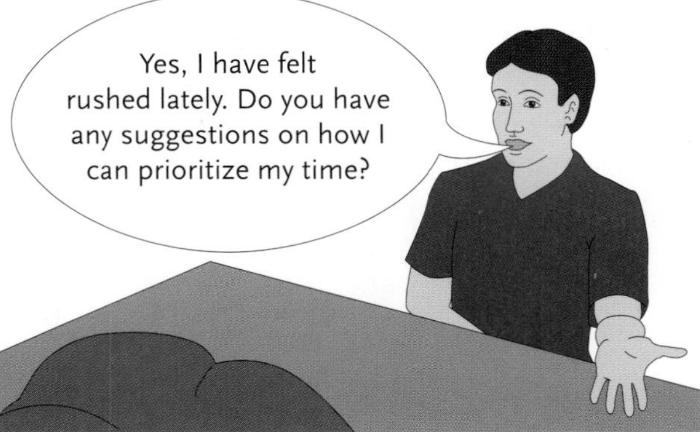

***Fig. 10-3.** Ask for suggestions when receiving constructive feedback.*

- Apologize and move on. If you have made a mistake, apologize as needed (Fig. 10-4). This may be to a supervisor, a resident, or others. Learn from the incident and put it behind you. Do not dwell on it or hold a grudge. Responding professionally to feedback is important for success in any job.

I'm sorry I've been late several times this month. I know it's inconvenient for you. I am making more of an effort to be on time, and I expect not to be late again.

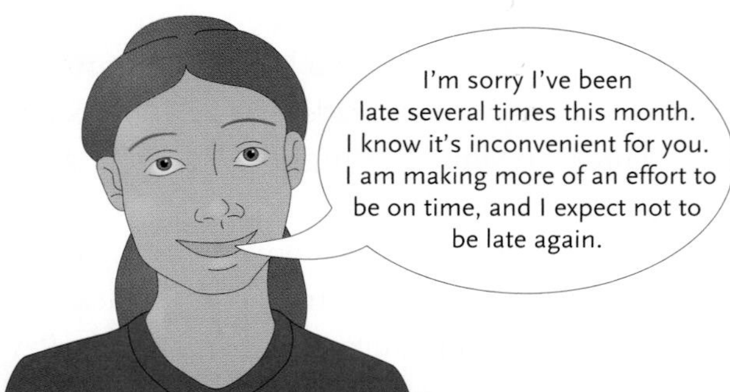

Fig. 10-4. *Be willing to apologize if you have made a mistake.*

Your evaluation will also cover overall knowledge, conflict resolution, and team effort. Flexibility, friendliness, trustworthiness, and customer service will also be considered. Evaluations are often the basis for salary increases. A good evaluation can help you advance within the company. Being open to feedback and suggestions for improvement will help you be more successful.

If you decide to change jobs, be responsible. Always give your employer at least two weeks' written notice that you will be leaving. Otherwise, your facility may be understaffed. Both the residents and other staff will suffer. Future employers may talk with past supervisors. People who change jobs too often or who do not give notice before leaving are less likely to be hired.

5. Discuss certification and explain the state's registry

To meet the requirements set forth in the Omnibus Budget Reconciliation Act (OBRA), states must regulate nursing assistant training, evaluation, and certification. OBRA requires 75 hours as the minimum level of initial training and a 12-hour minimum for annual continuing education (called *in-services*). Many states' requirements exceed the minimum hours. It is a good idea to know your state's rules.

After completing an approved training program, NAs are given a competency evaluation (a certification exam or test) so that they can be certified to work in a state. This exam usually has both a written and skills evaluation. You must pass both parts in order to be certified to work as a nursing assistant.

OBRA also requires that each state keep a registry of nursing assistants. This registry is maintained by a state department. Often this is the state's Board of Nursing or Department of Health. The registry contains NAs' training information and results of certification exams. It also has any findings of abuse, neglect, or theft by nursing assistants. Employers are able to access this list to check if you have passed the certification exam. They can see if your certification is current. They are also able to see if you have been investigated for or found guilty of abuse or neglect.

Each state has different requirements for maintaining certification. Learn your state's requirements. Follow them exactly or you will not be able to keep working. Once you are certified, you can lose your certification if you fail to follow your state's rules. This can occur if you do not work in long-term care for a period of time or fail to get the required number of continuing education hours. You can also lose certification due to criminal activities, including abuse and neglect.

6. Describe continuing education

The federal government requires that nursing assistants have a 12-hour minimum of continuing education each year. Many states may require more. In-service continuing education courses help you keep your knowledge and skills fresh. Classes also give more information about certain conditions, challenges in working with residents, or regulation changes. You need to be up-to-date on the latest that is expected of you.

Your employer may be responsible for offering in-service courses. However, you are responsible for attending and completing them. You must do the following:

- Sign up for the course or find out where it is offered.
- Attend all class sessions.
- Pay attention and complete all the class requirements.
- Make the most of your in-service programs. Participate (Fig. 10-5).

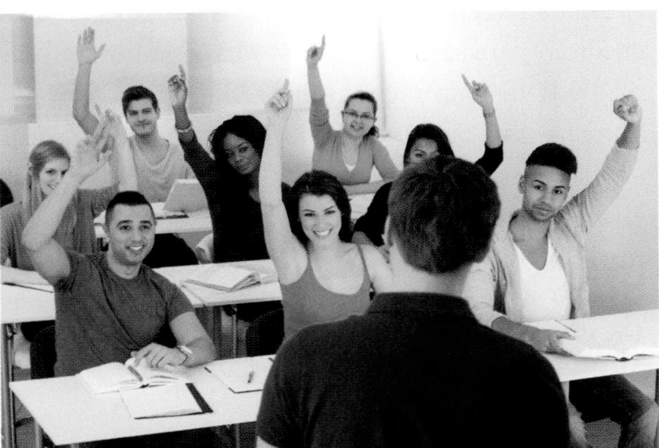

***Fig. 10-5.** Students should pay attention and participate during continuing education courses.*

- Keep original copies of all certificates and records of your successful attendance so you can prove you took the class.

7. Explain ways to manage stress

Stress is the state of being frightened, excited, confused, in danger, or irritated. It is often thought that only bad things cause stress. However, positive situations cause stress, too. For example, getting married or having a baby are usually positive situations. But both can cause enormous stress from the changes they bring to a person's life.

You may be thrilled when you get your new job. But starting work may also cause you stress. You may be afraid of making mistakes, excited about earning money or helping people, or confused about your new duties. Learning how to recognize stress and what causes it is helpful. Then you can master a few simple methods for relaxing and learn to manage stress.

A **stressor** is something that causes stress. Anything can be a stressor. Some examples include the following:

- Divorce
- Marriage
- New baby
- Parenthood
- Children growing up
- Children leaving home
- Feeling unprepared for a task
- Starting a new job
- Problems at work
- New responsibilities at work
- Feeling unsupported at work (not enough guidance and resources)
- Losing a job
- Supervisors
- Coworkers
- Residents
- Illness
- Finances

Stress is not only an emotional response. It is also a physical response. When a person has stress, changes occur in the body. The endocrine system makes more of the hormone adrenaline. This can increase nervous system response, heart rate, respiratory rate, and blood pressure. This is why, in stressful situations, your heart beats fast, you breathe hard, and you may feel warm or perspire.

Each person has a different tolerance level for stress. What one person would find overwhelming might not bother another person. A person's tolerance for stress depends on his personality, life experiences, and physical health.

Guidelines: Managing Stress

To manage stress in your life, develop healthy dietary, exercise, and lifestyle habits:

- G Eat nutritious foods.
- G Exercise regularly (Fig. 10-6). You can exercise alone or with others.

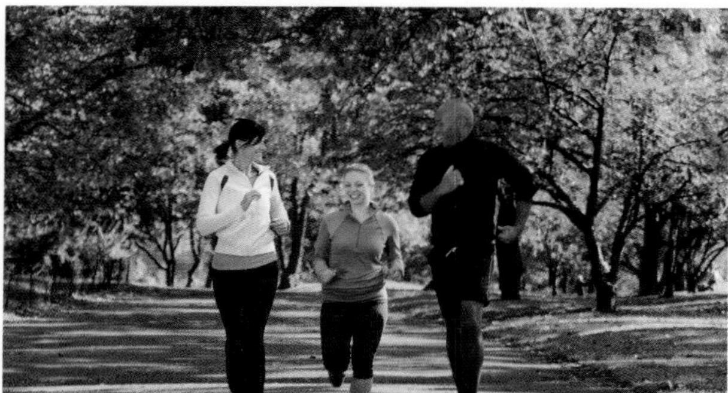

Fig. 10-6. Regular exercise is one healthy way to decrease stress.

- G Get enough sleep.
- G Drink only in moderation.
- G Do not smoke.
- G Find time at least a few times a week to do something relaxing, such as reading a book, sewing, watching a movie, or any of the following:
    - Being in nature
    - Doing something artistic (painting, drawing, writing, singing, etc.)
    - Doing yoga
    - Getting a massage
    - Listening to music
    - Meditating

Not managing stress can cause many problems. Some of these problems affect how well you do your job. Signs that you are not managing stress well include the following:

- Showing anger or being abusive to residents
- Arguing with your supervisor about assignments
- Having poor relationships with coworkers and residents
- Complaining about your job and your responsibilities
- Feeling work-related burnout (burnout is a state of mental or physical exhaustion caused by stress)
- Feeling tired even when you are rested
- Having trouble focusing on residents and procedures

Stress can seem overwhelming when you try to handle it yourself. Often just talking about stress can help you manage it better. Sometimes another person can offer helpful suggestions. You may think of new ways to handle stress just by talking it through with another person. Get help from one or more of these resources when managing stress:

- Your supervisor or another member of the care team for work-related stress
- Your family
- Your friends
- A support group
- Your place of worship
- Your doctor
- A local mental health agency
- Any phone hotline that deals with related problems (check online)

It is not appropriate to talk to your residents or their family members about your personal or job-related stress.

Developing a plan to manage stress can be helpful. The plan can include nice things you will do for yourself every day and things to do in stressful situations. Before making a plan, first answer these questions:

- What are the sources of stress in my life?
- When do I most often feel stress?
- What effects of stress do I see in my life?
- What can I change to decrease the stress I feel?
- What do I have to learn to cope with because I cannot change it?

When you have answered these questions, you will have a clearer picture of the challenges you face. Then you can come up with strategies for managing stress.

The Body Scan

A relaxation exercise can often help you feel refreshed and relaxed in only a short time. Below is a simple relaxation exercise. Try it out. See if it helps you feel more relaxed.

Close your eyes. Focus on your breathing and posture. Be sure you are comfortable. Starting at the balls of your feet, concentrate on your feet. Find any tension hidden in the feet. Try to relax and release the tension. Continue very slowly. Take a breath between each body part. Move up from the feet, focusing on and relaxing the legs, knees, thighs, hips, stomach, back, shoulders, neck, jaw, eyes, forehead, and scalp. Take a few very deep breaths. Open your eyes.

Look back over all you have learned in this program. Your work as a nursing assistant is very important. Every day may be different and challenging. In a hundred ways every week you will offer help that only a caring person like you can give.

Do not forget to value the work you have chosen to do (Fig. 10-7). Your work can mean the difference between living with independence and dignity and living without. The difference you make is sometimes life versus death. Look in the face of each of your residents. Know that you are doing important work. Look in a mirror when you get home. Be proud of how you make your living.

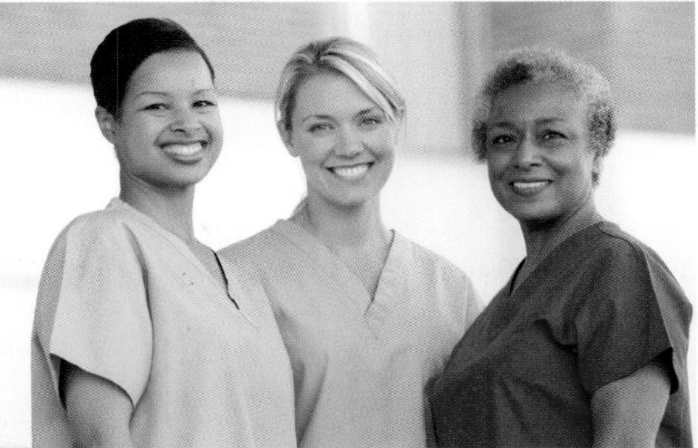

Fig. 10-7. *Value your work. Be proud of what you have chosen to do.*

Abbreviations

ac, a.c.	before meals
ad lib	as desired
ADLs	activities of daily living
amb	ambulate, ambulatory
amt	amount
ap	apical
as tol	as tolerated
ax.	axillary (armpit)
BID, b.i.d.	two times a day
BM	bowel movement
BP, B/P	blood pressure
BPM	beats per minute
BRP	bathroom privileges
BSC	bedside commode
$\bar{c}$	with
C	Centigrade
cath.	catheter
C. diff	*Clostridium difficile*
CHF	congestive heart failure
c/o	complains of
COPD	chronic obstructive pulmonary disease
CPR	cardiopulmonary resuscitation
CVA	cerebrovascular accident, stroke
DAT	diet as tolerated
DNR	do not resuscitate
DOB	date of birth
DON	director of nursing
Dx, dx	diagnosis
F	Fahrenheit
FF	force fluids
ft	foot
H_2O	water
h, hr, hr.	hour
HBV	hepatitis B virus
HOB	head of bed
HS, hs	hours of sleep
ht	height
HTN	hypertension
hyper	above normal, too fast, rapid
hypo	low, less than normal
I&O	intake and output
inc	incontinent
isol	isolation
IV, I.V.	intravenous (within a vein)
lab	laboratory
lb.	pound
LTC	long-term care
meds	medications
mL	milliliter
mm Hg	millimeters of mercury
MRSA	methicillin-resistant *Staphylococcus aureus*
N/A	not applicable
NKA	no known allergies
NPO	nothing by mouth
O_2	oxygen
OBRA	Omnibus Budget Reconciliation Act
OOB	out of bed
oz	ounce
$\bar{p}$	after
peri care	perineal care
per os, PO	by mouth
PPE	personal protective equipment
p.r.n., prn	when necessary
$\bar{q}$	every
q2h	every two hours
q3h	every three hours
q4h	every four hours
R	respirations, rectal
rehab	rehabilitation
RF	restrict fluids
ROM	range of motion
$\bar{s}$	without
SOB	shortness of breath
spec.	specimen
S&S, S/S	signs and symptoms
stat, STAT	immediately
T., temp	temperature
TB	tuberculosis
TID, t.i.d.	three times a day
TPR	temperature, pulse, and respiration
UTI	urinary tract infection
VS, vs	vital signs
w/c, W/C	wheelchair
wt.	weight

Glossary

abdominal thrusts: a method of attempting to remove an object from the airway of someone who is choking.

abduction: moving a body part away from the midline of the body.

abrasion: an injury that rubs off the surface of the skin.

absorption: the transfer of nutrients from the intestines to the cells.

abuse: purposeful mistreatment that causes physical, mental, or emotional pain or injury to someone.

active neglect: the purposeful failure to provide needed care, resulting in harm to a person.

activities of daily living (ADLs): daily personal care tasks, such as bathing; dressing; caring for skin, nail, hair, and teeth; eating; drinking; walking; transferring; and elimination.

acute care: 24-hour skilled care given in hospitals and ambulatory surgical centers for people who require short-term, immediate care for illnesses and injuries.

adaptive devices: special equipment that helps a person who is ill or disabled to perform activities of daily living; also called *assistive devices.*

adduction: moving a body part toward the midline of the body.

adult day services: care for people who need some help during certain hours, but who do not live in the facility where care is given.

advance directives: legal documents that allow people to choose what medical care they wish to have if they are unable to make those decisions themselves.

affected side: a side of the body that is weakened due to a stroke or injury; also called *weaker* or *involved side.*

ageism: prejudice toward, stereotyping of, and/or discrimination against older persons or the elderly.

Alzheimer's disease: a progressive, incurable disease that causes tangled nerve fibers and protein deposits to form in the brain, which eventually cause dementia.

ambulation: walking.

ambulatory: capable of walking.

amputation: the surgical removal of some or all of a body part, usually a hand, arm, leg, or foot.

angina pectoris: chest pain, pressure, or discomfort.

antimicrobial: an agent that destroys, resists, or prevents the development of pathogens.

anxiety: uneasiness, worry, or fear, often about a situation or condition.

apathy: a lack of interest in activities.

aspiration: the inhalation of food, fluid or foreign material into the lungs.

assault: a threat to harm a person, resulting in the person feeling fearful that he will be harmed.

assisted living: residences for people who do not need 24-hour skilled care, but do require some help with daily care.

assistive devices: special equipment that helps a person who is ill or disabled to perform activities of daily living; also called *adaptive devices.*

atrophy: the wasting away, decreasing in size, and weakening of muscles from lack of use.

autoimmune illness: an illness in which the body's immune system attacks normal tissue in the body.

battery: the intentional touching of a person without her consent.

bipolar disorder: a type of mood disorder that causes mood swings, changes in energy levels and the ability to function, periods of extreme activity, and periods of extreme depression.

bloodborne pathogens: microorganisms found in human blood, body fluid, draining wounds, and mucous membranes that can cause infection and disease in humans.

body mechanics: the way the parts of the body work together when a person moves.

bony prominences: areas of the body where the bone lies close to the skin.

brachial pulse: the pulse located inside the elbow, about one to one-and-a-half inches above the elbow.

cardiopulmonary resuscitation (CPR): medical procedures used when a person's heart or lungs have stopped working.

care plan: a plan developed for each resident to achieve certain goals; it outlines the steps and tasks that the care team must perform.

catastrophic reaction: reacting to something in an unreasonable, exaggerated way.

catheter: a thin tube inserted into the body to drain or inject fluids.

causative agent: a pathogenic microorganism that causes disease.

Centers for Disease Control and Prevention (CDC): a federal government agency that issues guidelines to protect the health of individuals and communities.

cerebrovascular accident (CVA): a condition that occurs when blood supply to a part of the brain is blocked or a blood vessel leaks or ruptures within the brain; also called *stroke*.

chain of command: the line of authority within a facility.

chain of infection: way of describing how disease is transmitted from one human being to another.

charting: documenting information and observations about residents.

Cheyne-Stokes: alternating periods of slow, irregular breathing and rapid, shallow breathing, along with periods of not breathing.

chronic: long-term or long-lasting.

cite: in a long-term care facility, to find a problem through a survey.

claustrophobia: the fear of being in a confined space.

clean: in health care, a condition in which objects are not contaminated with pathogens.

clean-catch specimen: a urine specimen that does not include the first and last urine voided; also called *mid-stream specimen*.

clichés: phrases that are used over and over again and do not really mean anything.

closed bed: a bed completely made with the bedspread and blankets in place.

***Clostridium difficile* (*C. diff*, *C. difficile*):** a bacterium that is spread by spores in feces that are difficult to kill; it causes symptoms such as diarrhea and nausea and can lead to serious inflammation of the colon (colitis).

cognition: the ability to think logically and clearly.

cognitive: related to thinking and learning.

cognitive behavioral therapy (CBT): a type of psychotherapy that is often used to treat anxiety disorders and depression and focuses on skills and solutions that a person can use to modify negative thinking and behavior patterns.

cognitive impairment: the loss of ability to think logically and clearly.

combative: violent or hostile.

combustion: the process of burning.

communication: the process of exchanging information with others by sending and receiving messages.

compassionate: being caring, concerned, considerate, empathetic, and understanding.

condom catheter: a type of urinary catheter that has an attachment on the end that fits onto the penis; also called *Texas catheter*.

confidentiality: the legal and ethical principle of keeping information private.

confusion: the inability to think logically and clearly.

conscientious: guided by a sense of right and wrong; principled.

conscious: the state of being mentally alert and having awareness of surroundings, sensations, and thoughts.

constipation: the inability to eliminate stool, or the infrequent, difficult, and often painful elimination of hard, dry stool.

constrict: to narrow.

contracture: the permanent and often painful shortening of a muscle or tendon, usually due to a lack of activity.

cultural diversity: the different groups of people with varied backgrounds and experiences who live together in the world.

culture: a system of learned beliefs and behaviors that is practiced by a group of people and is often passed on from one generation to the next.

culture change: a term given to the process of transforming services for elders so that they are based on the values and practices of the person receiving care; core values include choice, dignity, respect, self-determination, and purposeful living.

cyanotic: blue or gray, in reference to skin color.

dangle: to sit up with the legs hanging over the side of the bed in order to regain balance and stabilize blood pressure.

defense mechanisms: unconscious behaviors used to release tension or cope with stress.

dehydration: a serious condition that results from inadequate fluid in the body.

delirium: a state of severe confusion that occurs suddenly and is usually temporary.

delusions: persistent false beliefs.

dementia: the serious loss of mental abilities, such as thinking, remembering, reasoning, and communicating.

dentures: artificial teeth.

developmental disabilities: disabilities that are present at birth or emerge during childhood that restrict physical and/or mental ability.

diabetes: a condition in which the pancreas produces too little insulin or does not properly use insulin.

diabetic ketoacidosis (DKA): a complication of diabetes that is caused by having too little insulin in the body.

diagnoses: medical conditions determined by a doctor.

diastolic: the second measurement of blood pressure; phase when the heart relaxes or rests.

digestion: the process of preparing food physically and chemically so that it can be absorbed into the cells.

dilate: to widen.

direct contact: a way of transmitting pathogens through touching the infected person or his secretions.

dirty: in health care, a condition in which objects have been contaminated with pathogens.

disinfection: a process that destroys most, but not all, pathogens; it reduces the pathogen count to a level that is considered not infectious.

disorientation: confusion about person, place, or time.

disposable: only to be used once and then discarded.

disposable razor: a type of razor that is discarded in a biohazard container after one use; requires the use of shaving cream or soap.

diuretics: medications that reduce fluid volume in the body.

doff: to remove.

domestic violence: physical, sexual, or emotional abuse by spouses, intimate partners, or family members.

don: to put on.

do-not-resuscitate (DNR): a medical order that instructs medical professionals not to perform cardiopulmonary resuscitation (CPR) in the event of cardiac or respiratory arrest.

dorsiflexion: bending backward.

draw sheet: an extra sheet placed on top of the bottom sheet; used for moving residents in bed.

durable power of attorney for health care: a signed, dated, and witnessed legal document that appoints someone else to make the medical decisions for a person in the event she becomes unable to do so.

dysphagia: difficulty swallowing.

dyspnea: difficulty breathing.

edema: swelling caused by excess fluid in body tissues.

electric razor: type of razor that runs on electricity; does not require the use of soap or shaving cream.

elimination: the process of expelling wastes (made up of the waste products of food and fluids) that are not absorbed into the cells.

elope: in medicine, when a person with Alzheimer's disease wanders away from a protected area and does not return.

embolism: an obstruction of a blood vessel, usually by a blood clot.

emesis: the act of vomiting, or ejecting stomach contents through the mouth and/or nose.

emotional lability: inappropriate or unprovoked emotional responses, including laughing, crying, and anger.

empathy: identifying with the feelings of others.

enema: a specific amount of water, with or without an additive, that is introduced into the colon to stimulate the elimination of stool.

ergonomics: the science of designing equipment, areas, and work tasks to make them safer and to suit the worker's abilities.

ethics: the knowledge of right and wrong.

expiration: the process of exhaling air out of the lungs.

expressive aphasia: trouble communicating thoughts through speech or writing.

extension: straightening a body part.

false imprisonment: the unlawful restraint of someone that affects the person's freedom of movement; includes both the threat of being physically restrained and actually being physically restrained.

fecal incontinence: the inability to control the bowels, leading to involuntary passage of stool.

financial abuse: the improper or illegal use of a person's money, possessions, property, or other assets.

first aid: emergency care given immediately to an injured person by the first people to respond to an emergency.

flammable: easily ignited and capable of burning quickly.

flexion: bending a body part.

fluid balance: taking in and eliminating equal amounts of fluid.

fluid overload: a condition that occurs when the body cannot handle the amount of fluid consumed.

foot drop: a weakness of muscles in the feet and ankles that causes problems with the ability to flex the ankles and walk normally.

Fowler's: a semi-sitting body position in which a person's head and shoulders are elevated 45 to 60 degrees.

fracture: a broken bone.

fracture pan: a bedpan that is flatter than a regular bedpan.

full weight-bearing (FWB): a doctor's order stating that a person has the ability to support full body weight (100%) on both legs.

gait: manner of walking.

gait belt: a belt made of canvas or other heavy material used to help people who are weak, unsteady, or uncoordinated to walk.

gastrostomy: a surgically created opening into the stomach in order to insert a tube.

generalized anxiety disorder (GAD): an anxiety disorder that is characterized by chronic anxiety and worry, even when there is no cause for these feelings.

gestational diabetes: type of diabetes that appears in pregnant women who have never had diabetes before but who have high glucose levels during pregnancy.

glands: organs that produce and secrete chemicals called hormones.

glucose: natural sugar.

gonads: sex glands.

grief: deep distress or sorrow over a loss.

grooming: practices to care for oneself, such as caring for fingernails and hair.

hallucinations: false or distorted sensory perceptions.

hand hygiene: washing hands with either plain or antiseptic soap and water and using alcohol-based hand rubs.

hat: in health care, a collection container that can be inserted into a toilet bowl to collect and measure urine or stool.

healthcare-associated infection (HAI): an infection acquired within a healthcare setting during the delivery of medical care.

Health Insurance Portability and Accountability Act (HIPAA): a federal law that requires health information be kept private and secure and that organizations take special steps to protect this information.

hemiparesis: weakness on one side of the body.

hemiplegia: paralysis on one side of the body.

hepatitis: inflammation of the liver caused by certain viruses and other factors, such as alcohol abuse, some medications, and trauma.

hoarding: collecting and putting things away in a guarded way.

holistic care: a type of care that involves caring for the whole person—the mind as well as the body.

home health care: health care that is provided in a person's home.

homeostasis: the condition in which all of the body's systems are working at their best.

hormones: chemical substances created by the body that control numerous body functions.

hospice care: holistic, compassionate care given to people who have approximately six months or less to live.

hygiene: practices that keep bodies clean and healthy.

hypertension (HTN): high blood pressure, regularly measuring 130/80 mm Hg or higher.

impairment: a loss of function or ability.

incident: an accident, problem, or unexpected event during the course of care that is not part of the normal routine in a healthcare facility.

incontinence: the inability to control the bladder or bowels.

indirect contact: a way of transmitting pathogens from touching an object contaminated by the infected person.

indwelling catheter: a type of urinary catheter that remains inside the bladder for a period of time; also called *Foley catheter.*

infection: the state resulting from pathogens invading the body and multiplying.

infection prevention: the set of methods practiced in healthcare facilities to prevent and control the spread of disease.

infectious: contagious.

inflammation: swelling.

informed consent: the process in which a person, with the help of a doctor, makes informed decisions about his health care.

input: the fluid a person consumes; also called *intake.*

inspiration: the process of inhaling air into the lungs.

insulin: a hormone that works to move glucose from the blood and into the cells for energy for the body.

insulin reaction: a complication of diabetes that can result from either too much insulin or too little food; also known as *hypoglycemia.*

intake: the fluid a person consumes; also called *input.*

intravenous (IV) therapy: the delivery of medication, nutrition, or fluids through a person's vein.

involuntary seclusion: the separation of a person from others against the person's will.

involved side: a side of the body that is weakened due to a stroke or injury; also called *weaker* or *affected side.*

lateral: body position in which a person is lying on either side.

laws: rules set by the government to help people live peacefully together and to ensure safety.

length of stay: the number of days a person stays in a healthcare facility.

liability: a legal term that means someone can be held responsible for harming someone else.

living will: a document that outlines the medical care a person wants, or does not want, in case she becomes unable to make those decisions.

localized infection: an infection that is limited to a specific location in the body and has local symptoms.

logrolling: moving a person as a unit without disturbing the alignment of the body.

long-term care (LTC): care given in long-term care facilities for people who need 24-hour skilled care.

major depressive disorder: type of mood disorder that causes pain, fatigue, apathy, sadness, irritability, anxiety, sleeplessness, and loss of appetite, as well as other symptoms; also called *depression* or *clinical depression.*

malpractice: injury to a person due to professional misconduct through negligence, carelessness, or lack of skill.

masturbation: to touch or rub sexual organs in order to give oneself or another person sexual pleasure.

Medicaid: a medical assistance program for people who have a low income, as well as for people with disabilities.

medical asepsis: measures used to reduce and prevent the spread of pathogens.

Medicare: a federal health insurance program for people who are 65 or older, have certain disabilities or permanent kidney failure, or are ill and cannot work.

menopause: the end of menstruation; occurs when a woman has not had a menstrual period for 12 months.

mental health: the normal functioning of emotional and intellectual abilities.

mental health disorder: a disorder that affects a person's ability to function and often causes inappropriate behavior; confusion, disorientation, agitation, and anxiety are common symptoms.

metabolism: physical and chemical processes by which substances are broken down or transformed into energy or products for use by the body.

microbe: a living thing or organism that is so small that it can be seen only under a microscope; also called *microorganism.*

microorganism (MO): a living thing or organism that is so small that it can be seen only under a microscope; also called *microbe.*

Minimum Data Set (MDS): a detailed form with guidelines for assessing residents in long-term care facilities.

mode of transmission: the method of describing how a pathogen travels.

modified diets: diets for people who have certain illnesses, conditions, or food allergies; also called *special* or *therapeutic diets.*

MRSA (methicillin-resistant *Staphylococcus aureus*): bacteria (*Staphylococcus aureus*) that have developed resistance to the antibiotic methicillin.

mucous membranes: the membranes that line body cavities that open to the outside of the body, such as the linings of the mouth, nose, eyes, rectum, or genitals.

myocardial infarction (MI): a condition that occurs when the heart muscle does not receive enough oxygen because blood flow to the heart is blocked; also called *heart attack.*

nasogastric tube: a feeding tube that is inserted into the nose and goes to the stomach.

neglect: the failure to provide needed care that results in physical, mental, or emotional harm to a person.

negligence: an action, or the failure to act or provide the proper care, that results in unintended injury to a person.

nonintact skin: skin that is broken by abrasions, cuts, rashes, pimples, lesions, surgical incisions, or boils.

nonverbal communication: communication without using words.

non-weight-bearing (NWB): a doctor's order stating that a person is unable to touch the floor or support any body weight on one or both legs.

NPO: abbreviation meaning *nothing by mouth;* medical order that means a person should not have anything to eat or drink.

nutrient: a necessary substance that provides energy, promotes growth and health, and helps regulate metabolism.

nutrition: how the body uses food to maintain health.

objective information: information based on what a person sees, hears, touches, or smells; also called *signs.*

obsessive compulsive disorder (OCD): an anxiety disorder characterized by obsessive behavior or thoughts, which may cause the person to repeatedly perform a behavior or routine.

obstructed airway: a condition in which something is blocking the tube through which air enters the lungs.

Occupational Safety and Health Administration (OSHA): a federal government agency that makes rules to protect workers from hazards on the job.

occupied bed: a bed made while a person is in the bed.

ombudsman: a legal advocate for residents in long-term care facilities who helps resolve disputes and settle conflicts.

Omnibus Budget Reconciliation Act (OBRA): a law passed by the federal government that includes minimum standards for nursing assistant training, staffing requirements, resident assessment instructions, and information on rights for residents.

open bed: a bed made with linen folded down to the foot of the bed.

opposition: touching the thumb to any other finger.

oral care: care of the mouth, teeth, and gums.

orthosis: a device that helps support and align a limb and improve its functioning; also called *orthotic device.*

orthotic device: a device that helps support and align a limb and improve its functioning; also called *orthosis.*

osteoarthritis: common type of arthritis that usually affects the hips, knees, fingers, thumbs, and spine; also called *degenerative joint disease (DJD)* or *degenerative arthritis.*

osteoporosis: a disease that causes bones to become porous and brittle, causing them to break easily.

ostomy: a surgically created opening from an area inside the body to the outside.

outpatient care: care given to people who have had treatments, procedures, or surgeries and need short-term skilled care.

output: all fluid that is eliminated from the body; includes urine, feces, vomitus, perspiration, moisture that is exhaled in the air, and wound drainage.

oxygen therapy: the administration of oxygen to increase the supply of oxygen to the lungs.

pacing: walking back and forth in the same area.

palliative care: care given to people who have serious diseases or who are dying that emphasizes relieving pain, controlling symptoms, and preventing side effects.

panic disorder: a disorder characterized by a person having regular panic attacks or living with constant anxiety about having another attack.

paraplegia: the loss of function of the lower body and legs.

parenteral nutrition (PN): the intravenous infusion of nutrients administered directly into the bloodstream, bypassing the digestive system.

partial bath: a bath given on days when a complete bath or shower is not done; includes washing the face, hands, underarms, and perineum.

partial weight-bearing (PWB): a doctor's order stating that a person is able to support some body weight on one or both legs.

passive neglect: the unintentional failure to provide needed care, resulting in physical, mental, or emotional harm to a person.

pathogens: microorganisms that are capable of causing infection and disease.

pediculosis: an infestation of lice.

percutaneous endoscopic gastrostomy (PEG) tube: a feeding tube that is placed into the stomach through the abdominal wall.

perineal care: care of the genitals and anal area.

perineum: the genital and anal area.

perseveration: the repetition of words, phrases, questions, or actions.

personal: relating to life outside one's job, such as family, friends, and home life.

personal protective equipment (PPE): equipment that helps protect employees from serious workplace injuries or illnesses resulting from contact with workplace hazards.

person-centered care: a type of care that places the emphasis on the person needing care and his or her individuality and capabilities.

phantom limb pain: pain in a limb (or extremity) that has been amputated.

phantom sensation: warmth, itching, or tingling in a body part that has been amputated.

phobia: an intense irrational fear of or anxiety about an object, place, or situation.

physical abuse: any treatment, intentional or not, that causes harm to a person's body.

policy: a course of action that should be taken every time a certain situation occurs.

portable commode: a chair with a toilet seat and a removable container underneath that is used for elimination; also called *bedside commode.*

portal of entry: any body opening on an uninfected person that allows pathogens to enter.

portal of exit: any body opening on an infected person that allows pathogens to leave.

positioning: the act of helping people into positions that promote comfort and health.

postmortem care: care of the body after death.

posttraumatic stress disorder (PTSD): an anxiety disorder caused by experiencing or witnessing a traumatic experience.

posture: the way a person holds and positions his body.

pre-diabetes: a condition that occurs when a person's blood glucose levels are above normal but are not high enough for a diagnosis of type 2 diabetes.

pressure injuries: injuries or wounds that result from skin deterioration and shearing; also called *pressure ulcers, pressure sores, bed sores,* or *decubitus ulcers.*

pressure points: areas of the body that bear much of the body weight.

procedure: a method or way of doing something.

professional: having to do with work or a job.

professionalism: the act of behaving properly when working.

pronation: turning downward.

prone: a body position in which a person is lying on his stomach, or front side of the body.

prosthesis: a device that replaces a body part that is missing or deformed because of an accident, injury, illness, or birth defect; used to improve a person's ability to function and/or to improve appearance.

protected health information (PHI): a person's private health information, which includes name, address, telephone number, social security number, email address, and medical record number.

psychological abuse: emotional harm caused by threatening, scaring, humiliating, intimidating, isolating, or insulting a person, or by treating him as a child.

psychosocial needs: needs that involve social interaction, emotions, intellect, and spirituality.

psychotherapy: a method of treating mental health disorders that involves talking about one's problems with mental health professionals.

puree: to blend or grind food into a thick paste of baby food consistency.

quadriplegia: loss of function of legs, trunk, and arms.

radial pulse: the pulse located on the inside of the wrist, where the radial artery runs just beneath the skin.

range of motion (ROM): exercises that put a joint through its full arc of motion.

receptive aphasia: difficulty understanding spoken or written words.

rehabilitation: care that is given by specialists to help restore or improve function after an illness or injury.

reproduce: to create new human life.

reservoir: a place where a pathogen lives and multiplies.

Residents' Rights: numerous rights identified in the OBRA law that relate to how residents must be treated while living in a facility; they provide an ethical code of conduct for healthcare workers.

respiration: the process of inhaling air into the lungs and exhaling air out of the lungs.

restorative care: care given after rehabilitation to maintain a person's function, improve his quality of life, and increase his independence.

restraint: a physical or chemical way to restrict voluntary movement or behavior.

restraint alternatives: measures used in place of a restraint or that reduce the need for a restraint.

restraint-free care: an environment in which restraints are not kept or used for any reason.

rheumatoid arthritis: a type of arthritis in which joints become red, swollen, and very painful, resulting in restricted movement and possible deformities.

rotation: turning a joint.

routine urine specimen: a urine specimen that can be collected any time a person voids.

rummaging: going through drawers, closets, or personal items that belong to oneself or others.

safety razor: a type of razor that has a sharp blade with a special safety casing to help prevent cuts; requires the use of shaving cream or soap.

scalds: burns caused by hot liquids.

schizophrenia: a type of psychotic disorder that causes problems with thinking, communication, and the ability to manage emotions, make decisions, and understand reality.

scope of practice: defines the tasks that healthcare providers are legally allowed to do as permitted by state or federal law.

sexual abuse: the forcing of a person to perform or participate in sexual acts against her will; includes unwanted touching, exposing oneself, and sharing pornographic material.

sexual harassment: any unwelcome sexual advance or behavior that creates an intimidating, hostile, or offensive working environment.

sharps: needles or other sharp objects.

shearing: rubbing or friction that results from the skin moving one way and the bone underneath it remaining fixed or moving in the opposite direction.

shock: a condition that occurs when organs and tissues in the body do not receive an adequate blood supply.

Sims': a body position in which a person is lying on his left side with the upper knee flexed and raised toward the chest.

skilled care: medically necessary care given by a skilled nurse or therapist.

special diets: diets for people who have certain illnesses, conditions, or food allergies; also called *modified* or *therapeutic diets.*

specimen: a sample that is used for analysis in order to try to make a diagnosis.

sputum: thick mucus coughed up from the lungs.

Standard Precautions: a method of infection prevention in which all blood, body fluids, nonintact skin, and mucous membranes are treated as if they were infected with an infectious disease.

sterilization: a cleaning measure that destroys all microorganisms, including pathogens.

stoma: an artificial opening in the body.

straight catheter: a type of urinary catheter that is removed immediately after urine is drained or collected.

stress: the state of being frightened, excited, confused, in danger, or irritated.

stressor: something that causes stress.

subacute care: care given in hospitals or in long-term care facilities for people who need less care than for an acute illness, but more care than for a chronic illness.

subjective information: information that a person cannot or did not observe, but is based on something reported to the person that may or may not be true; also called *symptoms.*

substance abuse: the repeated use of legal or illegal substances in a way that is harmful to oneself or others.

sundowning: becoming restless and agitated in the late afternoon, evening, or night.

supination: turning upward.

supine: a body position in which a person lies flat on his back.

surgical asepsis: the state of being completely free of all microorganisms; also called *sterile technique*.

susceptible host: an uninfected person who could get sick.

sympathy: sharing in the feelings and difficulties of others.

syncope: loss of consciousness; also called *fainting*.

systemic infection: an infection that travels through the bloodstream and is spread throughout the body, causing general symptoms.

systolic: first measurement of blood pressure; phase when the heart is at work, contracting and pushing the blood out of the left ventricle of the heart.

tactful: showing sensitivity and having a sense of what is appropriate when dealing with others.

terminal illness: a disease or condition that will eventually cause death.

therapeutic diets: diets for people who have certain illnesses, conditions, or food allergies; also called *modified* or *special diets*.

transfer belt: a belt made of canvas or other heavy material that is used to help people who are weak, unsteady, or uncoordinated to transfer.

transient ischemic attack (TIA): a warning sign of a CVA/stroke resulting from a temporary lack of oxygen in the brain; symptoms may last up to 24 hours.

transmission: passage or transfer.

Transmission-Based Precautions: method of infection prevention used when caring for persons who are infected or may be infected with certain infectious diseases.

tuberculosis (TB): a highly contagious disease caused by a bacterium that is carried on mucous droplets suspended in the air; usually affects the lungs and causes coughing, trouble breathing, weight loss, and fatigue.

tumor: a cluster of abnormally growing cells.

unoccupied bed: a bed made while no person is in the bed.

urinary catheter: a type of catheter that is used to drain urine from the bladder.

urinary incontinence: the inability to control the bladder, which leads to an involuntary loss of urine.

validating: giving value to or approving.

verbal abuse: the use of spoken or written words, pictures, or gestures that threaten, embarrass, or insult a person.

verbal communication: communication involving the use of spoken or written words or sounds.

vital signs: measurements—temperature, pulse, respirations, blood pressure, pain level—that monitor the functioning of the vital organs of the body.

voids: urinates.

VRE (vancomycin-resistant *Enterococcus*): bacteria (*enterococci*) that have developed resistance to the antibiotic vancomycin.

wandering: walking aimlessly around the facility or facility grounds.

workplace violence: verbal, physical, or sexual abuse of staff by other staff members, residents, or visitors.

Index

abbreviations 24, 250
abdominal thrusts 38
abduction 235, 236, 237, 238, 239
abduction pillow 83, 129
abuse 14
- and OBRA 10
- and Residents' Rights 12, 13
- observing and reporting 15-16
- reporting of 15, 16
- sexual 14
- signs of 15-16
- types of 14

acceptance
- and cultural diversity 63
- as a psychosocial need 60
- as a stage of grief 72

accident prevention 31, 32-34
acquired immunodeficiency syndrome (AIDS), see also human immunodeficiency virus (HIV)
- and dementia 107
- and Residents' Rights 109
- care guidelines 108
- diet 108
- emotional support 108
- signs and symptoms of 107
- transmission of 107

activities director 6
activities of daily living (ADLs) 3
- and Alzheimer's disease 116-118

activity 60, 64
activity therapy 123
acute care 2
adaptive devices, see also assistive devices 5, 232, 233
adduction 235, 236, 237, 238, 239
ADLs, see activities of daily living
admission
- guidelines for 169-170

admitting a resident
- procedure for 170-171

adolescence 67
adult day services 2
adulthood 67-68
advance directives 72
- and Residents' Rights 73

affected side 143
ageism 68
aging
- myths of 68

aging, normal changes of 69
- for circulatory system 91
- for endocrine system 102
- for gastrointestinal system 98
- for immune system 106
- for integumentary system 79
- for lymphatic system 106
- for musculoskeletal system 80
- for nervous system 84
- for reproductive system 105
- for respiratory system 94
- for sense organs 89
- for urinary system 97

agitation
- and Alzheimer's disease 118-119

AIDS, see acquired immunodeficiency syndrome (AIDS)
AIDS dementia complex 107
airborne infection isolation room 58
Airborne Precautions 55
alarms, bed or chair 190
alignment
- and body mechanics 31
- and pain management 73, 185
- guidelines for 233
- in a chair or wheelchair 164

Alzheimer's disease (AD) 113
- and activities of daily living 116-118
- and nutritional problems 117-118
- and personal care 116-118
- and Residents' Rights 122
- communication guidelines 114-116
- diagnosis of 113
- difficult behaviors 118-122
- therapies for 122-123

ambulation 229
- and visual impairment 230
- procedure for assisting with 229-230
- with assistive devices 231-232

ambulatory surgical centers 2
a.m. care, see also personal care 124
American Cancer Society 77, 109
amputation 233
- guidelines for care 234

anger
- as stage of grief 72
- guidelines for communication 30

angina pectoris 92
- care guidelines 92-93

anti-embolic stockings 83, 146
- procedure for putting on 146-147

antimicrobial 49
anxiety 70
- and HIV/AIDS 108

anxiety disorders 70-71
apathy 15, 70
aphasia
- expressive 44, 85
- receptive 44, 85

appetite
- guidelines for promoting 219

appetite, loss of
- and depression 70
- and cancer 110
- and COPD 95
- and HIV/AIDS 108
- and neglect 16

arthritis
- care guidelines 81
- types of 81

artificial eye 234
artificial nails 49
asepsis
- types of 47

aspiration 148, 223
- and oral care for an unconscious resident 148-149
- prevention of 223

assault 14
assisted living 2
assistive devices 5
- for ADLs 232
- for bathing 129, 136
- for ambulation 230-231
- for dressing 87, 144
- for eating 219, 225, 226

atrophy 80, 189, 228, 234
autoimmune illness 81, 88
autopsy 113
axilla 129, 130, 173, 174
axillary
- procedure for measuring and recording temperature 179-180

backrest 128
back rub
- procedure for 133-134

bandages, elastic 208
bargaining
- as a stage of grief 72

barriers
- to communication 24-25
- to managing pain 185

base of support 31
bathing
- and Alzheimer's disease 116
- guidelines for 129
- importance of 129
- procedure for bed bath 129-133
- procedure for shower or tub 134-135

battery 14
bed bath
- procedure for giving 129-133

bed cradle 108, 128, 233
bedmaking
- closed bed 206
- guidelines for 203
- open bed 207
- procedure for occupied bed 203-206
- procedure for unoccupied bed 206

bedpan 152
- procedure for assisting with 152-154

bed sore, see pressure injury
benign prostatic hypertrophy 105-106
biohazard container 48, 142
bipolar disorder 70
bladder retraining
- guidelines for assisting with 239-240

bleeding
- procedure for controlling 40-41

bloodborne pathogens 57
blood pressure
- and hypertension 91-92
- diastolic 182
- normal range 173
- procedure for measuring 183-184
- systolic 181

body fluids 48, 49, 53, 55, 57
- and Standard Precautions 48

body language 21, 27, 73, 112, 185
body mechanics 31-32
body positions 157
body systems, see individual system, e.g., circulatory system
body temperature, see also temperature 174
bony prominences 125
boundaries, professional 13-14
bowel movement 99, 152
bowel retraining
- guidelines for assisting with 239-240

brachial pulse 180
BRAT diet 108
burns
- guidelines for preventing 33
- procedure for treating 41

call light 24, 201, 228
cancer
- care guidelines 109-110
- causes of 109
- treatments for 109
- warning signs of 109

cane
- guidelines for use 231
- procedure for assisting resident with 231-232
- types of 230

carbohydrates 209
cardiopulmonary resuscitation (CPR) 37
care plan 7
care team 5-6
cataracts 90
catastrophic reaction 119
catheter, urinary 196
- guidelines for care 196
- observing and reporting 196
- procedure for care of 196-198
- procedure for emptying drainage bag 198-199
- types of 196

causative agent 46
C. difficile 59
center of gravity 31
Centers for Disease Control and Prevention (CDC) 47
Centers for Medicare & Medicaid Services (CMS) 3, 11
central nervous system, see also nervous system
- observing and reporting 84-85

cerebrovascular accident (CVA) 44
- and transfers 86
- care guidelines 86-87
- communication guidelines 87
- dressing 86-87
- problems experienced afterward 85
- signs of 44

certification, maintaining 246
certified nursing assistant, see nursing assistant
chain of command 6
chain of infection 46
charting, see documentation
chart, medical 18, 19, 47
chemotherapy 45, 109, 110
Cheyne-Stokes respirations 75
childhood 66-67
choking, see also obstructed airway
- preventing 34
- procedure for clearing obstructed airway 38

chronic 1
chronic conditions 1, 3
chronic obstructive pulmonary disease (COPD)
- care guidelines 95-96
- observing and reporting 96

circadian rhythm 174
circulatory system
- common disorders 91-94
- NA's role in assisting with 91
- normal changes of aging 91
- observing and reporting 91
- structure and function 90

claustrophobia 71
clean 54
- and infection prevention 54

clean-catch specimen 194
- procedure for collecting 194

cliché 25
clinical depression 70
closed bed 206
Clostridium difficile 59
cognition 112
cognitive impairment 112
colostomy 100
combative behavior 29-30
combustion 199
communication 21
- and call light 24
- and cultural considerations 26
- and CVA 87
- barriers to 24-25
- nonverbal 21
- telephone 24
- using the senses 22-23
- verbal 21
- with residents with Alzheimer's disease 114-116
- with residents with special needs 26-30

communication boards 87
community resources 77
computers 19-20
confidentiality 17
- and HIPAA 17-18
- and Residents' Rights 12

conflict
- guidelines for resolving 244-245

confusion 111
congestive heart failure (CHF)
- care guidelines 93-94

constipation 80, 89, 99, 216
constrict 79
Contact Precautions 56
contracture 80, 88, 128, 157, 228
conversion table 191
coronary artery disease (CAD) 92
CPR 37
criminal background check 242
criticism, hostile 245
crutches
- procedure for assisting with 231-232

cues
- and helping with eating 225

cultural diversity 63
culture 26
- and communication 26
- and diet 213
- and language 63
- and pain 185
- and touch 26

culture change 3
cyanotic 38, 40, 208
dairy
- and MyPlate 212

dangle 161
- procedure for assisting resident to 162-163

death, see also dying
- and advance directives 72-73
- and grief after death 76
- and hospice care 76-77
- and Kübler-Ross' stages of grief 72
- care guidelines 73-74
- legal rights and 74
- physical changes after 75
- postmortem care 75-76
- signs of approaching 75

decubitus ulcer, see pressure injury
defense mechanisms 25
dehydration 216
- guidelines for preventing 216-217
- observing and reporting 217

delirium 111
delusions
- and Alzheimer's disease 120
- and schizophrenia 71

dementia, see also Alzheimer's disease 112

denial
- as a defense mechanism 25
- as a stage of grief 72

dentures 151
- procedure for cleaning 151-152

depression
- and Alzheimer's disease 120
- and HIV/AIDS 108
- and inactivity 65
- and loss of independence 62, 63
- and pain 184
- as stage of grief 72
- signs and symptoms of 70
- treatment for 71
- types of 70

development, human 66-69
developmental disabilities 69
diabetes 102
- and diabetic ketoacidosis 43
- and diet 214-215
- and insulin reaction 42-43
- care guidelines 103-104
- foot care 104
- signs and symptoms 103
- tests 104
- types 103

diabetic ketoacidosis (DKA) 43
diagnoses 1
diarrhea 100
- and *C. diff* 59

diastolic pressure 182
diet, see also nutrition
- diabetic 214-215
- fluid-restricted 214
- liquid 215
- low-fat 214
- low-protein 214
- low-sodium 214
- mechanical soft 215
- modified calorie 214
- pureed 215-216
- soft 215
- vegetarian 215

diet cards 34, 214, 220, 221
digestion 98
dignity
- and dying residents 74, 75
- and personal care 125
- and person-centered care 3, 62
- and Residents' Rights 11, 12, 63
- and sexual needs 61

dilate 79

dirty 54
- and infection prevention 54

disability
- and rehabilitation 227, 232, 234

disaster guidelines 36-37
discharging a resident
- procedure for 172-173

disease, see specific disease
disinfection 54
disorientation 32
- and falls 32
- as a sign of approaching death 75

displacement 25
disposable 55
disposable gloves 53
disruptive behavior
- and Alzheimer's disease 121

diuretics 92
documentation
- guidelines for 18-20

domestic violence 14
do-not-resuscitate (DNR) order 73
dorsiflexion 235
draw sheet 128
dressing
- and Alzheimer's disease 116-117
- and assistive devices 144, 232
- guidelines for assisting with 143-144
- guidelines for IVs 145-146
- procedure for resident 144-145
- with one-sided weakness 86-87

dressings
- procedure for non-sterile 207

Droplet Precautions 56
durable power of attorney for health care 73
dying, see also death
- care guidelines 75
- legal rights and 74

dysphagia 85, 222
eating
- and Residents' Rights 220, 226
- assistive devices for 219, 232
- guidelines for assisting with 220
- guidelines for special needs 225-226
- independence with 220
- procedure for assisting with 221-222

edema 218

elastic stocking
- procedure for applying 146-147

elimination 98

embolism 146

emergencies, medical, see also specific emergency 37-45

emesis 44

emotional lability 85

empathy 9

employment
- application 242
- job description 243-244
- job interviews 242-243
- job seeking 241
- references 241-242

endocrine system
- common disorders 102-104
- NA's role in assisting with 102
- normal changes of aging 102
- observing and reporting 102
- structure and function 102

epilepsy 43

equipment
- and isolation 56-57
- and resident's unit 201-202
- handling 54-55
- personal protective 50-54

ergonomics 163

ethics 10
- guidelines for ethical behavior 10

exercise
- and circulatory system 91, 93
- and diabetes 104
- and mobility 228-229
- and stress 102
- range of motion 80

expiration 94, 180

expressive aphasia 44, 85

extension 235

eyes and ears
- common disorders 90
- observing and reporting 90

face shields, see personal protective equipment

facility, healthcare
- types of 2

fact
- vs. opinion 22

fainting
- procedure for responding to 42

falls
- and incident reports 20
- prevention of 32-33

false imprisonment 14

family
- role of 65
- types 65

fats
- categories of 210

fecal impaction 99

fecal incontinence 99

feedback, constructive 245

feeding residents, see also eating
- procedure for 221-222

fingernail care
- procedure for 138-139

fire
- guidelines for safety 35-36
- potential hazards 199

fire extinguisher 35

first aid 37
- procedures for 37-45

first impression
- and admission 169

flammable 199

flexion 235

flossing teeth
- procedure for 150-151

fluid balance 191

fluid overload 218
- observing and reporting 218

fluid-restricted diet 214

food, see eating, nutrition

footboard 128

foot care
- and diabetes 104
- observing and reporting 139
- procedure for 139-140

foot drop 128

Fowler's position 157

fracture 32
- hip 82-83

fracture pan 152

fruits
- and MyPlate 211

gait 22, 32, 88

gait belt 86, 163

gastric tubes 224

gastroesophageal reflux disease 100

gastrointestinal system
- common disorders 99-100
- NA's role in assisting with 99
- normal changes of aging 98
- observing and reporting 99
- structure and function 98

gastrostomy 224

geriatric chair 188, 189

glands 79, 102

glaucoma 90

gloves
- procedure for doffing 53-54
- procedure for donning 53
- when to wear 53

goggles
- procedure for donning 52

gown
- procedure for donning and doffing 51-52

grains
- and MyPlate 211

grief 72

grooming, see also personal care 124
- and Alzheimer's disease 116-117
- guidelines for assisting with 138-152

hair
- procedure for combing or brushing 141-142
- procedure for shampooing 134-135

hallucinations
- and Alzheimer's disease 120
- and schizophrenia 71

hand and fingernail care
- procedure for giving 138-139

hand hygiene 49
- procedure for 49-50

handrolls 128

handwashing
- procedure for 49-50
- when to wash hands 49

head or spinal cord injuries
- guidelines for care 88-90

healthcare team 5-6

Health Insurance Portability and Accountability Act (HIPAA) 17

hearing aid 25, 26

hearing impairment
- care guidelines 26-27

heart attack, see myocardial infarction

height
- procedure for measuring and recording 187-188

Heimlich maneuver, see abdominal thrusts
hemiparesis 44, 85
hemiplegia 44, 85
hemorrhoids 99
hepatitis 57
- and HIV/AIDS 107
- vaccination for type B 58, 59

Hierarchy of Needs 60
high blood pressure 91, 182
HIPAA, see Health Insurance Portability and Accountability Act
hip replacement
- care guidelines 82-83
- observing and reporting 83

hoarding 121
holistic care 62
home health care 2
homeostasis 78
hormones 102
hospice care 2, 76
- goals of 77

hospitals 1, 2
human development
- stages of 66-68

human immunodeficiency virus (HIV), see also acquired immunodeficiency syndrome (AIDS)
- and Residents' Rights 109
- care guidelines 108
- diet 108
- emotional support 108
- transmission of 107

human needs, basic 60
hydration
- documentation 191, 216

hygiene 124
hypertension (HTN) 91
- care guidelines 92

ileostomy 100
immobility
- complications of 65

immune system
- common disorders 106-109
- NA's role in assisting with 106
- normal changes of aging 106
- observing and reporting 106
- structure and function 106

impairment
- hearing 26-27
- visual 27-28

inactivity 65, 80
inappropriate behavior 30
incident 20
- guidelines for reporting 20

incontinence 23
- fecal 99
- urinary 97

incontinence briefs 240
independence
- after CVA 86
- and Alzheimer's disease 113, 121
- and personal care 124, 125
- and psychsocial needs 60
- and Residents' Rights 11, 63
- loss of 62, 63
- promoting 62

indwelling catheter 196
infancy 66
infection 45
- healthcare-acquired 46
- localized 45
- systemic 45

infection prevention 45
- Airborne Precautions 55
- and equipment handling 54-55
- and glove use 52-54
- bloodborne pathogens 57
- *C. difficile* and 59
- chain of infection 46-47
- Contact Precautions 56
- Droplet Precautions 56
- employee's responsibilities 59
- employer's responsibilities 59
- hand hygiene 49-50
- MRSA and 58
- spills, handling 55
- Standard Precautions 47-49
- Transmission-Based Precautions 55-57
- VRE and 59

inflammation 81
informed consent 12
in-service education 11, 36, 59, 246
inspiration 94, 180
insulin 42, 43, 103, 104
insulin reaction 42
intake 190
intake and output (I&O) 191-192
integumentary system
- and pressure injuries 125-126
- NA's role in assisting with 79
- normal changes of aging 79
- observing and reporting 79-80
- structure and function 79

intellectual disability 69
interpreter 21
intravenous (IV) therapy 145, 200
- dressing resident with an IV 145-146
- observing and reporting 200

involuntary seclusion 14
isolation guidelines 56-57
job, see employment
job interview 242-243
Kaposi's sarcoma 107
knee replacement 83-84
Kübler-Ross, Elisabeth 72
language
- and communication 25
- and culture 26, 63
- and person-centered care 3
- and Residents' Rights 21
- body 21

lateral position 157
laws 10
lesbian, gay, bisexual, transgender, or queer (LGBTQ) residents 62, 169
liability 6
lice 141
licensed practical nurse (LPN) 5
licensed vocational nurse (LVN) 5
lift, see mechanical lifts
linen, see also bedmaking
- guidelines for handling 54-55

liquid diet 215
living will 72
localized infection 45
logrolling 160
- procedure for 161

long-term care (LTC) 1
loss
- of independence 62, 63
- types that residents may be experiencing 62

low-fat diet 214
low-protein diet 214
low-sodium diet 214

lymphatic system
- NA's role in assisting with 106
- normal changes of aging 106
- observing and reporting 106
- structure and function 106

masks, see personal protective equipment

Maslow, Abraham 60

massage, see also back rub
- procedure for giving 133-134
- skin care 127

masturbation 60

Material Safety Data Sheet (MSDS), see Safety Data Sheet (SDS)

meal trays 20, 34, 49, 57, 202, 215, 220, 225

mechanical lifts
- procedure for transferring 167-168

mechanical soft diet 215

Medicaid 3

medical emergency, see also specific emergency
- responding to 37-45

medical record, see documentation

medical social worker (MSW) 6

medical terminology 23-24

Medicare 3

menopause 82, 105

mental health 28

mental health disorder 28
- and communication 29
- care guidelines 71
- observing and reporting 71-72
- types of 70-71

mental retardation, see intellectual disability

metabolism 78, 209

methicillin-resistant *Staphylococcus aureus* (MRSA) 58

microbe 45

microorganism 45

military time 19

minerals 210

mode of transmission 46

modified calorie diet 214

mood changes 15, 71, 85, 228

mood disorders 70

mouth care, see oral care

mucous membranes 46, 47, 48, 49, 51, 53

multiple sclerosis (MS)
- care guidelines 88

musculoskeletal system
- common disorders 81-84
- NA's role in assisting with 80
- normal changes of aging 80
- observing and reporting 80-81
- structure and function 80

myocardial infarction (MI) 39
- care guidelines 93
- responding to 40
- signs and symptoms of 40

MyPlate 210-212

nail care
- procedure for providing 138-139

nasal cannula 199, 200

nasogastric tube 59, 175, 224

needs
- basic physical 60
- Maslow's Hierarchy of 60, 61
- psychosocial 60
- sexual 60-61
- spiritual 61-62

neglect 15
- types of 15

negligence 15

nervous system
- common disorders 85-89
- NA's role in assisting with 84
- normal changes of aging 84
- observing and reporting 84-85
- structure and function 84

nitroglycerin 92

non-sterile dressings 207

nonverbal communication 21, 25, 87

non-weight bearing 82

nothing by mouth (NPO) 216, 224

nurse 5

nursing assistant (NA, CNA)
- and scope of practice 7
- as member of care team 5
- educational requirements 10-11, 246
- legal and ethical behavior 10
- professionalism 8-9
- qualities of 9-10
- role of 4

nutrition
- and Alzheimer's disease 117-118
- and appetite 219
- and cancer 110
- and HIV/AIDS 108
- and Residents' Rights 213, 220
- cultural factors 213
- documentation 222
- identifying residents 220
- MyPlate 210-212
- special diets 213-216
- tube feedings 224
- unintended weight loss 218-219

nutritional supplements 216

objective information 22

OBRA, see Omnibus Budget Reconciliation Act

obsessive-compulsive disorder 71

obstructed airway 38

Occupational Safety and Health Administration (OSHA) 34, 50, 163

occupational therapist (OT) 5

occupied bed 203
- procedure for making 203-206

ombudsman 16

Omnibus Budget Reconciliation Act (OBRA) 10
- and activities 65
- and admission 170
- and nursing assistant training 10, 246
- and resident assessments 11
- and Residents' Rights 11-13
- and restraint use 190
- and state registry 11, 246
- and temperature of resident's environment 202
- and transfers or discharges 172

open bed 207

opinion
- vs. fact 22

oral care 147
- and cancer 110
- observing and reporting 147
- procedure for 147-148
- procedure for flossing teeth 150-151
- procedure for unconscious resident 148-149

oral reports 21, 23

oral temperature
- procedure for measuring and recording 175-177

orthosis 128

orthotic devices 128

osteoarthritis 81

osteoporosis 81

ostomy 100
- procedure for care 101

outpatient care 2
output 191
  procedure for measuring and recording urinary 191-192
oxygen therapy 199
  safety guidelines for 199-200
pacing 119
pain, see also vital signs
  and Alzheimer's disease 118
  and cancer 110
  and dying resident 73
  as a vital sign 184
  management of 185
  observing and reporting 185-186
  questions to ask resident 185
  scale 185
palliative care 77
panic disorder 70
paraplegia 89
Parkinson's disease
  care guidelines 88
partial bath 129
partial weight bearing 82
PASS acronym
  fire extinguisher use 35
passive neglect 15
pathogens 45
pediculosis 141
percutaneous endoscopic gastrostomy (PEG) tube 224
perineal care 53, 132
perineum 129
peripheral vascular disease (PVD) 94
perseveration 114, 121
personal care
  a.m. care 124
  bathing 129-133
  denture care 151-152
  dressing 143-145
  foot care 139-140
  grooming 138-147
  hair care 141-142
  nail care 138-139
  observing and reporting 125
  oral care 147-148
  p.m. care 124
  promoting dignity 125
  promoting independence 124
  shampooing 134-135
  shaving 142-143
  shower or tub bath 136-138
  toileting 152-157
personal protective equipment (PPE) 50-54
person-centered care 3, 6, 7, 8, 11, 26, 62, 64, 81, 108, 114, 138, 217, 240
phantom limb pain 233
phantom sensation 233
phobia 71
physical therapist (PT or DPT) 5
physician (MD or DO) 5
p.m. care, see also personal care 124
pneumonia 95, 107, 189, 223, 228
poisoning 34
policy 8
portable commode 155
  procedure for assisting with 156-157
portal of entry 46
portal of exit 46
positioning
  basic body positions 157
  logrolling 161
  moving resident to the side of the bed 158-159
  moving resident up in bed 158
  positioning a resident on his side 159-160
  sitting up on side of bed 162-163
positioning devices
  guidelines for 128
possessions, personal 12
postmortem care 75
  care guidelines 76
posttraumatic stress disorder 71
preadolescence 67
pre-diabetes 103
pressure injury 126
  and incontinence 97
  areas at risk 125-126
  guidelines for skin care 127-128
  observing and reporting 127
  stages of 126
pressure points 125
privacy
  and bathing 136
  and dressing 144
  and dying resident 74
  and ostomy care 101
  and personal care 124-125
  and Residents' Rights 12
  and sexual needs 61, 105, 106
  as a beginning step in care procedures viii
  guidelines for protecting 17-18
privacy curtain 124, 201
procedure 8
professional 8
professionalism 8
  in employment 8-9
projection 25
pronation 235
prone position 157
prostate gland 105
prosthesis 234
prosthetic devices
  care guidelines 234
protein
  and MyPlate 211-212
  basic nutrient 209
psychosocial needs 60
puberty 67
pulse
  common pulse sites 180
  normal range 173
  procedure for measuring and recording radial 181
pulse oximeter 184
pureed diet 215-216
quad cane 230
quadriplegia 89
quality of life 11, 12
RACE acronym
  and fire evacuation 36
radial pulse 180
  procedure for measuring and recording 181
radiation therapy 109
range of motion exercises 234
  procedure for 235-239
  types 235
rationalization 25
razors
  types of 142
receptive aphasia 44, 85
rectal temperature
  procedure for measuring and recording 177-178
references
  in employment 241-242
registered dietitian (RD or RDN) 6
registered nurse (RN) 5
registry of nursing assistants 11, 246
regression 25
rehabilitation 227

relaxation technique 190, 249
religion
  and spiritual needs 61-62
  food preferences 213
religious differences 64
reminiscence therapy 123
repression 25
reproductive system
  common disorders 105-106
  NA's role in assisting with 105
  normal changes of aging 105
  observing and reporting 105
  structure and function 104-105
reservoir 46
resident(s)
  as member of care team 6
  communicating with 24-30
  identification of viii, 34, 220
Resident Council 12
Residents' Rights 11
  guidelines for protecting 13
Residents' Rights boxes
  abuse and Alzheimer's disease 122
  admission 170
  advance directives 73
  bathing 136
  call lights 228
  clothing protectors 220
  communicating with residents 30
  culturally sensitive care 64
  denture care 151
  different languages 21
  dignity and independence 63
  food choices 213
  HIV and AIDS 109
  LGBTQ residents 169
  maintaining boundaries 13
  names 21
  ostomies 101
  person-centered care 3
  privacy curtains 201
  resident as member of care team 6
  residents with special needs 226
  responsibility for residents 5
  sexual abuse 61
  sexual expression 106
  specimens 192
  speech impairment 87
  transfers or discharges 172
resident unit 200-202
respiration 94, 180
  procedure for counting and recording 181
respiratory system
  common disorders 95-96
  NA's role in assisting with 94
  normal changes of aging 94
  observing and reporting 94-95
  structure and function 94
restorative care 227
  guidelines 227-228
  observing and reporting 228
restraint alternatives 190
restraint-free care 189
restraints 188
  monitoring 190
  problems associated with 189
restrict fluids 214
rheumatoid arthritis 81
rotation 235
safety
  and transfers 163
  and oxygen use 199-200
  during bathing 136
  general guidelines 31-34
Safety Data Sheet (SDS) 34-35
scalds 33
schizophrenia 71
scope of practice 7
seizures
  procedure for responding to 43
self-care
  and Alzheimer's disease 116
  importance of 4, 62
sense organs
  common disorders 90
  NA's role in assisting with 89
  normal changes of aging 89
  observing and reporting 89
  structure and function 88, 89
senses
  using to gather information 22-23
sexual abuse 14
sexual behavior, inappropriate 30
sexual needs 60-61
shampooing hair
  procedure for 134-135
sharps 48
shaving
  procedure for 142-143
shearing 126
shock 39
  procedure for responding to 39
shower
  procedure for giving 136-138
  safety guidelines 136
signs and symptoms 21, 22
Sims' position 157
sit up
  procedure for helping resident to 162-163
skeletal, see musculoskeletal system
skin, see also integumentary system
  observing and reporting 79-80
skin care
  and cancer 110
  and dying resident 73
  and incontinence 97
  guidelines for 127-128
sleep
  importance of 202
slide board 163
smoking
  as a fire hazard 35
  oxygen use 199
social behavior, inappropriate 121
soft diet 215
special diets 213
  types of 213-216
specimen 192
  collecting clean-catch 194
  collecting routine urine 192-193
  collecting stool 195
speech-language pathologist (SLP) 6
speech loss
  and stroke 86
sphygmomanometer 182
spills, handling 55
spinal cord injuries
  care guidelines 89
  types of 89
spirituality 60, 61, 64
spiritual needs, respecting 61
sputum 47, 58, 95, 196
Standard Precautions, see also infection prevention 47
  guidelines for 48
  importance of 47-48
sterilization 54
stockings, anti-embolic
  procedure for applying 146-147
stoma 100

stool specimen
procedure for collecting 195
straight catheter 196
stress 247
guidelines for managing 248
stressor(s) 247
stroke, see cerebrovascular accident
subacute care 2
subjective information 22
sundowning 119
supination 235
supine position 157
supplements, nutritional 216
supportive devices 160, 232
suppository, rectal 99
surgical asepsis 47
susceptible host 47
swallowing problems 222-223
systemic infection 45
systolic pressure 181, 182
tactful 9
teeth, see oral care
temperature, see also vital signs
normal range 173, 175
procedure for axillary 179-180
procedure for oral 175-176
procedure for rectal 177-178
procedure for tympanic 178-179
sites for measuring 174
terminal illness 1, 72
terminology, medical 24
therapeutic diet 213
thermometers 174
thickening consistencies 223
time management
for nursing assistants 244
toileting
and Alzheimer's disease 117
assisting with 152-157
transfer belt 163
transfer board 163
transferring a resident
from bed to wheelchair 165-166
using mechanical lift 167-168
transfers
and Residents' Rights 12, 172
one-sided weakness 86
within a facility 171-172
transient ischemic attack (TIA) 44
Transmission-Based Precautions 55
categories 55
guidelines for 56-57
triggers
and Alzheimer's disease 118, 119
trochanter rolls 129
tub bath
procedure for giving 136-138
safety guidelines 136
tube feeding
care guidelines 224
observing and reporting 224-225
tuberculosis 58
and HIV/AIDS 107
tubing
intravenous therapy 145-146, 200
oxygen therapy 199-200
urinary catheters 196-199
tube feedings 224-225
tumor 109
tympanic temperature
procedure for measuring and recording 178-179
uncircumcised penis
and bathing 132
unconscious resident
procedure for oral care 149
unit, resident's
care of 201-202
standard equipment in 201
unoccupied bed 206
procedure for making 206
urinal
procedure for assisting with 154-155
urinary incontinence 97
urinary output
procedure for measuring and recording 191-192
urinary system
common disorders 97-98
NA's role in assisting with 97
normal changes of aging 97
observing and reporting 97
structure and function 96
urinary tract infection (UTI) 97-98
urine specimens, collecting 192-194
USDA 210, 212
vaginitis 105
validating 122
validation therapy 122
vancomycin-resistant *Enteroccus* (VRE) 59
vegan diet 215
vegetables
and MyPlate 211
vegetarian diet 215
verbal abuse 14
verbal communication 21
violent behavior
and Alzheimer's disease 119
violent residents
responses to 29-30
vision impairment
and ambulation 230
and communication 27-28
and eating 225
common types of 90
vital signs
blood pressure 181-184
normal ranges 173
pain 184-186
pulse 180-181
reporting change 173
respirations 180-181
temperature 174-180
vitamins 210
walker
care guidelines 231
procedure for assisting resident with 231-232
wandering 119
washing hands, see also hand hygiene
procedure for 49-50
water
basic nutrient 209
procedure for serving 217-218
weight
procedure for measuring and recording 186-187
weight loss, unintended
guidelines for preventing 218
observing and reporting 218-219
wheelchair
guidelines for assisting with 163-164
procedure for transferring from bed to 165-166
wheelchair scale 187
withdrawal
as a sign of abuse 15
as a sign of depression 70
workplace violence 14